'This is a vital and important work. Facing traumatic experiences directly is often unbearable, and sometimes must be approached sideways, through fiction. In *Fiction in Documentary Film*, Bruce Eadie offers a sensitive and wide-ranging psychoanalytic interrogation of the way fiction and non-fiction intertwine in recent documentary films to make the representation and working-through of personal and historical trauma possible. This incisive and humane book challenges simplistic renderings of trauma, demonstrating the complexity of human struggles as they appear in film, fiction and "real" lives.'

Stephen Frosh, *author of* Those Who Come After *and* How to be Real. *Emeritus Professor of Psychology, Birkbeck, University of London*

'*Fiction in Documentary Film: A Psychoanalytic Exploration* is a highly original contribution to documentary studies. Drawing on Shakespeare's device of the play-within-the-play, Eadie argues that fiction sequences in documentary films about trauma can reveal truths that more conventional documentary devices cannot reveal. Referring to a very wide range of psychoanalytical material, and an equally wide range of writing on documentary film, Eadie demonstrates the role that can be played by fictional elements in documentary. Through his close analysis of key films, and drawing on a psychoanalytic understanding of trauma and affect, he presents a very significant new way of thinking about documentary's "fictionings" and about the role of such fictionings as a therapeutic tool.'

Elizabeth Cowie, *Professor Emeritus, Film Studies at the University of Kent*

Fiction in Documentary Film

Fiction in Documentary Film explores the use of fictional elements in contemporary documentaries about personal trauma.

Bruce Eadie argues that the documentary-making process can be a dynamic, therapeutic process, which bears comparison to the clinical practice of psychoanalysis. Traumas rooted in the past are reactivated in on-screen relationships, and fictions bring representational content to otherwise unrepresented aspects of traumatic experience. With reference to Freud, Winnicott, Bion and especially post-Lacanian French psychoanalytic thinkers, Eadie emphasises the theatrical, enacted, bodily and affective aspects of trauma and documentary. This book includes detailed case studies of *The Act of Killing* (2012) and *The Blonds* (2003).

Fiction in Documentary Film will be of great interest to academics and students of film, media and television, trauma and cultural studies and psychoanalysis, as well as those interested in the application of psychoanalytic ideas both inside and outside the clinic.

Bruce Eadie spent much of his career in television, making documentary films on challenging subjects often involving state-sanctioned violence, from forced sterilisation, to the death penalty, to French complicity in the Holocaust. In 1996, he won an EMMY for his film *Nuremberg* on the Nuremberg Trials. In recent years, he has returned to academic work, writing about museum cultures and documentary film. He is the film section editor of *The International Journal of Psychoanalysis*.

Psychoanalysis and Popular Culture Series
Series Editors: Caroline Bainbridge and Candida Yates
Consulting Editor: Brett Kahr

In partnership with the BPC Scholars' Network

This series builds on the work done since 2009 by the Media and the Inner World research network. It aims to consider the relationship between psychoanalysis and popular culture as a lived experience that is ever more emotionalised in the contemporary age. In contrast to many scholarly applications of psychoanalysis, works in this series set out to explore the creative tensions of thinking about cultural experience and its processes whilst also paying attention to observations from both the clinical and scholarly fields. The series provides space for a dialogue between these different groups with a view to evoking new perspectives on the values and pitfalls of a psychoanalytic approach to ideas of selfhood, society, politics, and popular culture. In particular, the series strives to develop a psycho-cultural approach by foregrounding the usefulness of a post-Freudian, object relations perspective for examining the importance of emotional relationships and experience. We nevertheless welcome proposals from all fields of psychoanalytic enquiry. The series is edited by Caroline Bainbridge and Candida Yates, with Brett Kahr as the Consulting Editor.

Other titles in the Psychoanalysis and Popular Culture Series:

Toy Story and the Inner World of the Child: Animation, Play, and Creative Life
by Karen Cross

How to be Intimate with 15,000,000 Strangers: Musings on Media Psychoanalysis
by Brett Kahr

Formative Media: Psychoanalysis and Digital Media Platforms
by Steffen Krüger

Fiction in Documentary Film: A Psychoanalytic Exploration
by Bruce Eadie

For more information about this series, please visit: https://www.routledge.com/The-Psychoanalysis-and-Popular-Culture-Series/book-series/KARNPSYPOP

Fiction in Documentary Film

A Psychoanalytic Exploration

Bruce Eadie

Routledge
Taylor & Francis Group
LONDON AND NEW YORK

Designed cover image: © Rachel Chaplin

First published 2027
by Routledge
4 Park Square, Milton Park, Abingdon, Oxon OX14 4RN

and by Routledge
605 Third Avenue, New York, NY 10158

Routledge is an imprint of the Taylor & Francis Group, an informa business

British Library Cataloguing-in-Publication Data
A catalogue record for this book is available from the British Library

ISBN: 978-1-041-10869-6 (hbk)
ISBN: 978-1-041-10868-9 (pbk)
ISBN: 978-1-003-65718-7 (ebk)

DOI: 10.4324/9781003657187

Typeset in Times New Roman
by codeMantra

Contents

Series preface

The application of psychoanalytic ideas and theories to culture has a long tradition, and this is especially the case with cultural artefacts that might be considered "classical" in some way. For Sigmund Freud, the works of William Shakespeare and Johann Wolfgang von Goethe were as instrumental as those of culturally renowned poets and philosophers of classical civilisation in helping to formulate the key ideas underpinning psychoanalysis as a psychological method. In the academic fields of the humanities and social sciences, the application of psychoanalysis as a means of illuminating the complexities of identity and subjectivity is now well established. However, despite these developments, there is relatively little work that attempts to grapple with popular culture in its manifold forms, some of which, nevertheless, reveal important insights into the vicissitudes of the human condition.

The 'Psychoanalysis and Popular Culture' book series builds on the work done since 2009 by the Media and the Inner World research network, which was generously funded by the UK's Arts and Humanities Research Council. It aims to offer spaces to consider the relationship between psychoanalysis in all its forms and popular culture that is ever more emotionalised in the contemporary age.

In contrast to many scholarly applications of psychoanalysis, which often focus solely on "textual analysis", this series sets out to explore the creative tension of thinking about cultural experience and its processes with attention to observations from the clinical and scholarly fields of observation. What can academic studies drawing on psychoanalysis learn from the clinical perspective and how might the critical insights afforded by scholarly work cast new light on clinical experience? The series provides space for a dialogue between these different groups with a view to creating fresh perspectives on the values and pitfalls of a psychoanalytic approach to ideas of selfhood, society and popular culture. In particular, the series strives to develop a psycho-cultural approach to such questions by drawing attention to the usefulness of post-Freudian and object relations perspectives for examining the importance of emotional relationships and experience.

In this context, *Fiction in Documentary Film* offers a rich and strikingly original contribution. Bruce Eadie develops a sustained inquiry into why contemporary documentary films that confront traumatic histories so often turn to fictionalised sequences, staged re-enactments or films-within-the-film, and how such devices work to open routes towards psychic meaning that might otherwise remain foreclosed. Drawing on Freud's reflections on construction, as well as on later psychoanalytic developments attentive to embodiment, affect and symbolisation, Eadie shows how fiction may function not as evasion but as a carefully crafted invitation to truth, understood as a process rather than a fixed object.

Working across an impressive array of examples and theoretical frameworks, this book explores the subtle entanglements between testimony, representation, memory, fantasy and witnessing. It treats documentary not simply as a vehicle for information, but as an active site in which trauma can be staged, replayed, negotiated and sometimes gently transformed. Particularly compelling is the argument that documentary filmmaking has clear parallels with aspects of psychoanalytic practice, while never collapsing into it. Instead, Eadie traces moments in which fictional interludes provoke reactions, identifications and reflections that may generate new symbolic possibilities for both protagonists and viewers.

The study is attentive to clinical thinking, film theory and cultural analysis, and it brings these domains into conversation with clarity and care. In doing so, it demonstrates how a psycho-cultural perspective can illuminate evolving media forms and the emotional worlds they touch. This volume therefore deepens our understanding of the imaginative labour involved in addressing trauma on screen and contributes significantly to ongoing discussions about the ethics and aesthetics of documentary work.

We are delighted to include this book in the Psychoanalysis and Popular Culture series, where it opens new avenues for thinking about fiction, non-fiction and the complex processes through which meaning is forged in contemporary visual culture.

Caroline Bainbridge and Candida Yates

About this book

This book is an attempt to explain why a number of recent documentaries that deal with traumatic personal histories include fictional interludes: fictional films within the non-fictional documentary frame. Again and again, those documenting trauma turn to fiction, deploying animated scenes, fantasy scenes, dream sequences, role reversals, within what is otherwise a factual genre: Ari Folman's *Waltz with Bashir* (2008); Rithy Panh's *The Missing Picture* (2013); Joshua Oppenheimer's *The Act of Killing* (2012); Albertina Carri's *The Blonds* (2003); Guy Maddin's *My Winnipeg* (2007); etc. It seems there is something in the nature of trauma that demands the deployment of fictions as a route to truths or meanings about the real, non-fictional world.

I borrow the idea of a 'bait of falsehood' that can take a 'carp of truth' as my central organising principle. It draws on a clinical technique first suggested in Freud's radical 1937 paper *Constructions in Analysis* – itself drawing on speculations in *Hamlet* about the power of enacted, embodied fictions – where a fiction acts as a bait to take an otherwise unavailable truth about the "real" world. It is a technique that recognises the profound difficulty in representing trauma whilst rejecting the idea that trauma is unrepresentable and beyond the reach of understanding.

These fictions, when viewed and reflected on by the protagonists in a documentary, are capable of producing psychic insights, "truths" or meanings for the documentary protagonist that might ameliorate the pain of traumatic experience. It is a contention that sees the documentary-making process as having the potential to be a dynamic, therapeutic process, which bears comparison with the clinical practice of psychoanalysis including the practice of self-analysis: an inter- and intra-personal exploration, where a trauma rooted in the past is revivified in current relationships and where it is necessary to deploy fictions to bring representational content to otherwise unrepresented aspects of traumatic experience. It is an argument that insists that certain documentaries do not just *show* something but *do* something. These films are records of a creative act playing out over time, in which things that happen in the filmic present transform (and can be seen and felt by the viewer to transform) fixed and intractable psychic patterns. To make this argument, I draw on film phenomenology and (especially) on post-Lacanian French psychoanalytic theory, developing a counter-transferential model for the emergence of psychic meaning in which viewer and viewed are mutually implicated.

Acknowledgements

I am deeply indebted to my partner, Rachel Chaplin, whose ideas and suggestions have had a profound and material impact on the final shape of this book. Hardly a day went by when I didn't engage Rachel in a discussion or dispute about some arcane detail of psychoanalytic theory or philosophy. I would also like to thank my two sons, Seth Eadie and Joel Eadie, for maintaining a genuine interest in what their father was writing and researching whilst simultaneously, with their sardonic wit, helping me to keep a much-needed sense of proportion. That this book has come into being at all is due to the prompting and encouragement of my old friend Professor Mandy Merck who, at all stages from inception through to delivery, believed in this project. I would also like to thank Birkbeck, University of London, for financing the research and writing of this book through the award of a generous scholarship. And finally, I owe a very special thank you to Silke Arnold-de Simine and Andrew Asibong at Birkbeck, for their unstinting generosity in sharing both their time and their ideas with me.

Prelude

A fictional film melodrama of 1912: Léonce Perret's *The Mystery of the Rocks of Kador*

Suzanne de Lormel is catatonic. An intertitle tells us she has suffered 'une démence'[1]; a catastrophic physical and mental collapse. She is mute and affectless – seemingly without will. She is led into a room, where she fails to notice the presence of her lover, Jean d'Erquy, whom she believes has been shot dead: the event that precipitated her *démence*.

The 'celebrated foreign alienist physician',[2] Professor Pierre Williams, guides her to a seat and positions her head so she is looking towards a cinema screen: '– Regardez, Suzanne…'. He is about to conduct the novel treatment he has set out in his pamphlet *Lecture to the Academy of Medicine on the Observations of Professor Williams Regarding the Application of the Cinematography to Psychotherapy.*[3]

The curtains are drawn and now we can see only Suzanne and the screen. Suzanne is to be shown a film, directed by Williams, that re-enacts the events that have so disturbed her: her lover's apparent murder on a lonely beach and her discovery of his "dead" body next to her in a rowing boat that has drifted out to sea. She gazes blankly as a film flickers into life. The inert Suzanne watches as her lover (who did not die at the beach and has since recovered), plays himself on the screen. He rows towards a beach in an isolated cove. Suzanne begins to stir, her blank gaze replaced by an intent stare of recognition. Landing his boat, d'Erquy is felled by a bullet from an unseen, would-be assassin and collapses beneath the towering cliffs of the rocks of Kador. Suzanne begins to breathe heavily. The wounded on-screen d'Erquy struggles up the beach and discovers "Suzanne" (who has been drugged by the same assassin) lying motionless in the sand; her role in this filmed re-enactment taken by an actress. D'Erquy drags her into the boat, where they both lose consciousness. The real Suzanne watching Williams's film (the film-within-the-film), becomes more disturbed and animated: her hands clasp her head; her breathing quickens further. As the boat floats out to sea with the apparently dead d'Erquy aboard next to an actress playing a now comatose Suzanne, the real Suzanne rises to her feet, approaches the screen and clasps her throat. She looks behind the screen as if searching for the source of the images.

DOI: 10.4324/9781003657187-1

The lights now come on in the room with the screen. A highly agitated Suzanne, both arms raised above her head, backs away from the screen and collapses. Revived with smelling salts, Suzanne comes-to in her lover's arms. She is now able to recognise him: she grasps his head in her hands, weeps, and kisses him. The *démence* has gone: '– Elle pleure…Elle est sauvée!' ('– She is crying…She is saved!') the intertitle informs us.

…one hundred years later…(almost)…

A documentary of 2007: Guy Maddin's *My Winnipeg*

All a dream, all a dream.
I need to wake up.
Keep my eyes open somehow.
I need to get out of here.
Out of here!
What if…
I film my way out of here?

These are the opening words of first-person narrator and director, Guy Maddin, in his autobiographical documentary *My Winnipeg*. Depressed and feeling trapped in isolated Winnipeg, Maddin hits on the idea of filming his way out of his depression and so out of Winnipeg (or *vice versa*). Maddin's means of escape is not merely the making of the documentary *My Winnipeg* but the making of a film within that film. He casts his mother to play his mother (although she ultimately pulls out to be replaced by a menacing, controlling Ann Savage reprising some of her famous *film-noir, femmes fatales* of the 1940s) and rents the house he grew up in to provide the set for the film-within-the-film. Narrator Maddin tells us:

> Only here can I properly recreate the archetypal episodes from my family history.
>
> Only here can I isolate the essence of what in this dynamic is keeping me in Winnipeg.
>
> And perhaps once this isolation through filmed re-enactment is complete, I can free myself from the heinous power of family and city and escape once and for all.
>
> […]
>
> It's 1963…ish. The time I believe most likely to conceal the key to all the memories and feelings which enervate me to this day.

Alas, there is to be no '– He is crying...He is saved!' moment for Maddin. Relentlessly ironic and sardonic about his current predicament and his traumatic childhood (his elder brother, Cameron, committed suicide when Guy was seven in 1963), Maddin displaces the film-within-the-film (the filmed re-enactment within *My Winnipeg*) to a rather peripheral role, building instead a humorous autobiographical portrait, which is simultaneously the biography of a city. But what was it that Maddin had hoped to achieve when he started on this film project that he describes as a 'docu-fantasia'? (Ebiri 2008).[4] How was a film-within-the-film – 'this strange plunge-back in time'[5] – this quasi-historical but ultimately fictional interlude within the documentary frame – going to release him from the enervating repetitions of childhood trauma?

Notes

1 All quotations in this brief synopsis of the film's climactic scene are taken from the film's intertitles (some translated). Original title of this French-made silent film: *Le Mystère des Roches de Kador.*
2 Despite the odd description, Williams is clearly modelled on psychiatrists and proto-psychoanalysts then working in Paris. In an earlier scene, the character d'Erquy has chosen Williams from a group of psychological experts listed in a telephone directory – the directory listings clearly visible to the viewer – all of whom (excepting Williams) were real, practising physicians (e.g. Henri Claude who introduced Freudian theories into French psychiatry and Pierre Janet who deployed psychotherapeutic techniques in cases of dissociation and traumatic memory). The fictional character, Williams, combines the new ideas of psychoanalysis with the new technology of film.
3 d'Erquy has been given a copy of this pamphlet in an earlier scene.
4 Interviewer (Bilge Ebiri): 'You've described *My Winnipeg* as a "docu-fantasia". Can you explain?' Maddin: 'That's just a label I threw on because I wanted to avoid arguments over whether it's a documentary or not. But it's a useful starting point. Rather than having to research facts, I just conducted all my research in my memory and in my heart. I got to rant, I got to squirt some bile.'
5 These are Maddin's words in voice-over in *My Winnipeg.*

Introduction

It is striking that in both Perret's fictional melodrama of 1912 and Maddin's documentary of almost a hundred years later, a fictional film-within-the-film plays such a similar role. The film-within makes, or in Maddin's case was initially expected to make, a radical intervention in a traumatic story and to have the power to alleviate the diegetic protagonist's symptoms and psychic pain *if* past events can be represented and understood.

Maddin's documentary addresses a real, traumatic personal history whilst in Perret's film the real world of Suzanne is a conceit (she and her story are fictional). Nevertheless, both films suggest that there may be parallels between the filmic and the psychoanalytic process. Can certain documentary films claim – as analysis claims – to be able to make an active, therapeutic intervention in a traumatic history? In what follows, the central question is whether a fictional film within a documentary can precipitate a psychic transformation in the diegetic protagonist's experience of trauma. *The Mystery of the Rocks of Kador* has been described as 'the first psychoanalytic film' (programme notes from the 'Pordenone Silent Film Festival', 1995, quoted in Bergstrom 1999: 15) in which '[p]sychoanalysis and cinema join forces to cure a female subject' (Bergstrom 1999: 15). Can the documentary filmmaking process make a similar intervention in the real world and real experience of a traumatised documentary protagonist?

In the last couple of decades, a few documentaries have explored the impact and continuing ramifications of traumatic events in the life of a protagonist who appears in the film and who also often directs it.[1] These films deploy fictional interludes (films-within-the-film or "fictional" films within the "non-fictional" frame of the documentary) that range from attempts to meticulously retell – to *re*-present – a past event to approximate as closely as possible to the known, assumed, remembered or part-remembered details of a historical occurrence (the role Professor Williams's film performs within the albeit fictional frame of *The Mystery of the Rocks of Kador*) through to fantastical sequences, often employing explicitly non-indexical representational techniques, such as animation, which could never be mistaken for straightforward re-enactments of past events.

The fictional interludes are deployed in what seems to be an attempt to prompt the emergence of meanings within the documentary diegesis for the documentary

DOI: 10.4324/9781003657187-2

protagonist: meanings that may or may not help to ameliorate (to lessen) the pain of the protagonist's current psychological experience of the trauma. We, as viewers, are witnesses to an evolving filmic present as the protagonist engages with an "other" (whether a "real" other, such as the director, or an other conjured from within the protagonist). These documentaries seem to *do* something and not just *show* something. Viewers of the documentary watch an active, self-reflexive process playing out over time – an active process that I will argue is set in motion and kept in motion by a desire for meaning in the wake of trauma. The changing perceptions or emerging meanings that are made possible by the very process of film production itself seem to echo the changing perceptions made possible by clinical psychoanalysis as a traumatic history is explored in a self-reflexive, evolving temporal process, in an encounter between a traumatised protagonist and an external (or internal in the case of self-analysis) other.

Of course, all of the films I look at in detail are complex cultural artefacts, art works, exercises in aesthetics and much else besides, but my focus here is on the therapeutic potential of the filmmaking process: how involvement in the act of making a film has been utilised by certain documentary filmmakers and documentary protagonists to work through a traumatic past. I want to understand what Ari Folman meant when he described the process of making *Waltz with Bashir* (2008), as 'four years of therapy' (Folman in interview quoted in Schäuble 2011: 210).

This condensed description begs more questions than it answers; questions which will need to be teased out. The questions fall into three areas.

First, how has trauma been theorised in psychoanalysis and in post-structuralism (the two major accounts[2]) and to what extent can trauma be represented and understood? This opens up profound epistemological and ontological issues about the possibility of meaning and "truth" in relation to trauma (indeed the possibility of meaning or truth at all). Where post-structuralism forecloses on the possibility of meaning (and indeed representation), psychoanalysis deploys strategies for the recovery of meaning through dynamic inter- and intra-personal encounters (and the intense identifications generated in these encounters), *and* through the construction of fictions (to represent the apparently unrepresentable). These encounters and fictions are the focus of my two more specific areas of questioning below.

The second area concerns documentary practice and how documentary makers have expanded the boundaries of what we understand by documentary to the point where it is capable of approaching the complex psychological phenomenon of trauma; developments that seem to mirror aspects of clinical psychoanalytic practice, particularly the attempt to gain access to the past through an examination of the structure of experience in the present as it plays out in current relationships with external or internal others (a phenomenological approach to the generation of knowledge).

The third area concerns the potentially creative power of fictions to open up a route to understanding trauma. Again, there seems to be a parallel between psychoanalytic practice and documentary practice. Both deploy fictional representations of trauma in an effort to find or create a meaningful account of an overwhelming past and, perhaps, through understanding, to ameliorate the debilitating impact of the trauma in the life of the analysand or documentary protagonist (as Professor Williams's fictional film-within-the-film succeeds in doing for Suzanne in *The Mystery of the Rocks of Kador*).

In what follows, I will point to *parallels*, *echoes* and *mirrorings* between psychoanalytic practice and a certain sort of documentary filmmaking but, in doing so, I am not suggesting that filmmakers are trying to "do" psychoanalysis. Rather, I want to draw attention to the similarities of approach to the psychological complexities of trauma: the generation of fictions in the face of trauma's tendency to blank or evade representation; the use of fictions to start a process of reflection; the necessity of that process taking place within inter- (and intra-) personal exchanges in a dynamic "present" playing out over time; and an underlying assumption that representation leading to understanding (symbolisation) might be part of a process that starts to lessen the pain of a traumatic experience (a process of "working through"). Perhaps there is something in the nature of trauma itself that demands these responses. A few filmmakers do explicitly compare their practice to that of psychoanalysis: Perret in *The Mystery of the Rocks of Kador* (1912); Rithy Panh in *The Missing Picture* (2013); and Jean Rouch and Edgar Morin in statements they have made about their method of filmmaking. But, more generally, the parallels perhaps reflect the cultures or intellectual *milieux* in which these films were produced: cultures saturated with psychoanalytic categories and forms of thinking. Each of the directors of the films at the heart of this study is from a country where psychoanalysis has a deeply rooted cultural presence: Rouch and Morin from France, Panh from Cambodia but educated in France, Maddin from Canada, Oppenheimer from the United States, Carri from Argentina and Folman from Israel.

The approach adopted in this book is, broadly, "psycho-cultural", both in the application of clinical and theoretical psychoanalytic ideas to a popular cultural object (documentary film); and in the combination of these psychoanalytic ideas with those drawn from media and cultural studies[3] (here, especially, film phenomenology). And, in common with other psycho-cultural approaches to cultural objects, the arguments that follow draw on object-relations psychoanalysis, here particularly the work of Donald Winnicott. Winnicott's notion of the child's transitional object is used to conceptualise the meanings that emerge for the documentary viewer and for the traumatised documentary protagonist in their engagement with the documentary film; meanings that are simultaneously both created and found, both constructed and reconstructed, both fiction and truth.

The argument is set out over six chapters, with the last two chapters devoted to two detailed case studies of individual documentaries: Joshua Oppenheimer's *The Act of Killing* (2012) and Albertina Carri's *The Blonds* (2003). Across all the chapters, this is an exploration of the power of filmic fictions (things that never happened) to transform documentary protagonists' experience of real trauma (things that really happened). This transformed experience is not measured extra-diegetically[4] but rather is to be grasped in the marks and traces that remain legible in the filmic text and so available to the viewer.

Notes

1 The appearance in the film is sometimes not in picture but just in voice (or in an actor's voice-over of the protagonist/director's words) especially where animation is extensively employed: for example, Rithy Panh's *The Missing Picture* (2013) and Ari Folman's *Waltz with Bashir* (2008) – two films where the traumatised protagonist is also the director.

2 There is, of course, a third major account from American psychiatry, that of post-traumatic stress disorder (PTSD) but PTSD lacks philosophical elaboration (it is not grounded in theories of representation and reference) and so does not concern us here. For further discussion of PTSD, see Chapter 3.

3 The work of Caroline Bainbridge and Candida Yates has been central to both the definition and promotion of the notion of the "psycho-cultural" (Bainbridge and Yates 2014: 1–6; Bainbridge and Yates 2011: i–ii; Bainbridge 2019: 65).

4 That is, it is not measured using extra-filmic methodological techniques, such as interviewing protagonists after the event about their experience of participating in a film-making process.

Chapter 1

Models for the film-within-the-film and interpretive framework

Freud, Hamlet and the play-within-the-play as a 'bait of falsehood'

Sitting behind the formal chapter-by-chapter structure of this book, and threading its way through all the chapters, is the idea of the dramatic device of the play-within-the-play that Shakespeare deploys in *Hamlet*. It offers a way to theorise the fictional films-within-the-film of documentary makers attempting to represent and understand traumatic personal histories. In 1937, Shakespeare's dramatic device is taken up by Freud to explain a radically new method of approaching the most intractable cases of trauma, which come without memory, without representation.

Two models for the fictional film-within-the-film in Shakespeare's Hamlet

Hamlet offers at least two models of a fiction – a fictional play-within – performing an active, creative role in uncovering hidden "truths" about the "real" world: truths that are prompted into existence by the provocation of the play-within and which reveal themselves in the real world of the play-without.[1] The first is a quasi-historical re-enactment of past events and the second is an *out-and-out* fiction.

The first model – which we see performed as a play directed by Hamlet which he calls *The Murder of Gonzago* or *The Mouse-trap* (Act III Scene II) – closely follows what Hamlet believes to be real, non-fictional, historical events that have taken place in Elsinore: the murder of his father by his uncle Claudius. The play could be viewed as a reconstruction of the historical events. Hamlet hopes that in performing the play in front of his uncle, his uncle will reveal the truth not in words but in a spontaneous bodily 'blench'[2] or in being 'struck [...] to the soul'[3]; that is, in involuntary affective and somatic reactions to watching a performance of his crime. And this is what happens; Claudius storms out of the production in anger. It is only later in the play-without that Claudius is able to articulate (to provide a meaningful account of) his involuntary, essentially non-representational response to the play-within. His initial response is revealing but affective and performative and awaits reflection and interpretation.

DOI: 10.4324/9781003657187-3

But we should also be aware that this apparently historical account is inextricably bound up with imaginings, conjectures and unconscious reworkings, which render the present theatrical re-articulation of the past closer to fiction than the *re*-presentation of historical truth (or render it at most a quasi-historical *re*-presentation). Hamlet seems to recognise this himself when he says: 'I'll have these players / Play something like the murder of my father' (Act II Scene II). It is at best, only 'something like' the supposed historical event. After all, *The Murder of Gonzago* tells the story *not* of a brother murdering a brother who is King and marrying the brother's wife but *instead* it tells of 'one Lucianus, nephew to the King' (Act III Scene II) who murders his uncle. As Hamlet is nephew to the current king, Claudius, one is forced to speculate about the meaning of this transposed relationship. Perhaps the play-within is less a restaging of the traumatic past and more a revenge fantasy in which Hamlet (with Lucianus as his double) murders his usurping uncle. Or it could be read as an Oedipal fantasy in which a nephew murders his uncle and goes on to marry his aunt: a reading in which "nephew", "uncle" and "aunt" are thin disguises for son, father and mother. In taking *The Murder of Gonzago* as a model for those films-within in documentaries that re-enact past events, we must be aware of its fictionalisation of the past and how the past is distorted by a complex set of present psychic imperatives and identifications. Restagings of the "past" in the filmic present reveal the structure of experience in the present; they are a *present experience of the past* and inseparable from fantasy and projections.[4]

The second model is intentionally fictional and makes no pretence of being a re-enactment of real events. Polonius, wanting to know what his son Laertes is up to whilst away from home, instructs his servant Reynaldo to conceal his identity and then to tell Laertes's friends a series of scurrilous lies about his son (which Polonius calls 'forgeries', 'slight sullies' and 'taints' (Act II Scene I)). Polonius hopes that on hearing the lies, Laertes's friends will correct Reynaldo's stories and in so doing will inadvertently reveal the truth about what Laertes is really up to. Reynaldo is to play a part in a drama conceived and directed by Polonius although it is a drama which we, as the audience of *Hamlet*, never see. Polonius describes the lies Reynaldo is to tell as a 'bait of falsehood' designed to take the 'carp of truth'.[5] A fiction (a 'falsehood') is constructed in order to uncover a truth about the real world.

Two models for the fictional film-within-the-film in psychoanalysis

The two models in *Hamlet* for flushing out a truth about the real world are mirrored closely in the two models that Freud offered for approaching trauma. In the most familiar model – which Freud described as his archaeological method[6] – trauma is to be understood through a careful *reconstruction* of the historical events that seem to lie at the root of the trauma. But like Hamlet's theatrical production before his uncle, it is a reconstruction of the past in a dynamic present and subject to distortions, uncertainties, forgettings, fantasies and unconscious projections and so, to some degree, a fictionalisation.

The second model – which Freud calls a *construction* – was articulated late in his career. In a short paper, *Constructions in Analysis* (1937b),[7] Freud came to consider the most intractable cases of trauma – where the trauma comes without conscious registration or memory and yields no representations through the normal analytic procedures of free association, dreams, etc. He turned to Polonius's 'forgeries' as a model for a radical (even revolutionary) analytic procedure. With no conventional interpretation possible, its place must be taken by what Freud's calls a 'construction', which he equates with Polonius's 'bait of falsehood'; a coherent fictional narrative that the analyst invents.[8] It is ostensibly an entirely fictional account, constructed to fit the gaps and absences in the analysand's account and to conform to the analyst's intuitive grasp of the nature of the trauma (it is grasped in the analyst's counter-transference although Freud does not use the term in this paper). If the construction is productive, then (as Freud put it): 'to borrow the words of Polonius, our bait of falsehood had taken a carp of truth' (1937b: 262). Freud also offers some advice as to how the analyst will know that the 'carp' has been taken: a failed construction will leave the patient 'untouched',[9] implying that if confronted with a successful construction, the patient will be *touched*. However we interpret a *touch*, it seems that Freud did not expect the fictional narrative to prompt a considered, conscious and articulated response from the patient but rather was looking for non-verbal, somatic and affective clues as to the construction's productiveness.

What unites Freud's models of reconstruction and construction – and what unites Hamlet's play which is 'something like' the murder of his father and Polonius's 'bait of falsehood' – is that both seek to generate a "truth" (what I will call a meaning) in the real world through the catalyst of a fiction which is performed and witnessed. The fiction is the bait or mouse-trap, truth the quarry. Both methods generate meaning in a dynamic present encounter with a fiction and both generate meaning indirectly. Neither Hamlet nor Freud expect their fictions to prompt the immediate emergence of meaning or the instantaneous revelation of the truth but rather hope that the fiction will provoke a reaction – a *blench* or a *touch* – from the fiction's intended recipient.

Two models for the fictional film-within-the-film in documentary

The fictional films-within in documentaries that seek to explore traumatic personal histories appear to perform a similar function both to the plays-within in *Hamlet* and to the constructions and reconstructions of clinical psychoanalysis. The traumatised documentary protagonists in *The Blonds* and *The Act of Killing* recreate events from the traumatic past and stage filmic fantasies that never occurred in the real world. These representations of the trauma provoke somatic and affective responses in the protagonists (*blenches* and *touches*) and generate intense identifications as they witness their own films-within; responses that in turn require reflection and interpretation in the framing documentary for meaning to emerge.

The complex projections, role reversals and doublings of the fictional plays-within in *Hamlet*, hint at the immensely creative and creatively destabilising function of the play-within – the fictional construction or reconstruction – in documentary and in analysis.

Post-Lacanian French psychoanalysis

My theoretical approach to the fictions of documentary is informed by a particular version of psychoanalysis which, for the most part, could be described as post-Lacanian "French" psychoanalysis.[10] Insights derived from this body of thought are deployed in three contexts. First, in interpreting the body: its blenches and touches, its symptoms, its performances. Secondly, in providing a means to resolve contradictions between apparently conflicting understandings of representation and meaning. Thirdly, in insisting that meaning emerges in and through a dynamic counter-transferential encounter. This entangled, meaning-making process is what the French analyst-theorist, Alain Gibeault, describes as the process of symbolisation.

Interpreting the body: psychoanalysis as theatre and the body as a stage

Post-Lacanian French psychoanalysis has placed a particular emphasis on the theatrical, enacted, embodied, somatic and affective (often non-linguistic) aspects of the analysand's encounter with trauma (Birksted-Breen and Flanders 2010: 1–51). It is an approach to the analytic encounter which, although rigorously conforming to the Freudian notion of analysis as the talking cure, believes that the talking may only become possible once non-representational, performative and somatic aspects of the analysand's traumatic experience have been recognised and made into objects for reflection and interpretation – that is, they must first achieve representation. André Green encourages the analyst to be aware of a disparate array of clues, many non-linguistic, including 'thing-representation, word-representation, affect, corporal [*sic*] states, acts, and so forth' which he describes as the 'heterogeneity of the signifier' (Green in interview in Kohon and Perelberg 2017: 119). It is only in recognising that these non-representational states and actions are indeed signifiers of the trauma (and not mute facts in the here-and-now) that the analysis can move towards interpretation and symbolisation; towards a meaningful account in words.

Recently, a number of psychoanalytic practitioners, who work with severely traumatised patients, have stressed the importance of the body in finding representational form for non-symbolised traumatic experience. Sverre Varvin, a psychoanalyst specialising in violence-induced trauma, argues that

> Treatment must address this [disturbance of symbolisation caused by trauma] and provide a setting where experiences that have been insufficiently symbolised

> (expressed in somatisation, acting, non-verbal characteristics of speech, procedural aspects of transference, etc.) can be placed in context through a process of historisation [*sic*].
>
> (Varvin 2003: 5)

Varvin rejects the notion that trauma is unrepresentable and compares bodily manifestations of trauma to Bion's thoughts without a thinker; that is 'wild', disorganised traces of traumatic experience that can be brought back within the representational sphere.

This approach to trauma seems particularly suited to documentary, which gives access to the bodies and actions as well as the words of protagonists and provides a stage for the performance of traumatic experience in the fictionalised films-within (and indeed in the documentary frame). André Green explicitly compares the analytic encounter to theatre (1979: 3–4) and Joyce McDougall takes theatre, plays, playing, acting, acting out, staging, performing, etc., as more than just metaphors for the analytic encounter: the analytic encounter *is* a form of theatre (McDougall 1986, 1989). As Birksted-Breen and Flanders remind us, the

> metaphor of the theatre is a recurring theme in French psychoanalysis. Psychoanalysis is conceived of and represented as a three-dimensional space, a theatre where unconscious scenes are staged. The […] patient and analyst are, in a sense, both spectators to this stage.
>
> (2010: 43)

Like analysis, documentary provides a stage on which the protagonist can perform whilst the protagonist's body (like the analysand's body) provides a stage on which the psyche can perform its distress through somatisation.

That said, this approach to the analytic encounter was not invented in France – it is evident in the first analytic case studies – but has received persistent and sustained elucidation in French psychoanalytic thinking. The first (proto-)psychoanalytic patient, 'Anna O' (Bertha Pappenheim), described her inner psychic reality – her daydreams, fantasies and other free associations – as her 'private theatre' (Breuer 1955 [1893]: 22, 41). By bringing these private productions to her analysis with Josef Breuer, these inner private plays were given a semi-public performance where, arguably, as part of an inter-personal transaction, they could reveal formerly concealed meanings. Anna O's description of her fantasy life as theatre is echoed in Laplanche and Pontalis's definition of fantasies as 'scripts of organised scenes which are capable of dramatisation, usually in a visual form […] in which the subject has his [*sic*] own part to play and in which permutations of roles and attributions are possible' (1988 [1967]: 318). Laplanche and Pontalis are referring here specifically to the role-play Freud sees in the fantasies of the child in *A Child Is Being Beaten* (1919a); an essay I will return to in Chapter 5 in relation to Anwar Congo's role-playing in the documentary *The Act of Killing* (2012).

One of the theatrical aspects of analysis, *acting out*, is still frequently considered to be an impediment to the progress of an analysis as the past, rather than being remembered, is dissipated in actions which the analysand does not associate with the past. But Green recognises the repetition of the past in action ('acts') as one of those heterogeneous signifiers that demand attention and, for McDougall (1986: 110–3), understanding these acts is central to the analytic process.

'Acting out' has a rather confused and confusing history in psychoanalytic literature that can be traced back to the coining of the term 'agieren' by Freud[11] in his case study of 'Dora' (Ida Bauer) (1905 [1901]). Dora both acts out in the transference with Freud aspects of a past relationship with someone identified in the case study as 'Herr K' and also breaks off her treatment with Freud. As a consequence, since 'Dora' acting out has been used to denote either a performative aspect of the transferential relationship (acting out past relationships repetitively in the present in place of remembering those relationships)[12] or the action of bodily flight from something that is proving too difficult psychically.[13] McDougall considers both manifestations of acting out as both are enactments – non-verbal bodily communications – between the analytic pair which carry the analysis beyond talking into the realm of the bodily and the performative. For McDougall, acting out (discharging or expelling psychic distress into the external world) is a valuable clue to understanding the analysand's psychic state and a clue which can ultimately be brought back within the representational sphere (the web of words that is the talking cure) by turning it into an object for consideration by the analytic pair (1986: 110–3). Repetition compulsion – a morbid, melancholic response to loss and trauma revealed in acting out – becomes another potential route to insight.

Acting out in both its forms is a performance that documentary can capture. In Albertina Carri's *The Blonds* (2003), the director, feeling trapped and controlled by other people's accounts of her traumatic past, replicates that experience in the rigid control she exerts over the actor-double who plays the part of Albertina Carri in the film-within. And perhaps the famous scene in *Shoah* (1985), where Abraham Bomba attempts to end the interview with director Claude Lanzmann, was an attempted acting out in the second sense (for a transcription of this interview, see Lanzmann 1995). Placed in an intolerable situation by Lanzmann – cutting hair in a barber's shop in Jerusalem whilst being asked to recount the story of how in Treblinka he cut the hair of women about to be gassed – Bomba is overwhelmed perhaps by guilt and certainly by the horror of the past. He seeks flight. In his book, *The Play Within the Play: The Enacted Dimension of Psychoanalytic Process*, psychoanalyst Gil Katz (2014) relates acting out in the sense of flight to Claudius storming out of Hamlet's production of *The Murder of Gonzago*. Claudius *acts* rather than confront his own past as it is presented to him in the fictionalised form of the play-within. Katz argues (as McDougall had done) for the performative, bodily act of acting out in both senses to be embraced by psychoanalysis as a valuable heuristic tool – not as an obstruction in the path of a successful analysis.[14]

Eugene Mahon, in reviewing Katz's book, succinctly summarises Katz's contention

> The more the enacted dimension in adult psychoanalytic process can be considered a playful extension of childhood ludic experimentation rather than a destructive force that can threaten, even destroy, the analytic frame, the more likely we are as practitioners to embrace its therapeutic potential and understand its anarchic energies [...] this play within a play is a piece of theatre that analysts must now study and incorporate into their thinking.
>
> (2016: 1263)

I am making a similar case for documentary. Documentary's film-within-the-film, where the protagonist can watch back and react to their own embodied performances, offers a similar heuristic and therapeutic potential within the filmmaking process that Katz and McDougall seek to explore within the analytic process. Acting out as bodily flight, ludic play or the repetition of the structure of past relationships in the present of the analytic encounter can be incorporated into documentary when the documentary encounter is pursued as a self-consciously reflexive process.

And when the body is not acting and acting out it is often *acted on*; the body itself becomes a stage for the trauma. The French psychoanalytic tradition has been highly attuned to the corporeal and psychosomatic manifestations of trauma – the body's rigidities, ailments, malfunctions, symptoms, affects – where trauma remains unrepresented except as it is "written" on the body.[15]

For McDougall '[t]he body speaks no known language, yet it serves, time and again, as a framework for communicating the psychic scenes of the internal theatre' (1986: 53). In the 'psychosomatic theatre' the 'psyche appears to have given up the struggle, letting the soma stage its own essentially wordless show' (1986: 11–2). By paying attention to the body, McDougall allows unrepresented aspects of traumatic experience to enter the analysis, where they can be recognised by the analyst, discussed by the analytic pair, and so acquire representational form (that is, be seen to be representations). Having been recognised as signifiers (things that stand in for something that is absent) rather than as mute bodily facts, the analysis can then pursue a signified; the possibility of finding a meaningful account of the body's wordless performance as part of a process of symbolisation.

Documentary, like analysis, is able to stage past traumas not only in the present of the telling (through voice) but through the presence of the body of the traumatised protagonist which is available to the viewer and, in certain documentaries, through the device of the film-within-the-film which the protagonist watches, to the traumatised protagonist as well. Both viewer and protagonist are able to view the body's performance captured on film, to recognise that what is embodied might be a mute representation of something that is not present (something psychic that is missing). In McDougall's account (and potentially in documentary), the body is a silent signifier of psychic trauma and by recognising this, a process can begin that might unearth previously hidden or unavailable meanings.

Perhaps the most radical (or the least "classical") way in which French psychoanalysis has tried to exploit the theatrical aspects of the analytic encounter is by incorporating the techniques of the separate but related discipline of psychodrama into psychoanalysis, where circumstances demand. When conventional representations in words seem to be entirely absent, a number of French practitioners have turned to psychodrama to construct representations through dramatic (re-) enactments.[16]

> [F]or many French psychoanalysts, only neurotic patients are suitable for psychoanalysis. This [...] was Lacan's view, since there was no analysis outside of language only the neurotic patient is capable of the symbolic activity required for the analysis of "signifiers". To non-neurotic patients (psychosomatic, borderline or psychotic) French analysts will propose either psychotherapy face to face in order to avoid regression and potential disintegration, or a very French form of treatment, psychodrama [...] Sometimes this comes as a prelude to a classical analysis.
>
> (Birksted-Breen and Flanders 2010: 41)

The practice of *psychodrame psychanalytique individuel*[17] begins with the work of Evelyne Kestemberg, René Diatkine and Serge Lebovici in the immediate post-war period, with Didier Anzieu (2004 [1957]) credited with making psychodrama 'truly psychoanalytic' (Birksted-Breen et al. 2010: 477). More recently, Marilia Aisenstein (2017: 191–4) has been an influential and enthusiastic advocate of psychodrama in certain "difficult" cases as a prelude to classical analysis, and Nadine Amar (1988, 2005) has promoted psychodrama's re-enactments as giving 'access to representability' as 'the fiction created by the [psychodrama] play lifts certain inhibitions and facilitates access to unconscious conflicts' (Amar 2005: 78).

When Jacob L. Moreno devised psychodrama in Vienna in the 1920s, he drew on categories developed within psychoanalysis. Psychodrama attempts to harness the 'spontaneity-creativity' (Schact 2007)[18] of theatrical improvisation in the hope that this will reveal buried, disowned, unrecognised, unacknowledged or unknown parts of the self and give representational form to psychic residues that have evaded representation in words. It is frequently used today in the treatment of abuse and trauma in children who might be unable to express themselves through purely talking therapies (Bannister 2007) and so has echoes of Klein's introduction of *play* into child analysis. The spontaneity hoped for from psychodrama mirrors, through action as well as speech, the spontaneity hoped for from free association in the talking cure. In part, the practice of psychodrama – which involves role-playing in a group setting – can be seen as a controlled and creative use of acting out; acting out that might come to be seen as a representation of something missing when, in the final segment of the psychodrama session known as *integration*, the group reflects upon the performances that have been witnessed.

In documentary, the enacted dramas of the film-within give documentary access to exactly this route to representation, with the watching back of the film-within by the protagonist (or director-protagonist) mirroring the integration session that concludes a psychodrama session. Psychodrama, whether within classical analysis or in documentary, addresses one of the most intractable problems of traumatic experience: its escape from representation as trauma returns as either *aporia*, where memory is missing but disturbance is present, or as a so-called *veridical memory*, experienced not as memory but as the event happening in the present. Both these manifestations of trauma come without understanding (as all the major theoretical accounts of trauma attest).

The psychodrama of documentary or of analysis may precipitate the recovery of a lost memory but is perhaps more likely to unearth identifications (projections, introjections, historic hatreds, empathies, etc.) that reveal the structures of past relationships and the complex interactions between the protagonist's internal and external worlds: identifications that may reveal something of the trauma if they can become an object for consideration by analyst-analysand or documentary protagonist. Equally, the psychodrama may precipitate affective and somatic reactions in the protagonist/analysand (either within the drama or in reflecting upon the psychodrama after its conclusion) which are themselves not yet representations but, again, if they can become objects for consideration might precipitate a process that leads to a representation in words.

The performative practices that have been experimented with in documentaries treating traumatic histories bear similarities to the five core techniques of psychodrama. First there is *mirroring*, where the participant acts out an experience and is then replaced on stage by another participant who re-enacts the scene allowing the original participant to view their own action – their own psychic play – like an outsider. *Doubling* is a similar technique but it attempts to enact what is unspoken and repressed. The original participant will mount a performance and then their place will be taken by a double, who attempts to make conscious and give form to under-expressed material in the original performance. In psychoanalytic terms, it is an attempt to unearth the latent content of the original performance; content that appears to the double to have been repressed. Both mirroring and doubling are deployed throughout Albertina Carri's autobiographical documentary *The Blonds* (2003) where the director has herself played by an actor-double. Thirdly, there is *role-playing* where the participant plays the role of a person (or object) who is or has been of significance. In psychoanalytic terms, it gives scope for the participant to take the role of one of their own internal objects. Fourthly, there is *soliloquy*, where a participant articulates their normally unexpressed thoughts to the group. There are obvious connections here to the analysand's speech in analysis and to the practice of self-analysis where, as Didier Anzieu insists, the practice can only be effective if it is communicated to 'someone else' – to an outsider (1986 [1959 & 1975]: 569). That *someone-else* is manifested by the other members of the psychodrama group or in documentary by the director and film crew through conversation or interview, or even in solitary, imaginative reflection by the protagonist on how the putative (implied) documentary audience might eventually respond to what they see and hear in the psychodrama. Finally, there is *role reversal*, where one participant attempts to portray another participant, who in turn attempts to portray the first participant; they swop roles. Role-playing and role reversal are used again and again by Anwar Congo in the short films he devises and which are shown within the frame of Joshua Oppenheimer's documentary, *The Act of Killing* (2012).

All five techniques could be viewed as differing means to produce a play-within-a-play; a psychodrama play within the frame of the protagonist's everyday life. Each protagonist puts on stage and in front of an audience, a spontaneously scripted aspect of their life, which can then be recast, re-scripted and re-staged by others. Documentary is able to offer a similar opportunity to present a personal psychodrama to an audience within the diegesis as part of the filmmaking process and indirectly to an imagined viewer of the completed film.

Representation and meaning as simultaneously created and found

Beyond the *mechanics* of post-Lacanian French psychoanalysis (that is, its techniques and its attention to a heterogeneous range of signifiers which include bodies and affects as well as words), certain practitioners offer a synthesis of some of the apparent dichotomies in classical Freudian psychoanalysis. Dichotomies that express themselves in analytic practice, in the apparent objectives of analysis, and in its theory (theories) of meaning. In skeletal form: do we construct or reconstruct our representations of trauma? Do certain traumas have their roots in seduction (historical sexual assault) or unconscious fantasy? Is analysis process or archaeology? Is analysis a phenomenological enterprise concerned with the structure of experience in the present or is it a historical enterprise that finds its answers in the events of the past? Do we provoke meaning through representations that are 'something like the murder of my father' as Hamlet proposes or do we provoke it through the outright fiction of Polonius's 'bait of falsehood'? Do we create or find meaning? Does meaning emerge newly created like Aphrodite rising from the waves or do we have to find it like a Sleeping Beauty who needs to be awoken (André Green's two-part simile (1986b: 293))?

César and Sara Botella see Freud's work breaking into two not fully integrated phases. For the Botellas, the bulk of Freud's writing from around 1900 to 1937 deals with the recovery of memories in the face of neurotic conditions and follows the archaeological method of recovering the past. The answer is to be *found* in the past. This middle phase of his writing is bookended by a more radical Freud (in his writings of 1900 and before and from 1937) who constructs representations to take the place of pasts that have gone missing in the face of catastrophic trauma, producing psychotic or borderline states in the sufferer. The answer must be *created*. The Botellas see this radical early/late phase as a quest for representation whether or not it can be linked to the past, with constructions (essentially imaginative fictions) based on dreamwork not as wish fulfillment, but as a form of work that brings something into being that had never existed (Botella and Botella 2005, 2013). In the *Constructions* paper, Freud himself did offer some sort of bridge (synthesis) between the two techniques (and the two forms of representation) from these two theoretical phases:

> Quite often we do not succeed in bringing the patient to recollect what has been repressed. Instead of that, if the analysis is carried out correctly, we produce in

> him an assured conviction of the truth of the construction which achieves the same therapeutic result as a recaptured memory.
>
> (1937b: 265–6)

César Botella takes this notion further suggesting that it is not just the outcomes (the therapeutic results) that are the 'same' but that the techniques of construction and reconstruction themselves are often indistinguishable: the construction being a reconstruction of a memory without recollection (without content) and the reconstruction (following Winnicott's work), being a regression to a structure of dependence and not strictly a recollection of past events at all (Botella 2014: 911–6). I have followed this synthesis in my readings of fictions in documentary by refusing a too rigid distinction between reconstructed and constructed fictions.

More central to my purposes is André Green's reworking of Winnicott's ideas about play, the transitional object and potential space (see for example, Green 1978a, 1978b) that allow me to view the meaning that emerges from both the analytic and the documentary process as being simultaneously, and inseparably, both created and found, both constructed and reconstructed, both fiction and truth. A crude distinction between "fictional" and "true" meanings is discarded (as we can never know if we possess the truth), replacing it with a pragmatic evaluation of meaning. Not, is it *true*? but does it lessen the pain of traumatic experience and help to work through the trauma?

Symbolisation: meaning emerging out of a counter-transferential encounter

Finally, I draw on French psychoanalytic theorists when I argue that the representations and subsequently the meanings that emerge in both documentary and analysis, emerge in – and out of – a mutual, entangled, counter-transferential space. I am not suggesting that it is only in post-Lacanian French psychoanalysis that counter-transference has a central place (far from it), but simply acknowledging that I have turned to Green, to César and Sara Botella, to Michel Neyraut and to other French analyst-theorists when thinking about counter-transference. As the elements of transference and counter-transference are often so hard to distinguish, I sometimes follow the practice of using the conjoined term *transference/counter-transference* with its nod towards that mysterious entity that Thomas Ogden (2004) calls the 'analytic third' or, to de-personify the notion, the *co-transference* that exists between the analytic actors.

Sara and César Botella (2013) develop the embryonic ideas outlined in *Constructions in Analysis* and make explicit what Freud left unsaid. In cases where representations have gone missing or only ever registered as fragments, representation (and subsequently understanding) can be achieved through *regredient dreaming*; the grasping of the trauma (the intuiting of the trauma) in the transferential/counter-transferential space that exists between the analyst and the analysand through the creation of an imaginative fiction.[19] André Green reaches a similar conclusion when considering similarly intractable cases of trauma. What is required is 'another system of reference which gives pride of place to the countertransference. [...] The analyst ought to either use his imagination, or resign' (1986b: 294).[20] Once again, an imaginative fiction that emerges out of the counter-transference gives representational form to the trauma and can potentially, through a temporal process, lead to the emergence of meaning for analysis's "diegetic protagonist", the analysand.

In considering documentaries about personal traumatic histories, there is an additional location for meaning to emerge. As viewers, we witness the intra-diegetic struggle for meaning as the protagonist engages with others within the diegesis (the struggle the Botellas and Green describe within the analytic setting) but we also experience our own struggle for meaning as we engage with the documentary object and the characters in the diegesis, and this engagement generates its own set of identifications and empathetic encounters. Although my main focus is the meanings that are created or found by the diegetic protagonist, the meanings that we (the viewer) create or find are generated in a similarly entangled counter-transferential space. In what follows, I sometimes bracket out meaning for the viewer in order to focus on the meanings that become available to the diegetic protagonist. But we must always be aware that it is we, as viewers, who ascribe meanings to the protagonist. After all, the protagonist only exists for us as light on a screen and sound on tape and so the two *loci* for the emergence of meaning are ultimately inseparable as the meanings we find or create as viewers include the meanings we intuit and assign to the diegetic protagonist.

Green does provide some indication of how this interaction between the extra-diegetic viewer and the filmic text might work, in one of his rare forays into applied psychoanalysis. In a paper, 'The Unbinding Process' originally published in 1971, Green examines the reader's engagement with a literary text (and I think his speculations about the reader of literature can be transferred across to the viewer of documentary): '[T]he analyst [that is, the reader] reacts to the text as if it were a product of the unconscious. The analyst [reader] then becomes the *analyzed* of the text. It is within himself-as-text that he must find an answer'. Green is describing a counter-transferential process in which the analyst *as reader* must excavate his/her unconscious response to the text (as the text awakens 'both an idea and an affect in the reader') and then proceed to interrogate that response in a process that moves towards interpretation (an 'interpretation that he [the reader] must give himself of the effects of the text in his own unconscious'). Green calls this process an 'exercise in self-analysis' (1980 [1971]: 18).[21] The text is analysed by the reader and the reader is analysed by the text in a radical two-way movement, with the reader ultimately producing a text that is his/her own 'construction' (1980 [1971]: 21).

This extra-diegetic process and the process I am attempting to describe *within* the documentary diegesis (my main focus) is a counter-transferential process of symbolisation. It starts with a fictional representation, which substitutes for the missing trauma and acts as a catalyst or provocation or bait or trap, setting in motion a process which, if productive, leads to symbolisation: the emergence of a meaningful account of the trauma. Again, it is in French psychoanalytic theory that I find a description of this process that most closely mirrors the processes I discern in certain documentary films. French psychoanalyst, Alain Gibeault, provides a succinct description of the process, beginning with the creation of an essentially fictional representation:

> We can define symbolization as the operation by which something comes to represent something else for someone. While it may appear as the substitution of one object for another, it is primarily the result of a process that assumes both the ability to represent an absent object and a subject capable of knowing that the symbol is not the symbolized object. In this sense it promotes the ability to fantasize and the organization of mental space.

Gibeault then describes how meaning emerges:

> Aside from allowing one term to substitute for another [i.e. a form of fictionalisation or metaphorisation], symbolization designates back and forth flow of meaning between subject and object, between mental reality and external reality, between past and present. This is the effect of the symbolization process, which makes possible a system of intra- and intersubjective exchanges.
>
> (Gibeault 2005: 1712–4)

For Gibeault, meaning emerges out of counter-transferential entanglements organised around fictions that substitute for the traumatic content that has gone missing. The meaning-making process is both a temporal and an inter-/intra-personal one, in which barriers between apparently separate entities dissolve: barriers between self and other, between past and present.

Documentary theory

In 'theorizing documentary'[22] – and here in placing my work within the scholarly literature on documentary – I have been informed by two bodies of theory: by film phenomenology and by psychoanalytically informed approaches to documentary. There is overlap between the two bodies of theory even if expressed in different technical language, and both bodies of theory dovetail with the approaches to documentary I derive directly from psychoanalytic theory.

Both groups of scholars insist that the documentary object differs from the fictional film; it is a non-fictional object (even when deploying fictions and fictionalisations) and as such demands a different sort of engagement, can be asked different questions and gives access to different meanings about the world than those available in fictional films. Both groups maintain that something unique and potentially meaningful is created in the present of the filming. And both groups have imported approaches developed in relation to fictional films, repurposing and redeploying these theoretical approaches for documentary.

Phenomenological approaches to documentary

The application of film phenomenology to documentary has offered me three approaches that I adopt in pursuing my argument.[23] First, it recognises that documentary gives the viewer access to a unique, embodied encounter[24] that creates something new and potentially meaningful in the filmic present. Secondly, it offers a way to theorise the complex entanglements that characterise the interaction between subject and object, between viewer and film (including the diegetic protagonist's interaction with the internal film – documentary's film-within-the-film); an interaction that I then conceptualise as *counter-transferential*. The film (and the film-within-the-film) cannot be grasped objectively, as separate from its viewer, as *a thing-in-itself*: it is grasped in the flow and counter-flow between an experiencing-subject (the viewer) engaging with – and acted-on by – an experienced-object (the film or a protagonist within the film) (Sobchack 1999; also see gloss of Sobchack's work in: Ferencz-Flatz and Hanich, eds., 2016: 22). In Vivian Sobchack's words: 'objective phenomena [the film] and subjective consciousness [of the perceiving viewer] are entailed in an *irreducible correlation*.' [...] 'a film and its spectator [are] two active and differently situated viewers viewing in intersubjective, dialectical, and dialogic conjunction' (2009: 436, 443; Sobchack's italics). Neither subject nor object exists in isolation, each is always in dialogue with the other in – to borrow Gibeault's phrase – a 'back and forth flow of meaning between subject and object' (2005: 1713). This encounter is inseparable from the viewer's fantasies, projections, introjections, identifications, whether that viewer is *us* as the viewer of the documentary or the intra-diegetic viewer who watches the fictional films-within. The film comes to the viewer through the filter of his or her senses, conceived broadly to include the psychology of the perceiving mind. And finally, film phenomenology as described by Vivian Sobchack (1999, and also 1992), has encouraged me in my belief that documentary offers us a glimpse into the real lives of protagonists beyond or behind the screen. That is, for all its fictions and for all the entanglements between viewer and viewed (or, more accurately, *because of* what these fictions and entanglements reveal), documentary can tell us something about the real world and the real lives of documentary protagonists that exist independently of the film.

Psychoanalytic approaches to documentary

In common with phenomenological approaches to documentary, psychoanalytic approaches to documentary were rare until the 1990s (Renov 2004 [1996]: 93),[25] when a few scholars began to repurpose and redeploy predominantly Lacanian approaches to fictional films developed in the late 1960s and 1970s,[26] and to explore the complex subjective and psychological mechanisms at work both in documentary reception and in documentary production.

Beginning in the 1990s, Michael Renov and Elizabeth Cowie reconsider the nature of documentary reception, challenging the dominant conception of documentary as an exclusively sober, realist genre that satisfied a demand in the viewing public for rational, objective, informative accounts of a real, non-fictional world. Renov and Cowie question both "halves" of this equation: the nature of the documentary object and the nature of the viewer's engagement with that object.[27]

Cowie (1999: 19–20) argues that documentary had never been straightforwardly realist and had always encompassed elements of fantasy. She questions the conventional distinction between the supposedly separate cinematic traditions spawned by Louis Lumière and Georges Méliès (a realist, "scientific", empirical tradition and a tradition of filmic fantasy) and so, as Stella Bruzzi puts it in her review of Cowie's *Recording Reality, Desiring the Real*, 'collapses some of the differences between fictional and nonfictional cinema' (Bruzzi 2015b: 384–7). This collapsing of boundaries through the exploration of fantasy is explicitly espoused by the documentary makers I consider in what follows: fantasy does not creep into the documentary frame unacknowledged and unnoticed as an unwanted alien incursion but is deployed as a way – perhaps the only available way when trauma is in play – to uncover certain "truths" about the real world.

Renov and Cowie also question the nature of the viewer's engagement with this more complicated documentary object, by introducing the notion of a documentary viewer 'incited by unconscious drives as had been argued for the audience of the fiction film' (Renov 2004 [1996]: 93). Neither Renov nor Cowie abandons the conventional notion of a documentary viewer animated by epistemophilia and intellectual curiosity but argue that this knowledge-seeking viewer is also animated by unconscious desires; desires which Renov and Cowie theorise through Lacanian categories.[28] As viewers we are not simply disinterested, rational observers of the world presented in the documentary but are subject to unconscious forces as we, for example, identify with 'the social actors in the documentary as stand-ins for ourselves' (Cowie 1999: 31). There is an entanglement between viewer and viewed which not only requires acknowledgment but which, if explored and interrogated, might afford us a deeper understanding of what unfolds on the screen.

Other scholars have sought to deploy insights gleaned from psychoanalysis *inside* the filmmaking process: a shift of focus from the psychology of documentary reception to that of documentary production. Rather than explore the play of fantasy and desire in the documentary viewer who (at least nominally) sits *outside* the film and responds to – and identifies with – what unfolds on screen, the focus shifted to the unconscious forces that "incite" the documentary maker and the documentary protagonist who exist *inside* the film.[29]

Diane Waldman and Janet Walker made early incursions into this field in their seminal editors' introduction to *Feminism and Documentary* (1999b). They saw a powerful parallel between the analyst-analysand encounter in clinical psychoanalysis and the encounters between characters in the documentary diegesis: in both encounters, something of the absent past re-emerges and 'is made operative in actions and resistances in the present' (1999b: 25). In this transferential model, meaning emerges in the filmic or analytic present in and through the inter-personal relations between the diegetic "actors". A similar agenda is pursued by psychotherapist Emanuel Berman, following interviews he conducted with documentary makers. Berman began to consider the unconscious motivations that affect the director's choice of subject and that continue to animate the filmmaker throughout the filmmaking process. Berman was particularly interested in the relationship that develops between director and protagonist during filmmaking: an inter-personal process that he felt was akin to the inter-personal processes at play in analysis: 'the process of transference and counter-transference' (Berman quoted in Chanan 2007: 216; see also: Berman et al. 2003).

But perhaps unsurprisingly, it is two film scholars who are also filmmakers who have most energetically pursued this line of enquiry, deploying insights derived from their reading of Lacan in an attempt to understand what drove their own filmmaking practice. Alisa Lebow (2008) explores the unconscious forces at play in the filmmaking process as she considers the desire of the filmmaker in making the film and in her characterisation of filmmaking as an active, creative attempt to come to terms with loss: an argument she pursues in part through a consideration of her own experience in making the autobiographical (or, to use her preferred term, 'first-person') film, *Treyf* (Lebow and Madansky 1998). It is Agnieszka Piotrowska, though, who most extensively explores the "internal", psychological mechanics of filmmaking (again, in part, through an examination of her own filmmaking practice).[30] At the heart of Piotrowska's account (2014) is the complex relationship between the documentary director and protagonist, which is cast as an unequal transferential relationship of love which inevitably ends in betrayal. It is a relationship that begins (or at least begins in the imagination) from the moment the idea of the film first enters the director's head and, for the protagonist, from the moment when they are first contacted by the director, and it persists throughout the production of the film. This entangled, transferential relationship profoundly influences the shape, content and tone of the finished documentary but leaves few concrete traces. As Piotrowska writes: 'Very often the actual mechanics of the documentary encounter are concealed from the viewer and hard to investigate' (2014: 11).

I want to make a similar incursion "inside" the documentary to the one Piotrowska and Lebow make, in order to investigate the unconscious mechanics of the documentary-making process. But it takes a particular sort of documentary text for the traces of these internal mechanics to remain legible and available to the viewer; that is, for these mechanics not to be concealed or only to become available retrospectively and "extra-textually" in director's or protagonist's reminiscences. In certain films, the viewer is afforded privileged access to the complex psychological factors at play during the production of the documentary, circumventing the lack of visibility that Piotrowska identifies. Reflexive films (that unmask the mechanics of the filmmaking process) and especially self-reflexive films (where the documentary itself becomes a subject of the documentary) can give the viewer this privileged access to the desires and identifications that drove the diegetic protagonists during the making of the film. The device of the film-within-the-film – a fiction within the documentary created by, watched by, and reflected-on by the diegetic protagonists – has the power to provoke or catalyse responses within the diegesis that facilitate our access to these complex psychological mechanics, revealing the inter-personal processes through which the diegetic protagonists struggle towards a meaningful account of a traumatic history.

In what follows, I want to build on these psychoanalytic readings of both documentary reception and documentary production. My principal focus of attention is the intra-diegetic emergence of meaning in the filmic present as protagonists respond to fictional representations of trauma within an inter- or intra-personal frame playing out over filmic time. To achieve this, I am influenced by the work of those who have written about the psychology of documentary production. But as the meanings we assign to the protagonists cannot be separated from the meanings we as viewers make through our engagement with the filmic text (that is, we cannot evade the possibility that we have created – invented – the meanings that we assign to protagonists), my readings draw on the work of those who have examined documentary reception through a psychoanalytic lens and this must involve an examination of our own identifications, projections and affective responses as viewers to watching the film.

Afterword on Lacanian approaches to documentary

Where I differ from most of those who have developed psychoanalytic approaches to documentary reception and production is that my readings are not rooted in Lacanian theory. That said, my readings are not anti-Lacanian and I acknowledge that it is "Lacanians" who have opened up this field and who have written about it with deep insight. But I have chosen to draw instead on a different body of psychoanalytic theory – post-Lacanian French psychoanalytic theory – because I have found it more closely addresses the phenomena that documentary (and especially documentary that explores trauma) seems to make available. Of course, the talking head has been a basic component of documentary at least since Rouch and Morin made *Chronique d'un été* (1961), and words and speech are the basic transactional material of Lacanian psychoanalysis.[31] But documentary gives us much beyond language even if we apply quite a broad definition of language – and sometimes language is not available.

In cases of profound trauma both in analysis and in documentary – with representational capacities fractured or disabled – a linguistic transaction may, at first, not be possible (even if the ultimate goal – meaning – will take linguistic form if it is ever to be achieved). We might instead be presented with the shattered fragments of traumatic experience that manifest themselves only as bodily epiphenomena (somatisation, acting out, affect, physical paralysis, etc.) or as the bizarre objects of Bion's theoretical speculations (Bion 1957). These manifestations of trauma are at the very least extra-linguistic (perhaps non-linguistic) and suggest that parts of the psyche are alien to the structuring influence of language.[32] Profound traumatic experience seems to create psychic states that are variously described as psychotic, schizophrenic or borderline and which fail to manifest themselves in those linguistic forms that are available in the face of neurosis.

Post-Lacanian French psychoanalysis, which emphasises the embodied, theatrical, somatic and affective[33] (non-linguistic) aspects of the analysand's presentations in analysis, seems to provide a good theoretical fit with the heterogeneous range of signifiers[34] that the physical presence of the traumatised protagonist makes available in documentary. As viewers we must pay attention to the embodied, corporeal manifestations of trauma which protagonists exhibited during the filmmaking process. We must pay attention to the *blenches* and *touches* generated in the protagonist's confrontation with the fictional representations of the film-within.

And finally, in my preferred version of psychoanalysis – following the Freud of *Constructions in Analysis*, the Botellas, André Green, Berman in his speculations on the documentary encounter, and many post-Lacanian French analysts – a fundamental interpretive tool (perhaps *the* fundamental interpretive tool) of the psychoanalytic encounter is the counter-transference, *if* the feelings generated in the counter-transference can be made into an object of enquiry. Many of the documentary theorists who pursue a psychoanalytic approach to documentary, make transference a central component of their interpretive strategies but I would argue that even more fundamental is the counter-transference which, following the argument of Michel Neyraut (2010: 218–32), is either indistinguishable from the transference or precedes it and takes precedence over it (the transference is only activated in the context of the counter-transference). Lacan often expressed a negative view of the impact of counter-transference on an analysis, describing it as 'the sum of the prejudices, passions, perplexities, and even insufficient information of the analyst at a certain moment in the dialectical process of the treatment' (Lacan 1966: 225). I agree with Lacan to the extent that *unacknowledged* and *unexamined* counter-transference is an impediment to an analysis (and interpreting it is difficult as counter-transference both elucidates unconscious phenomena and simultaneously resists interpretation (Neyraut 2010: 226)). But if the analyst applies a rigorously self-reflexive approach to his or her counter-transference – constantly interrogating and questioning what is felt and perceived – then the counter-transference can be more than a marker of the analyst's failure or a product of an early phase of the analysis (which will fade away as the analyst begins to grasp the true nature of the analysand's psychic landscape). Before the 1960s, Lacan expressed an interest in counter-transference as indicative of 'the desire of the analyst' (as a subject not only supposed to know but a subject supposed to desire) but from the early 1960s, Lacan became openly hostile to the suggestion that analysts should work in the counter-transference (Evans 1996: 31) – a symmetrical relationship – insisting it was sufficient to speak of the different ways analyst and analysand were implicated in the powerfully asymmetrical relationship of the transference (Lacan 1991 [1960–61]: 233). For me, it is the very symmetricality of the counter-transferential relationship that allows it to be psychoanalysis's most powerful heuristic tool and a highly productive conceptualisation of the identificatory entanglements of subject and object in life, in film and in analysis. It is central to my readings of my two case studies in Chapters 5 and 6.

Notes

1 The device of the play-within-the-play in Shakespeare, and before Shakespeare in Thomas Kyd's plays (e.g. *The Spanish Tragedy* of c.1587), are themselves examples in theatrical form of the literary device of the story-within-the-story which dates back to the birth of literature, where the inner story is used to entertain, to provide a moral example or to be of symbolic or psychological significance to the characters in the outer story and where often the "fictional" inner story is a vehicle for revealing a "truth" in the outer story.

2 'I'll observe his looks; / [...] if he but blench, / I know my course' (*Hamlet*: Act II Scene II).

3 'I have heard / That guilty creatures sitting at a play / Have by the very cunning of the scene / Been struck so to the soul that presently / They have proclaim'd their malefactions' (*Hamlet*: Act II Scene II).

4 Lacan described this same process in analysis: 'history is not the past' but 'is the past in so far as it is historicised in the present [of the analysis]' – it is a 'present synthesis of the past which we call history' (Lacan 1988: 12, 36).

5 Polonius (to Reynaldo): 'Your bait of falsehood takes this carp of truth; / And thus do we of wisdom and of reach, / With windlasses and with assays of bias, / By indirections find directions out' (Act II Scene I).

6 Freud first compared psychoanalysis to archaeology (with both practices said to uncover something hidden or buried) in his 1896 essay *The Aetiology of Hysteria* (1896: 192). Freud continued to make this comparison throughout his career (Thomas 2009).

7 Freud describes both reconstruction (the archaeological method) and construction in this paper.

8 An idea first put forward by Freud in his 1919 essay *A Child Is Being Beaten* but not fully worked through until the 1937 *Constructions in Analysis* essay.

9 'no damage is done if [...] we make a mistake and offer the patient a wrong construction [...] What in fact occurs in such an event is [...] that the patient remains as though he were untouched by what has been said and reacts to it with neither a "Yes" nor a "No". This may possibly mean no more than that his reaction is postponed; but if nothing further develops we may conclude that we have made a mistake and we shall admit as much to the patient [...] [A]n opportunity will arise when some new material has come to light which allows us to make a better construction and so to correct our error. In this way, the false construction drops out, as if it had never been made; and, indeed, we often get an impression as though, to borrow the words of Polonius, our bait of falsehood had taken a carp of truth' (Freud 1937b: 260–1).

10 A heterogenous collection of analyst-theorists (not necessarily French nationals) working in France or influenced by ideas emerging from "French" psychoanalytic institutions. See the edited volume: Dana Birksted-Breen, Sara Flanders, and Alain Gibeault, eds. 2010. *Reading French Psychoanalysis*.

11 Conventionally translated into English as *to act out* or *acting out* (this is the translation adopted in the English *Standard Edition* of Freud's work).

12 As Freud puts it in *Remembering, Repeating and Working-Through* (1914a: 150–1): 'we may say that the patient does not remember anything of what he has forgotten and repressed, but acts it out. He reproduces it not as a memory but as an action; he repeats it, without, of course, knowing that he is repeating it' and so 'the compulsion to repeat [...] replaces the impulsion to remember.'

13 This is confirmed by Laplanche and Pontalis: 'The term "acting out" enshrines an ambiguity that is actually intrinsic to Freud's thinking here: he fails to distinguish the element of actualisation in the transference from the resort to motor action which the transference does not necessarily entail' (1988 [1967]: 4).

14 Despite Katz's call to embrace acting out, a recent study of analytic practice reveals that many practising analysts from a variety of schools still consider acting out to be an impediment to an analysis (a position that the authors of the study do not share) and the study concludes that still: '[t]he rule of psychoanalysis is "speech not action"' (Bohleber et al. 2013: 518). See also Wilhelm Skogstad's 2015 paper 'Speaking through Action, Acting through Speech: Acting and Enacting in the Analytic Process'.

15 Psychosomatics is institutionalised in France in the *École psychosomatique de Paris,* whose members have included many leading analyst-theorists. Individual "French" analysts who have stressed the centrality of psychosomatics to analysis include Joyce McDougall, Pierre Marty, Didier Anzieu, Michel Fain, Christian David and Michel de M'Uzan.

16 The practice has attracted its most extensive theoretical elaboration by analysts in France but has been deployed in other countries, for example in (Albertina Carri's) Argentina since the early 1960s.

17 Psychoanalytic psychodrama is a group activity but differs from psychodrama in that the working group is made up of several analysts and one protagonist (hence the label 'individuel') rather than one specialist working with a group of non-specialists.

18 Moreno described his new practice as the 'theatre of improvisation' and the 'theatre of spontaneity' (Schact 2007) as knowledge is generated in a dynamic, theatrical present (a phenomenological epistemology).

19 There are parallels to Bion's notion that '[t]he analyst must be able to dream the session' (1992: 120).

20 Green makes it clear that this creative use of the counter-transference is an elaboration of what Freud implied but never fully realised, as he adds that '[h]ere we have evidently reached the limits of Freudian practice and theory' (1986b: 294).

21 Throughout this paper, Green refers to the 'analyst' but he is always concerned with the analyst *as reader* (and is merely signalling his belief that analysts make particularly acute readers of literary texts). Notwithstanding, this paper is about the reader and the act of reading a text (not about the analyst *qua* analyst).

22 I borrow this term from Renov: it is the title of his 1993 monograph.

23 Vivian Sobchack (along with Alain Casebier) was central not only to the revival of phenomenological approaches to film in the 1990s (much neglected since the 1960s in the face of semiotic approaches to film) but in the application of film phenomenology to documentary.

24 As regards *embodied* approaches to documentary, I have drawn on the work of Vivian Sobchack (see for example, 1992, 1996, 1999, 2004, 2009, etc) and Linda Williams (see for example, 1991, 1993, etc) in particular (beginning with a number of articles published in the 1990s). The spectator's body and the protagonist's body become key elements in cinematic perception and interpretation.

25 Renov makes this point in his 2004 introduction to the republication of his 1996 essay 'Charged Vision' where he also reflects on the call he made for a psychoanalytic approach to documentary in *Theorizing Documentary* (1993).

26 Theoretical approaches developed by scholars, such as the Christian Metz, Roland Barthes, Ann Kaplan, Laura Mulvey and others writing in the journals *Screen, m/f, Cahiers du Cinéma* and elsewhere.

27 Renov began setting out his ideas in *Theorizing Documentary* (1993) and the essay 'Charged Vision' (2004 [1996]) and continues to pursue these ideas in, for example, his 2015 essay 'Documentary and Psychoanalysis: Putting the Love Back in Epistephilia'.

Elizabeth Cowie entered the fray with her 1999 essay 'The Spectacle of Actuality' and explores this field at book length in *Recording Reality, Desiring the Real* (2011).

28 In Cowie's account (1999: 19), there are twin motivational desires: 'On the one hand there is a desire for reality held and reviewable for analysis as a world of materiality available to scientific and rational knowledge [...] On the other hand there is a desire for the real not as knowledge but as spectacle'.

29 In the reflexive and self-reflexive films I consider here, the documentary maker has a presence within the diegesis (as well, of course, as having an extra-diegetic existence as the unseen maker of the film which is common to all documentaries).

30 Piotrowska's and Lebow's accounts of their own practice differ markedly in that Lebow was the director of a first-person film whilst Piotrowska's films have always been third-person films (with a separate director and protagonist). I consider these two modes of address in Chapter 4.

31 For Lacan: 'psychoanalysis is understood in theory and practice to be a linguistic enterprise. Words are its medium, the process is a discourse, words produce the illumination which is its product. More radically, Lacan claimed that the unconscious is structured like a language' (Birksted-Breen and Flanders 2010: 31).

32 This is the implication of Freud's introduction of the tripartite division of the psyche in 1923 in *The Ego and the Id*. The Id stands outside representation and language.

33 With Lacan, there is 'the virtual elimination of affect from the psychoanalytic field' (Birksted-Breen and Flanders 2010: 32). André Green concurs: 'affect has no place in it [Lacan's work]' (Green 1999: 99). The only affect which does find a place in Lacan's thought is anxiety to which he devoted his 1962–63 seminar but it is clearly singled out as the only affect that does not *deceive* and so the only one which deserves attention. And, even in admitting anxiety as an affect worthy of attention, Lacan set limits to its legitimate range, confining it to the anxiety that we do not know what we are for the other.

34 André Green coined the phrase the 'heterogeneity of the psychoanalytic signifier' to counter Lacan's conception of an unconscious structured like a language and composed homogeneously of linguistic signifiers (Green 1999: 299; Kohon and Perelberg 2017: 119).

Chapter 2

The fictionality of fiction and the non-fictionality of non-fiction

My argument in this and succeeding chapters depends upon maintaining some sort of distinction between fiction and non-fiction both in documentary *and* more broadly. In this chapter, I ask to what extent can documentary – a highly constructed form and not a simple window on reality – be said to be non-fictional *and* what makes the filmic interlude (the film-within-the-film) fictional? Before considering the fictionality of the fictional interlude, I first want to consider the non-fictionality of the documentary frame.

The non-fictionality of documentary

Non-fiction claims a fidelity to something beyond itself; it refers to something independent of the non-fictional narrative that exists or existed. Fiction makes no such claim. It is a product of the imagination and although it must work with elements we recognise from a real world beyond the imagination, the most it can claim is to be *like* the real world.[1] Despite the appeal of this commonsense definition, it is grounded in claims about referentiality, which are deeply contested. In recent decades, poststructuralist theorists have stressed the fictionality of all forms of narration (and indeed of all forms of meaning-making) including those that make referential claims like historiography and documentary. The binary of fiction/non-fiction is collapsed into fiction. This is deeply problematic for documentary, which has been defined since its inception as cinema's non-fictional form. 'Documentary arises, with Grierson and Dziga Vertov, in response to fiction' according to Bill Nichols (1994: 94). It is the fiction film's binary other and documentary is routinely defined as non-fiction film.

The blurring of the fiction/non-fiction boundary

Even for critics, like Nichols, who are not convinced by the post-structuralist case, the division between fiction and non-fiction in documentary is extremely difficult to draw: 'One of the most blurred of recent boundaries lies precisely between fiction and nonfiction' (1994: x). Nichols uses the word 'recent' as, in common with numerous critics[2] from a number of theoretical backgrounds, there seems to be a consensus that documentary has been expanding the range of filmic devices and representational

DOI: 10.4324/9781003657187-4

forms that it is able to draw on in creating its narratives: devices and forms that were once more commonly associated with fictional narratives or at least more with declaredly subjective narratives than had been common in documentary. This process has only accelerated since Nichols wrote about it in *Blurred Boundaries* in 1994.

I have included the notion of subjectivity alongside fictionality not because the two can be directly mapped on to each other but because their binary opposites, objectivity and non-fictionality, have been frequently paired together in descriptions of the nature of documentary film. Recently, Nichols (2017) noted the increasing prevalence of documentaries that adopt a reflexive mode (documentaries that are self-conscious about their own constructedness) or a performative mode (emphasising the subjective or expressive aspect of the filmmaker's own involvement in the subject). Michael Renov (2008) has written about a particular sort of subjective approach in tracing the revolutionary impact of the rise of the autobiographical documentary in the 1990s,[3] claiming '*the VERY IDEA of autobiography reinvents the VERY IDEA of documentary*', whilst noting the reluctance of 'some documentary scholars' to accept the autobiographical impulse within the tradition of non-fiction as, for them, it compromises the non-fiction enterprise. For Renov, the opposite is true. Autobiographical documentary gives documentary access to non-fictional private truths and inner realities; subjective, psychological truths on the 'psychoanalytic model' (2008: 41–2; Renov's capitals and italics).[4]

In recent years, documentary makers addressing traumatic histories have adopted modes of representation *more commonly* associated with fictional film: animation, sequences using toys, dioramas with clay models, re-enactment, the use of actors (who sometimes take the place of the principal protagonist who is also present in the diegesis) and dream, fantasy and hallucinatory sequences.[5] Of course, none of these devices or representational techniques are entirely new to documentary. The first animated documentary[6] even predates Grierson's coining of the term 'documentary' in 1926 (Grierson 1966); and the use of the term *docu-fiction*, which has come to prominence since the millennium to describe an apparently "new" form of documentary, has been traced back to 1980 by Jean-Pierre Candeloro (2000), with examples of the sub-genre extending back (in all but name) to the birth of documentary and Robert Flaherty's *Moana* of 1926. And documentary and fiction film have a long history of borrowing and counter-borrowing of filmic styles and tones of voice. What I think is new in the last twenty years or so is a new permissiveness in the range of filmic devices, representational forms and subjective modes of address (including the autobiographical), that documentary filmmakers can adopt and mix together. Perceptions have shifted as to what documentary *is*, what documentary is *allowed to be*, before it crosses an invisible but nonetheless powerful taxonomic boundary and is no longer considered to be a documentary by either its makers or its audience.

Non-fictionality as ethical contract

For all the greater range of representational styles and more subjective voices that are now permissible in documentary, and even the inclusion of fictional interludes within the frame of the documentary, there remains a sense amongst viewers of documentary that they are not watching fiction and that they can distinguish between the fictional interlude and the non-fictional frame. There is an unspoken contract between documentary viewers and documentary makers that for all the blurring of boundaries between fiction and non-fiction, what is being presented is in essence non-fictional and that the documentary film affords us access to a real world beyond the film, even if that real world is mediated and constructed by the documentary maker and cannot be grasped directly but only approached obliquely and subjectively.

Documentary maker, Jean Rouch, invoked this contract when asked in interview about the nature of *cinéma vérité*:

> [I]t would be better to call it cinema-sincerity [...] you ask the audience to have confidence in the evidence, to say to the audience, "This is what I saw. I didn't fake it, this is what happened ... I look at what happened with my subjective eye and this is what I believe took place ... It's a question of honesty."
>
> (Rouch quoted in: Levin 1971: 135)

Carl Plantinga makes a similar point claiming that producers and viewers of documentary make 'an *implicit contract* to view a work as documentary' (1987: 46; Plantinga's italics) whilst Elizabeth Cowie argues, that for all its 'deformations' and 'fabrications', documentary film 'sets out a contract with its audience by its self-declaration as a documentary. Its fabrications do not thereby make it not non-fiction' (2011: 45).

I want to build on this idea of an honest, ethical contract between documentary maker and documentary viewer and place it within the broader frame of a phenomenological account of documentary, which teases out the consequences of contracting to perceive the object as non-fictional. It allows me to construct an account of how the act of perceiving the object as non-fictional changes how the object is understood (it changes the meanings that can be drawn from the object). This is crucial to my contention that in documentary we can witness the emergence of new meanings in the real lives of documentary protagonists *within* the diegesis. It allows me to advance an argument about the non-fictionality of documentary's fictions as they give access to non-fictional meanings. That said, I will return to the problem of fiction (invented) and non-fiction (real) at the end of the next chapter, not in the context of the object of study but at a profounder metaphysical level where I will suggest that we can never know if the meanings we draw from the world are created (fictional) or found (non-fictional).

A phenomenological account of non-fictionality

My approach takes its cue from Vivian Sobchack's 1999 essay 'Toward a Phenomenology of Nonfictional Film Experience', where, rather than treating all film as text to be decoded, Sobchack distinguishes between filmic objects on the grounds of the different ways they are experienced by the viewer based on inherent differences between different genres of film as intentional objects. Sobchack frames her argument in opposition to what she calls 'that foundational theory of cinematic identification based on Lacanian psychoanalysis' (1999: 241) but it is an argument which also stands in opposition to non-Lacanian post-structuralist approaches to the film object.[7] Post-structuralism

> treats the spectator's phenomenological sense of the "real" as it relates to cinematic representation of *any* kind as essentially phantasmatic in nature and does not seem to allow for the structural differences that distinguish our engagement with cinematic images we regard as documentary representations of "the real" from those we regard as real representations of a "fiction".
>
> (1999: 241: Sobchack's italics)

In short, we experience what we take to be documentary in a different way to how we experience a fictional film and make very different judgements about that experience. It is a different model of 'cinematic identification', opening up moral and affective connotations that flow from 'the charge of the real' (1999: 242).

Drawing on the work of Jean-Pierre Meunier,[8] Sobchack posits three broad categories of filmic object: the fiction film, the documentary and the *film-souvenir* (or *home movie* in English parlance). All screen objects in all these categories of film are equally physically absent and only have presence as images and recorded sound but 'this fundamental absence characteristic of all cinematic representation is always *modified* by our personal and cultural knowledge of an object's existential position as it relates to our own' (1999: 242; Sobchack's italics). The fiction film exists only on the screen and we glean our meanings from the relation between objects on the screen. As Sobchack puts it, the horizon of our attention 'is nearly isomorphic with the screen' (1999: 245) and, I would add, it is a form of experience very readily susceptible to the post-structuralist approach that examines the play or relation of on-screen signifiers. But in our experience of documentary, and more so of the *film-souvenir*, we look both *at* the screen and *through* the screen; we are dependent upon the screen for knowledge but are 'also aware of an excess of existence not contained by it' (1999: 246). Sobchack illustrates this difference with a description of the moment when we are watching a character in a fictional film walking through a crowded city and suddenly wonder if the people on the street know they are in a movie. In this *moment of wondering*, the viewer has switched from looking at the fiction *on* the screen to perceiving the images as documentary in nature and so looking *through* the screen to another reality behind it (1999: 246). Michael Renov (2004: 248, footnote 6) makes a similar point when describing the moment in Haskell Wexler's 1969 fictional feature *Medium Cool*, where the soundman shouts 'Look out, Haskell, it's real!' as a tear-gas canister lands amongst the film crew during the filming of a riot intended for inclusion in the fictional diegesis. The camera shakes and wobbles at this point as the historical real bursts into the feature filmmaking and we see through the screen to a world beyond.

The nature of the intentional filmic object changes what we ask (and what we can ask) of the film and so changes the meanings that might emerge.[9] The sort of questions we might ask about "Sol Nazerman", the pawnbroker and Auschwitz survivor who is the central character in Sidney Lumet's 1964 fictional feature *The Pawnbroker*, are very different from the sort of questions we can ask about Marceline (Marceline Loridan-Ivens), the interviewer/interviewee and Auschwitz survivor in Jean Rouch and Edgar Morin's 1961 documentary *Chronique d'un* été. We can ask *on-the-screen* questions about Nazerman and *through-the-screen* questions about Marceline.[10]

Christian Ferencz-Flatz and Julian Hanich (2016: 22) identify a shift in Sobchack's focus of attention between 1992 (when she published *The Address of the Eye*) and 2004 (when she published *Carnal Thoughts*), a shift from *film-as-intentional-object* to *film-as-experiencing-subject*, a shift that took the focus of attention from *noema* to *noesis* (in Husserlian terms[11]), from the 'act matter' (what is thought about) to the 'act quality' (the mental act of liking, judging or meaning by the viewer). Both these facets of Sobchack's approach to film are valuable as they refuse a simple division between object and subject, with the object always being an *experienced-object* and with the subject always being an *experiencing-subject*. The 1999 essay 'Toward a Phenomenology of Nonfictional Film Experience' that I refer to above was written during the transitional phase in Sobchack's thought and combines both facets of her thinking. But, for two reasons, my particular interest here is in what that essay says about the noematic content – the *experienced-(non-fictional)-object*. First, by highlighting the object as it is experienced, Sobchack rescues the non-fictional film from post-structuralism's tendency to co-opt it to fiction whilst fully acknowledging the subjective nature of that experience. Secondly, in her description of the object as experienced, Sobchack opens up a space *through* or *behind* the screen; a space that allows us access to aspects of the life of the on-screen protagonist beyond the screen. It is a theoretical position that helps to substantiate my contention that certain documentaries that deal with traumatic histories can give us access to *diegetic meanings*: meanings that emerge for the on-screen protagonists through the filmmaking process; meanings whose emergence might have a reparative or curative impact in the protagonists' lives in and beyond the film, even though we as viewers are dependent upon the screen for knowledge. I am distinguishing these diegetic meanings (meanings whose emergence the viewer witnesses through consideration of the noema) from the meanings that become available directly to the viewer – the *experiencing-subject* – which we might call the film's *extra-diegetic meanings* (or noetic meanings).

If this seems fanciful in the case of documentary film, it can be argued by analogy to the psychoanalytic case study. The analytic case study may be dismissed (or indeed celebrated) as a fictional text but many readers take the text (the *experienced-object*) as a means of access to aspects of the real life of the analysand; a real life that has or had its existence beyond or behind the text. It is this perception of the case study as *experienced-object*, that makes it available for certain sorts of counter-readings; readings that were not foregrounded in the original text as published but which use the material presented in the original text to construct or recover new meanings in the life of the diegetic protagonist. This is precisely what Nicolas Abraham and Mária Török (1986) do with Freud's 'Wolf Man' case (1918); they re-imagine the Wolf Man's (Sergei Pankejeff's) trauma by taking the words used by Pankejeff in his analysis with Freud, and as reported by Freud in his text, and re-interpret them in the light of Pankejeff's multi-lingual background. When Pankejeff's words spoken in German to Freud are translated into his native Russian, they suggest puns and homophones that were not available in German and seem to give us access to relationships and events that were meaningful to Pankejeff but which bypassed Freud.[12] If published analytic case studies open up a space *beyond* or *behind* the text in the life of the analysand (to borrow Sobchack's terms), the documentary film offers the same opportunity – perhaps even a heightened opportunity – as documentary gives us access to the voice, the body and the affective responses of the protagonist played out in live relationships in the filmic present, providing us with revealing and intimate glimpses of a life lived on and beyond the screen.[13]

Elizabeth Cowie writes about these glimpsed moments. If Sobchack's account considers the documentary *as a whole* as the intentional object that gives us access to a real world beyond, then Elizabeth Cowie takes a more nuanced approach arguing that it is only at certain moments that we directly glimpse the real world. They are the documentary viewer's 'Look out, Haskell, it's real!'-moments. Such a moment is

> never fully intended for us by controlling authors or fully interpretable, but instead, as "found" reality, it is always in excess of the documentary narration. Documentary is an organized statement, an "utterance" of the recorded audiovisual, but it can never fully determine [...] the meaning of the utterance, for there is always some aspect that exceeds the intention of the filmmakers, which we refer to "reality". In this lies the specificity of the documentary as nonfiction.
>
> (Cowie 2011: 29)

It is these moments in documentary film that allow the viewer to see through the screen to a real, non-fictional life beyond, to see through the mediated text.

The fictionality of the fictional film-within

If the argument that follows depends upon making some sort of distinction between fiction and non-fiction in documentary (to understand the role of the fictional interlude within the documentary frame) then it is necessary to consider the fictionality of the fictional interlude alongside the non-fictionality of the frame. The role of the fiction will be considered at length in the next chapter when I examine how psychoanalysis has deployed fictions in an effort to *open up* a traumatic history and to allow a meaningful account to emerge for the traumatised protagonist. But some preliminary comments are necessary about what is meant by fiction. Just how fictional are the fictions of documentary?

Many fictional interludes borrow aesthetic forms commonly associated with fictional representations (animation, use of toys, theatrical re-enactment) but this is no guarantee of fictionality. Both Ari Folman in *Waltz with Bashir* (2008) and Rithy Panh in *The Missing Picture* (2013) use animation both in fictional interludes and to depict historical events whose veracity we are not asked to question. So, instead of looking at the form of the representation, it might be more helpful to look at the content. Sometimes the fictional interlude brings to the screen fantasies, hallucinations and internal conversations that have played in the mind of the traumatised protagonist. But they can also take a less fantastical form, such as the replaying of past events in the filmic present, with the role of the traumatised protagonist taken by a substitute (a double). These are not out-and-out fictions but they certainly entail degrees of fictionalisation. And all these films-within are fictional to the extent that they diverge from anything that ever happened in the real world in a way that a historian would recognise.

But the interludes are not fictional in the sense that *anything goes*. They are "real" in one of three ways. They are fictions in search of a non-fictional historical "truth" where the historical account is difficult to recover (often as a result of traumatic disruptions of memory) and can be seen as an attempt to re-imagine a historical event which is out of reach. Or secondly, they are entirely invented but may evoke powerful affective responses in the traumatised protagonist. This response is the measure of the truth of a fiction that Freud (1937b) proposes in *Constructions in Analysis*; a fiction with the power to have a positive transformatory impact on an analysand's current experience of a real, non-fictional traumatic past. Those fictions without affective force are revealed as *fictional fictions* or *untrue fictions*, and are forgotten and fall away. Or thirdly, they reproduce real imaginings or fears or hallucinations that play, or have played, in the mind of the protagonist.

Castoriadis and Rancière question the definition of fiction

Many philosophic accounts of reality would not categorise these "events" as real even though these interludes seem to be attempting to reproduce a present or past *psychic* reality. This suggests that they are only unreal or fictional in a limited sense. Here I want to re-purpose an argument that the philosopher and psychoanalyst Cornelius Castoriadis deployed about the nature of being to critique the way many philosophers have approached and described reality:

> Remember that philosophers almost always start by saying: "I want to see what being is, what reality is. Now, here is this table. What does this table show to me as characteristic of real being?" No philosopher ever starts by saying: "I want to see what being is, what reality is. Now, here is my memory of my dream last night."
>
> (Castoriadis 1997: 5)

Following Castoriadis, I would argue for the 'reality' of these fictions, or describe them as *true fictions* or, better, as reproductions (*re*-presentations) of psychic realities. Castoriadis's argument coincides with (and is likely derived from) Martin Heidegger's (1962 [1927]) distinction between the *factual* (the ontic or *factum brutum*) and the *factical* (or existential-ontological). The factual lends itself to empirical validation (or at least has that potential) whilst the factical has a reality in lived experience but not in the external, historical world. The factical, whilst not conventionally factual, is certainly not straightforwardly fictional.

For Jacques Rancière (2006: 34), these fictions of documentary are more truthful than the fictions of fiction film. 'Documentary film, film devoted to the "real", is [...] capable of greater fictional invention than "fiction" film, readily devoted to a certain stereotype of actions and characters'. The truthfulness of documentary's fictions flows from the genre's devotion to the real and Rancière's belief that '[t]he real must be fictionalized in order to be thought'. They are fictions of the "real".

Reality fictions in Waltz with Bashir

The two "fictions" or films-within at the heart of Ari Folman's animated, autobiographical documentary, *Waltz with Bashir* (2008) – the second fiction being precipitated by the first – both fall into the category that Castoriadis has sought to reposition as elements of reality and seem to pass Rancière's truthfulness test. The film opens at night in Tel Aviv with a pack of ferocious dogs running through the streets. It is a frightening scene and begins without any accompanying explanation or context. It emerges that the scene reproduces a recurring nightmare of Ari Folman's friend, Boaz Rein, who Folman had known since they both served as teenagers in the Israeli Army occupying Beirut during the Lebanon War of over twenty-five years before. In the scene following the nightmare, Rein meets Folman to ask if his description of the ferocious dogs sparks any memories for Folman. Rein is convinced it is connected in some way with their experiences in the Lebanon War and believes it to be a disguised dream-memory related to the Israeli army's practice, before a night-time attack, of killing the dogs which prowled the outskirts of Lebanese villages (something Rein was often asked to do). Folman tells Rein that not only does the description of the nightmare not spark any memories but that he is surprised to realise he has virtually no memories at all of his time in Lebanon and Beirut. An actual meeting between Rein and Folman (which is reproduced in animation in the film) is the event which prompted Folman to make *Waltz with Bashir*. The film that emerges is an unfolding filmic record of Folman's quest to recover this "lost" past, as Folman visits friends, former soldiers and a psychologist in his attempt to both remember and try to understand why he cannot remember.

As the film progresses, aspects of Folman's youthful army experiences come back to him, sometimes as a result of others recalling events at which Folman was present. Folman's abiding recovered "recollection", sparked by his engagement with his friend's nightmare, is a not a recollection at all but a kind of recurrent waking hallucination (which Folman describes in voice over as a 'flashback')[14] in which Folman sees himself and other young Israeli soldiers emerging naked from the sea off Beirut against a bizarrely illuminated urban backdrop. Folman's desire to understand his hallucinatory vision takes over as the driving force of the film's narrative and does eventually lead Folman to recover a memory of his involvement as a bystander during the Christian Phalangist massacre of Palestinian men in the Sabra and Shatila suburbs of Beirut; the bizarre illumination of the scene in the hallucination perhaps recalling the flares that were used to illuminate the sky and assist the Phalangists in finding hiding Palestinians at night. It is a deeply troubling memory for Folman, especially as the child of Holocaust survivors, as he remembers he had *stood by* and allowed mass murder to occur.

It is the two fictions – Rein's nightmare and Folman's hallucination – which open a route to understanding the traumatic past for Folman. Both are fictions in a strict historical sense but both are very real aspects of the present psychic reality of two veterans of the Lebanon War and fit with Castoriadis's expanded phenomenological conception of reality which includes 'Now, here is my memory of my dream last night'. Meaning emerges for Folman not solely in recovering a lost or repressed memory of a specific time and place but in constructing an account which could explain *why* that memory had been lost or repressed. *Waltz with Bashir* is a complex text with memory (or lack of memory) of events in Lebanon haunted by another "memory": a second-generation, post-memory of the Holocaust. Meaning emerges for Folman when he unmasks the unconscious forces that had impelled him to forget the past; something about – or associated with – that past was "unthinkable". It is a palimpsestic memory as Max Silverman (2018) describes: 'a hybrid of traces', with memory as an 'act of construction in the present' involving a 'conjunction of different pasts' (some of which might more properly be described as his parents' pasts).[15] The *ontic* fiction but *factical* reality of the dream and hallucination in *Waltz with Bashir* are not meaningful in themselves but begin a process that uncovers a trauma that was itself hidden (the film does not offer the viewer any insight into what effect *not* remembering his youthful military experiences had on Folman in the period before the filmmaking process began). It is ironic that the quest for Folman began not as an attempt to understand a traumatic past which was troubling him; his initial amnesia seemingly acted as a successful defence against trauma. But once prompted by his friend's nightmare, the desire to know, to understand and to produce a meaningful account of the past, became a driving obsession.

That the use of "fictions" in documentary seems to be driven in the main by documentary makers, like Folman, trying to explore traumatic pasts is perhaps a product of the nature of trauma itself (the subject of the next chapter). The three broad categories of fictional interlude that documentaries have employed (categories that can in practice overlap) could be summarised as psychic realities (representations of *factical* "events"), fictions that provoke strong affective responses and so hint that some "truth" is at least in play or fictions that attempt to represent historic events that are lost or obscured. The label *fictional* retains value for its clarity (and for this reason, I will continue to use it in what follows but always with the provisos set out here). But these films-within are not fictional in the sense of *fictitious* (untrue or a lie) but closer to *fictive*[16]; they emerge from the imagination or perhaps the unconscious or are provocations that have the power to reconfigure understandings of what might be conventionally described as the "real" world. Perhaps better still, we could think of them as alternative frames of experience that interact with and modify other frames of experience, which appear more straightforwardly non-fictional. It is in the dynamic encounter between the frames, that insights ("truths", meanings) become available. This technique is deployed to great and sometimes bewildering effect in Albertina Carri's *The Blonds* (the subject of Chapter 6) where there are frames, nested within frames, nested within frames, as Carri tries to understand her traumatic past.

The non-fictionality of documentary despite its fictions

So, to return to the question I asked at the beginning of this chapter about the fictionality of fiction and the non-fictionality of non-fiction, I am arguing that fictions of a sort can be introduced into documentary – inner frames of experience can be explored – without compromising the perception of the documentary *as a whole* as non-fictional. These documentaries remain non-fictional intentional objects despite the inclusion of interludes which are fictional according to many conventional accounts.

Recent work by philosophers working in the analytic tradition is reaching similar conclusions about literary texts. Fictive utterance theorists like Gregory Currie (1990), writing in the 1980s and 1990s, broke texts into discrete parts labelling some parts fictional and some non-fictional. But recently, Stacie Friend (and others) have advocated an approach that looks at the text as a whole and concludes that a text can be non-fictional even if discrete passages within that text are fictional.

> [T]he reason fictive utterance theories have so much trouble accounting for the distinction between works of fiction and non-fiction is that they are reductionist: they seek to reduce fictionality to properties possessed by the parts of a work or a single dimension of the work. [...] the right way to distinguish between fiction and non-fiction focuses attention, not on how the parts of a work add up to the whole, but instead how the whole work is embedded in a larger context, and specifically in certain practices of reading, writing, criticizing, and so on.
>
> (Friend 2012: 187)[17]

Amongst documentary scholars, Linda Williams was one of the first to appreciate the role fictions were beginning to play in documentary from the 1980s as filmmakers, such as Claude Lanzmann in *Shoah* (1985) and Errol Morris in *The Thin Blue Line* (1988), introduced "fictional" interludes into the "factual" frame of documentary and openly owned the idea that 'documentary truth is [...] subject to manipulation and construction' (Williams 1993: 12). For Williams, this positive development did not entail having to reclassify documentary as fictional but instead rescued documentary from being forced into one or the other position within a false dichotomy.

> Instead of careening between idealistic faith in documentary truth and cynical recourse to fiction, we do better to define documentary not as an essence of truth but as a set of strategies designed to choose among the horizon of relative and contingent truths. The advantage, and the difficulty, of the definition is that it holds onto the concept of the real – indeed of a "real" at all – even in the face of tendencies to assimilate documentary entirely into the rules and norms of fiction.
>
> (Williams 1993: 14)

Like Sobchack, Williams implicitly rejects the post-structuralist claim that the quest for a referent (through documentary) – a truth about the real world – is 'essentially phantasmatic'.[18] And writing more recently, Elizabeth Cowie (2011) has argued that a *desire for the real* is perfectly congruent with the documentary project with all its fabrications, and that documentary can be a route to knowledge about the real world even if the relation between film and world is complex.

For Williams, the introduction of fictions into documentary is not a roadblock on the route to knowledge of the real world but rather a crucial new path to that knowledge.

> My goal [...] is to get beyond the much remarked self-reflexivity and flamboyant auteurism of these documentaries, which might seem Rashomon-like, to abandon the pursuit of truth, to what seems to me their remarkable engagement with a newer, more contingent, relative, postmodern truth – a truth which, far from being abandoned, still operates powerfully as the receding horizon of the documentary tradition.
>
> (Williams 1993: 11)

Williams not only champions the deployment of fictions within documentary as a possible route to understanding a real world beyond the screen, she also tries to define the nature of the "truth" or knowledge that can emerge from a documentary-making process that deploys these fictional elements. She calls this emergent knowledge a 'postmodern truth' and 'relative and contingent truths'. I will return to these speculations at the end of the next chapter where I consider the epistemological status of the meanings (or "truths") we glean from documentary.

Notes

1 Fiction film and documentary maker, Lindsay Anderson, made the same distinction when defining documentary (in 1971): 'If the material is actual, then it is documentary. If the material is invented, then it is not documentary' (quoted in: Minh-Ha 1990: 78).

2 Including (but certainly not limited to) Janet Walker, Alisa Lebow and Stella Bruzzi. Michael Renov was one of the first scholars to identify these changes in documentary practice and has published several essays on the subject (for example, Renov 1999).

3 In a later essay (2015: 148), Renov makes it clear he was thinking particularly about documentaries of the late 1980s and early 1990s that dealt with the personal experience of AIDS, familial dysfunction and gendered and racial oppression. Amongst these first-person (autobiographical) filmmakers, Renov includes Issac Julien, Marlon Riggs, Su Friedrich, Gregg Bordowitz, Richard Fung, Rea Tajiri, etc.

4 Film autobiography pre-dates the 1990s but Renov argues that it then fell 'outside the consensual limits of documentary' (2008: 44). I will return to autobiography in Chapter 4 when considering the authorship of the fictions that operate within the documentary frame: those created by a third-person director versus those created by a first-person director/protagonist.

5 For example: Albertina Carri's *The Blonds* 2003; Guy Maddin's *My Winnipeg* 2007; Ari Folman's *Waltz with Bashir* 2008; Joshua Oppenheimer's *The Act of Killing* 2012; Rithy Panh's *The Missing Picture* 2013. For further discussion of the rise of fiction in documentary, see Eadie (2020).

6 Conventionally this is thought to be Winsor McCay's *The Sinking of the Lusitania* (1918) but in her recent book, Donna Kornhaber (2020) suggests the title should go to a short animation designed to solicit donations for the Second Boer War.

7 Sobchack is here writing in opposition to Lacanian approaches to film that date from the late 1960s and 1970s and the tendency in post-structuralism to co-opt documentary as a form of fiction, and not in opposition to more recent Lacanian approaches to documentary (discussed in Chapter 1).

8 Sobchack credits the Belgian psychologist and film critic, Jean-Pierre Meunier, as the pioneer of this approach as outlined in his neglected 1969 book *Les structures de l'experience filmique: L'identification filmique*, which in turn draws on Maurice Merleau-Ponty's existential phenomenology.

9 Working in a different philosophic tradition (contemporary analytic aesthetics), Stacie Friend has recently advanced an argument about written texts that is very close to Sobchack's argument about film: 'the classification of a work as fiction or non-fiction can make a genuine difference to appreciation. Labelling a work in one way or the other has an effect on how we read it, primarily by directing our attention to different aspects of the work'. Friend regrets that 'there are relatively few studies that look at the effects on reading strategy of the fiction/non-fiction distinction specifically' (Friend 2012: 200–2).

10 In other areas of scholarship in the humanities, similar phenomenological distinctions are made on the basis of the nature of the intentional, experienced object. F. R. Leavis is meant to have joked that fellow literary critic, A. C. Bradley, asked illegitimate questions about fictional characters in literary texts, such as asking 'How Many Children Had Lady Macbeth?' of the character in the Shakespeare play (2015 [1606]). But historians can perfectly legitimately ask this same question of the historical figure of Lady Macbeth, the wife of the eleventh century Scottish King, Mac Bethad mac Findláich, who Shakespeare is drawing on. With Shakespeare's Lady Macbeth we can ask only *in-the-text* questions (as the intentional object is fictional); with the wife of Mac Bethad mac Findláich we can ask *through-or-behind-the-text* questions (as the intentional object is or was "real"). The questions that can be asked are dependent on the object's ontological status (existential status in Sobchack's usage). Questions that are illegitimate in relation to a fictional object may well be legitimate in relation to a non-fictional object. The story of the jibe Leavis directed at Bradley is recounted in Britton (1961).

11 The reference here is to Husserl's *Ideas: General Introduction to Pure Phenomenology* (2013 [1913]).

12 Abraham and Török are not alone in reworking the Wolf Man case by re-interpreting the information presented in Freud's case study to try to unearth what was meaningful for the "real" Pankejeff beyond or behind the text (meanings that had evaded Freud), for example, Jacques Lacan in his seminar of 1951–52.

13 Andrew Tracey has made similar claims for the images and sounds of the 'Essay Film' which he sees as 'part of a matrix of meaning that extends beyond the screen' (Tracey et al. 2013, 2019).

14 In much post-structuralist trauma theory, flashbacks are described as veridical memories; literal, mental imprints of historic events (see Chapter 3). I have called this "flashback" a hallucination to avoid association with the notion of veridical memory. Ruth

Leys (Leys and Goldman 2010: 666), Thomas Trezise (2013) and several other critics hostile to trauma theory argue that memory is *never* veridical and Folman himself is clear that his "flashback" is to an event that never occurred in the real world.

15 For Silverman's use of the figure of the palimpsest to highlight the hybrid, 'impure' nature of memory, see his monograph *Palimpsestic Memory* (2013). Specifically re-*Waltz with Bashir*, see also Claire Launchbury's essay 'Animating Memory' in a collection edited by Silverman and Griselda Pollock (Launchbury 2013: 193–202).

16 In relation to documentary, Janet Walker (2013: 20) says it was Michael Renov who was the first scholar to introduce the notion of the 'fictive' (Renov 1993: 7).

17 Friend says one cannot establish either *necessary* or *sufficient* conditions that could be used to delineate a work of fiction from a work of non-fiction and we should think of them instead as genres: that is socially agreed-upon conventions that develop (and change) over time. Carl Plantinga (2005: 105) defines the non-fictionality of documentary in similar terms – not something with necessary or sufficient conditions but rather as a set of 'central tendencies'.

18 Sobchack (1999: 241) rejects the idea that the quest is 'phantasmatic', and Williams resists (like Fredric Jameson whom she quotes) the tendency of post-structuralism to bracket the referent and efface the past altogether 'leaving us with nothing but texts' (Jameson 1984: 64, quoted in Williams 1993: 14).

Chapter 3

The peculiar case of trauma and the demand for fiction

Three accounts of trauma

Broadly, three accounts of trauma co-exist today. Each came into being in response to what might be described as a major cultural or societal trauma. The psychoanalytic account arose within late nineteenth-century psychiatry in response to patients presenting a variety of debilitating symptoms that seemed to have their origins in the stresses and strains of modern urban life including (after World War One) the strains of modern industrialised warfare. In the wake of World War Two and, in particular of the Holocaust, a second account emerged within post-structuralist philosophy and cultural theory; an account further elaborated since the 1990s by Cathy Caruth and others in what has come to be known as trauma theory. The third account, that of post-traumatic stress disorder (PTSD), emerged from American psychiatry in the 1970s in response to symptoms being presented by combat veterans of the Vietnam War. Despite each account arising out of a particular set of historical circumstances, none of them limits what might be called the precipitators of trauma to the events that brought the account into being. There is broad unanimity across the three accounts as to the sort of life experiences that are likely to precipitate trauma: witnessing or being subject to violence, sexual assault, accident, sudden bereavement, loss of a love object, etc.

There is also broad unanimity as to the likely effects of trauma (its symptoms): the generation of disturbing thoughts, feelings or dreams, which cause mental and physical distress or sometimes just a debilitating feeling of blankness. All these symptoms seem to entail disruptions of memory[1] and the ability to represent the trauma, from the absence of representation (aporia) accompanied by distressing negative affect, through partial recall or recall that displaces or screens the traumatic events, to vivid, flashback memories that *seem* to replay the past in the present. Where psychic manifestations are absent (or in addition to psychic manifestations), trauma can manifest itself somatically as physical ailments. All three accounts also agree on the "late" registration of trauma, with symptoms striking retrospectively (*Nachträglichkeit* to use Freud's term).

But, at this point, the three accounts begin to diverge. Only the psychoanalytic and post-structuralist accounts are grounded in theories of representation

DOI: 10.4324/9781003657187-5

and reference; the PTSD account is practically focused and looks to ameliorate symptoms by managing their effect. Both the post-structuralist and psychoanalytic accounts universalise trauma, seeing it as fundamental to the human condition (unlike the PTSD account which sees trauma as only ever affecting a portion of the population). Beyond this, the psychoanalytic and post-structuralist accounts also diverge. Psychoanalysis seeks to provide a meaningful account of the trauma, which might help to lessen its negative psychic (and physical) symptoms; whilst the post-structuralist account sees trauma as both beyond representation and understanding, and the psychic consequences of trauma as perpetual and unshiftable. The experience of trauma is reconceived as a terrible, post-modern sublime, "real" and veridical, and unreclaimable to meaning. It is at this point of divergence that psychoanalysis deploys fictions: fictions which are created or found (constructed or reconstructed), giving representational content to the formerly unrepresented trauma and beginning a process that might lead to a meaningful account of the trauma. And crucially, this process takes place over time, in an inter-personal encounter (both these contexts are refused in the post-structuralist account). And it is, as I hope to establish, in parallel circumstances that fictions are deployed in documentary in the form of fictional films-within, as documentary makers try to find or create a meaningful account of a traumatic personal history.

Psychoanalysis and the many roles of fiction

In psychoanalysis, trauma is everywhere and fictions are everywhere. As psychoanalysis developed, Freud came to see trauma not merely as an individual reaction to specific, unbearable events but as a universal component of normal individual and indeed group development. And in all these arenas, fictions played a role: fictions (in the shape of unconscious fantasy) could precipitate trauma, fictions (such as screen memories) could obscure the underlying trauma, fictions could describe and explain both individual and societal trauma and fictions could play a therapeutic role in the process of "recovery" from trauma.

Freud (in collaboration with Josef Breuer) began the work which became psychoanalysis with much more limited ambitions. Freud and Breuer struggled to understand the roots of hysteria in their largely female patients. Freud's distinctive contribution was to trace hysterical symptoms (which were both psychic and physical) back to a "real" world event – sexual seduction. In his 1896 essay *The Aetiology of Hysteria*, Freud argued that 'at the bottom of every case of hysteria there are *one or more occurrences of premature sexual experience*' (1896: 203; italics in the *Standard Edition* translation); the so-called seduction theory. But within two years, this exogenous (real-world) precipitator of trauma had been remodelled as an endogenous precipitator through the notion of unconscious fantasy. In a letter of September 1897 to his colleague Wilhelm Fleiss, Freud wrote that he no longer believed in 'my *neurotica*' (his seduction theory) as 'there are no indications of reality in the unconscious, so that one cannot distinguish between truth and fiction that has been cathected with affect' (Freud and Masson 1985: 264; italics in the

Masson translation). The notion of fiction and its complex relation to truth was to remain at the heart of psychoanalysis both in its attempts to describe trauma[2] and in the therapeutic strategies it developed to treat trauma. A fiction which elicits a powerful affective response becomes a route to the truth, just as the fictional production of Hamlet's *The Murder of Gonzago* – through the affective response it precipitates in Hamlet's uncle Claudius – starts a process through which the truth is revealed.

As Freud's ideas developed, trauma was not only furnished with an endogenous cause in unconscious fantasy, but he came to see it as a universal component of ordinary development; an idea he explored in *Beyond the Pleasure Principle* in 1920 as he observed his grandson's struggle to come to terms with the originary trauma of maternal separation (1920: 14–7). And, in his highly speculative work of 1939, *Moses and Monotheism*, trauma is given a further universalising twist. Not simply the individual but society (culture) itself is seen to have its roots in trauma. Psychological trauma, once recognised, had become all-pervasive, whether it was a response to something outside the individual (in the form of violence, physical injury, sexual assault, the vicarious trauma of witnessing damage inflicted on others or the experience of loss) or from within (as the individual struggled to cope with disturbing sexual fantasies). Trauma had the power to explain both individual and group development, with the construction of creative fictions being of pivotal importance in both explaining and in gradually coming to terms with these traumas.

The effect of trauma on the sufferer's ability to represent and to understand what had happened to them was complex and Freud returned to it again and again; perhaps it was *the* task of the new discipline of psychoanalysis. Early case studies often recorded the complete absence of any conscious representation of the trauma, and understanding could only come through the analyst's attempt to trace the bodily registration of the trauma (psychosomatic symptoms) back to a forgotten event (seen first of all in Breuer's work with 'Anna O' (Breuer 1893 [1955]: 21–47)). Where a representation did exist, whether in dream or hallucination or screen memory, it often obscured (in effect, *fictionalised*) the historical cause of the trauma. Freud's fullest attempt to explain traumatic memory was perhaps in *The Interpretation of Dreams* of 1900–01; symbolisation is disrupted by traumatic memory and symptom-formation is subject to complex metaphoric and metonymic displacements that need careful interpretation and translation if something of the originary trauma is ever to be recovered (Luckhurst 2008: 45–6). Trauma disrupts time, destroying or fracturing the narratives of our lives and interfering with our capacity to know or represent what it is that troubles us. Trauma is experienced on a spectrum from amnesia or *aporia* (where the trauma seems to make no registration in the conscious mind), through to searingly vivid, hypermnesic, perhaps hallucinatory registration (which comes with no conscious understanding), to mis-remembered, mistaken, repressed, displaced or disguised registration.

Two accounts of a fictional construction/reconstruction of trauma: **Constructions in Analysis** *and the* **fort-da** *vignette*

But psychoanalysis did not simply present the difficulties inherent in traumatic memory. It tried to restore representation and understanding in the belief that this would lessen the impact of the trauma through *catharsis* (not as Breuer conceived it in conjunction with hypnosis, but in its broad modern sense of release or partial release from the emotional pain of trauma and the grip of hysteria), or, in certain cases, simply release the sufferer from the grip of physical symptoms. Most of these attempts involved the restaging of the apparent representational, affective or emotional traces of the past in the present of the analytic encounter. But Freud also indicated that where a restaging was not possible – where the traces of the past were apparently absent – the analyst would need to mount a completely new production and to imagine the missing traces and to stage them for the analysand. Two short pieces of writing by Freud help to explicate these ideas: the late essay *Constructions in Analysis* (1937b), and the *fort-da* game of Freud's grandson (1920: 14–17), described in *Beyond the Pleasure Principle* (1920: 1–64).

Both these texts make it clear that the creation of an analytic play-within-the-play – a fictional or quasi-fictional construction or reconstruction of a traumatic history – is not enough on its own to act as a catalyst that might help meaning to emerge. The fiction must be set both within a temporal frame *and* in the context of an inter-personal encounter, where the traumatised protagonist is able to reflect upon the fiction with an *other* (with an outsider to their particular traumatic history). Of the two accounts I have chosen, *Constructions in Analysis* foregrounds the importance of another mind reflecting on the fiction (helping to create it), whilst in the *fort-da* vignette the temporal comes to the fore, emphasising the role of repetition (of returning again and again to the fiction) as part of the process through which meaning can coalesce.

In *Constructions in Analysis*, Freud outlined a method for approaching the most impenetrable manifestations of trauma, where the original traumatic event appears to be entirely forgotten by the analysand (or never registered) leaving the analyst to imaginatively produce a representation – a construction – of the missing representation and offer it to the patient.

> The analyst has neither experienced nor repressed any of the material under consideration; his task cannot be to remember anything. What then is his task? His task is to make out what has been forgotten from the traces which it has left behind or, more correctly, to construct it.
>
> (1937b: 258–9)

Although Freud assigns authorship of the fiction to the analyst, it is clear that it arises out of a mutual, inter-personal space (a counter-transferential space). César and Sara Botella (2013: 104) take a similar tack, moving even deeper into this territory with their notion of *regredience*; a meeting of the psyches of analyst and analysand outside the normal representational sphere, offering the possibility of 'approaching unrepresentable zones of infantile pre-history, thereby permitting the analysand to appropriate a new capacity for experiencing and giving shape, in the form of affects and representations, to his [*sic*] nameless and shapeless distress' (2013: 107). In cases of adult trauma, the unrepresentable zone is not that of infantile pre-history but a zone that is unrepresentable because of the shattering impact of trauma. The fiction – the representation – is the product of an intense *inter-personal* encounter in the analysis; the mutual entanglement (and even the loss of boundaries) between two psyches in identification.

For the Botellas, the analyst's regredient construction, like a dream, is visual first[3] and so suggests the creative potential of deploying dream-like sequences and visual fantasies in documentary. Both Freud and the Botellas place an outsider to the trauma, the analyst, in a pivotal creative position. But the broad implication of both Freud's *Constructions* paper and the Botellas speculations is that the fantasies and fictions arise out of an entangled, counter-transferential encounter where authorship is always mutual with the traumatised protagonist signalling the importance of the fiction through their affective and/or somatic response to it.

The analyst's task in relation to the analysand in the case of an unrepresented trauma may have echoes in Bill Nichols's and Werner Herzog's description of the new techniques that documentary makers have employed in recent years to bring what could not be represented by conventional documentary means to 'a condition of visibility' (Nichols 2016: 108)[4] that reveal an 'ecstatic truth' (Herzog 2005). For Nichols, this new

> form of knowing presupposes finding the means to bring to a condition of visibility that which has escaped notice. It sets out to identify what may attain visibility and yet still cannot be seen since what is seen is a trace, sign, symptom or consequence of that which remains beyond the net of words and the reductive aspects of naming.
>
> (2016: 108)

Herzog (2005) says in a radio interview:

> In great moments of cinema you are hit and struck by some sort of enlightenment, by something that illuminates you, that's a deep form of truth and I call it ecstatic truth, the ecstasy of truth, and that's what I'm after in documentaries and feature films.

These ecstatic moments in films register affectively and somatically – the viewer is 'hit and struck' at the moment of ecstatic revelation. Nichols concurs with Herzog (repeating his phrase): 'Hit and struck. This is a form of knowledge or a way of seeing that is closer to a paradigm shift than an accretion of information, the laborious process of conventional learning, mystery solving, or the marshalling of evidence' (Nichols 2016: 107).

The notion of being hit and struck mirrors the language Shakespeare uses in *Hamlet* to describe the impact the fictional play-within might have on the diegetic audience: they will be 'struck so to the soul', that a hidden truth will be revealed.[5] Nichols and Herzog are concerned with the impact on the extra-diegetic audience when the hidden attains visibility. For Freud, the Botellas, Shakespeare, and for my argument here, the affective impact of bringing something deeply traumatic to a condition of visibility is in its impact on the intra-diegetic audience: the analysand in the analytic setting (or as described in the analytic case study); the character in the play-without watching the play-within; or the traumatised protagonist in the documentary responding to the film-within. This is a crucial difference but the mechanism through which the *truth is revealed* (or what I would more cautiously describe as *the process through which meaning emerges*) is the same whether it is revealed to the extra- or intra-diegetic audience. It is signalled in the affective and somatic responses of those who witness what has been made visible, what was formerly without shape or form. That this affecting representation might be fictional rather than historically accurate (that is not built out of the traditional materials of documentary-making which Nichols describes as the 'accretion of information, the laborious process of conventional learning, mystery solving, or the marshalling of evidence') is not the standard by which it should be judged. The standard for Herzog's 'ecstatic truth' is not whether it is reached through factual or fictional representations but in its affective impact on the viewer and what is revealed to the viewer in that moment.

A second account that Freud offers of attempting to overcome trauma through fiction is no more than a vignette in *Beyond the Pleasure Principle*. It emphasises the importance of time and repetition in dealing with trauma and is less focused on the importance of the inter-personal encounter, which is at the heart of the account in *Constructions in Analysis*.[6] In his description of his grandson's game of *fort-da* in *Beyond the Pleasure Principle*, Freud deals with trauma at the opposite end of the spectrum from that dealt with in *Constructions*; the quite normal and universal trauma of every human infant as he or she learns to bear the initially overwhelming trauma of the "loss" of the mother and enters the world of representation.

Freud's grandson, Ernst (aged eighteen months), throws away and out of sight a small wooden reel shouting 'fort' ('away') only to immediately drag the reel back to himself by means of a string, shouting 'da' ('there'). Ernst repeats the game again and again. The game can be interpreted as the child's struggle to overcome and *work through* the originary, ontogenic trauma and discover that the mother is *other* and separate and may be absent. The absence of the mother is at first experienced as an absolute, overwhelming, irreparable loss ('nameless and shapeless distress' to borrow the Botellas's phrase) as the tiny infant exists in an all-encompassing and inescapable present with no concept of time (or indeed space). Gradually the infant learns that the *loss* is not permanent but is an *absence* and that the mother will return. Ernst's game is the working through in play of the deeply unpleasurable experience of the loss of the mother; he repeats the loss ('fort') but, in his retrieval of the reel ('da'), the loss is reformulated as *temporary absence*. The flood of affect experienced by the infant when the mother disappears is gradually overcome through the repetition in play, in fictional make-believe, of the unpleasurable, terrifying loss, through the substitution of the real mother for a meaningful, symbolic representation of the lost object, now felt to be separate but not vanished.

My reading of Ernst's game as the child's successful attempt to come to terms with a traumatic "event" through the invention and repetition of a fiction puts a particular gloss on Freud's account in *Beyond the Pleasure Principle* (1920: 1–64). Freud does not specifically call Ernst's experience of maternal absence a trauma but he does place the *fort-da* vignette immediately after an extended discussion of various trauma-inducing events from horrific railway accidents to the traumatic neuroses of soldiers who had participated in 'the terrible war that has just ended' (1920: 12). The precise placement of the *fort-da* vignette within *Beyond the Pleasure Principle* strongly suggests that Freud saw Ernst's experience as traumatic.[7]

Within the *fort-da* vignette itself, Freud concerns himself not explicitly with trauma but with the pleasure principle and attempts to understand why Ernst would repeat and repeat in his play – in fiction – what was such a deeply unpleasant experience, and asks: 'How then does his repetition of this distressing experience as a game fit in with the pleasure principle?' (1920: 15). His answer is that the repetition brings with it a *bonus of pleasure*. There are two parts to this process. At first the trauma of the mother's non-existence is overwhelming. It prompts an instinctual renunciation, which is not a choice but a response to brute exigency: the mother is not there so the absence/non-existence must be accepted – it is simply a fact. But the game, in repeating the trauma and the renunciation, has a pleasurable aspect.

> At the outset he was in a *passive* situation – he was overpowered by the experience; but, by repeating it, unpleasurable though it was, as a game, he took on an *active* part. The efforts might be put down to an instinct for mastery that was acting independently of whether the memory was in itself pleasurable or not.
>
> (1920: 16; italics in the *Standard Edition* translation)

Freud adds that the game might yield another pleasurable bonus if we think of the game as the child taking revenge on the mother in fictional form; throwing away the reel-mother who had abandoned him. With either interpretation, the child has gained the pleasure of agency ('mastery') and is no longer just the hapless, helpless victim. In fact, the child's very ability to reproduce the trauma in a fictional account – to represent the trauma at all – might be dependent upon its yield of pleasure:

> [T]he child may, after all, only have been able to repeat his unpleasant experience in play because the repetition carried along with it a yield of pleasure of another sort but none the less a direct one.
>
> (1920: 16)

The fiction of the game in *Beyond the Pleasure Principle* is not only the repetition of a hidden trauma but also the working through of that trauma. Something is salvaged from a terrible situation. In parallel, I will argue that in documentary, the construction of certain films-within by the traumatised protagonist are a repetition of a trauma (a repetition where the trauma perhaps achieves representational form for the first time; where the hidden attains visibility) but that this unpleasurable repetition might carry with it a bonus of pleasure: mastery of the past; perhaps revenge; and very often (I believe) a pleasurable mastery that comes from meaning, from understanding something of the trauma for the first time.

Freud's recognition of the profound seriousness of his grandson's play later received systematic elaboration in Melanie Klein's innovative work with children where Klein introduced play – games with toys – into the analytic space and encouraged the child to stage scenarios using toys as characters in "fictional" productions (see for example, Klein 1984 [1932]). With small children lacking the verbal dexterity required for free association – the talking cure – Klein's games were designed as an alternative method of unlocking the structure of the unconscious mind.[8] Within classical psychoanalysis, the use of toys remains the preserve of the child analyst and so perhaps its potential to unlock the unrepresentable traumatic pasts of adults (unrepresentable in the sense of not available in words) has not been fully explored.[9] But some recent documentary makers have not had the same reluctance. In *The Missing Picture* (2013), Rithy Panh stages an elaborate series of miniature plays in which clay figurines take a variety of roles, tapping into the unrealised potential *for adults* of Klein's use of toys in her work with children. Panh has indicated that it was only when he stumbled upon the idea of staging his past in elaborate scenarios with "toys" that the making of a film about his traumatic childhood became possible.[10] Similarly, in her autobiographical documentary *The Blonds* (2003), Albertina Carri creates animated scenarios with Playmobil figures and Playmobil sets to give representational and dramatic form to her childhood trauma. Both Panh and Carri stage elaborate plays, substituting their particular toys for Ernst's cotton reel and piece of string.

Comparisons might be drawn with Art Spiegelman's (1992) exploration of second-generation, post-Holocaust trauma through his use of cartoon characters, which invoke both fictional play and the dream-like quality of the Botellas's regredient constructions, in his graphic novel *Maus II*. For Michael Rothberg, these playful, dream-like fictions are perhaps the only way to represent the unreal or unimaginable reality of the death camps arguing that 'the historical trauma of the Nazi genocide [...] *de-realizes* human experience and thus creates a need for fiction' (2000: 206; Rothberg's italics).

Beyond the central role of the child's capacity for creative play and for producing creative fictions to represent the trauma, four crucial ideas are encapsulated in the short *fort-da* vignette (ideas that all re-emerge in Albertina Carri's *The Blonds*).

First, the originary trauma is worked through as the child moves into the world of representation; the representation is the comforting *idea* of the mother that exists (as what we now might call an internal object) even when the *real* mother is absent.

This representation of the mother is not a simple, indexical copy of the mother (Ernst does not play with a photograph of his mother which he hides and then retrieves) but a complex metaphorical substitution, where a wooden cotton reel stands in for the absent and present mother (it is a meaningful, symbolic representation where signifier and signified eventually, through repetition, form a unitary sign). The *reel* mother stands in for the *real* mother. A fictionalised account is created in play that reproduces (but also alters) the real, non-fictional world, and the trauma is contained.

Secondly, the child's ability to substitute a mental conception – an idea – for the real mother, does not happen in an instant but instead the traumatic event and the resolution to the trauma must be repeated again and again ('fort' – 'da', 'fort' – 'da', 'fort' – 'da') for the terror of the trauma to be contained.

Thirdly, the child's entry into the representational world marks the child's entry into the temporal world, as the child comes to recognise *absence* rather than *loss*; this recognition implies an ability to think that at a future moment the mother will return and an ability to remember that at a past moment the mother was once present.

Fourthly, this recognition marks the child's entry into the spatial world too as it entails an understanding that when the mother is absent she still exists, somewhere else, not simply as a representation but as a physical reality in another place (the string attached to Ernst's reel is the physical manifestation of this concept).

Rosine Perelberg argues (following Freud) that it is in this developmental moment that 'the whole of psychic reality, in its positive and negative aspects, is structured in terms of time and space' (2008: 2). It happens through fictional representation and in relation to an emergent temporally and spatially separate "other": 'The constitution of the individual takes place in the context of the time-space created in the relationship with the mother (and her body)' (2008: 21).

In the *fort-da* vignette, Freud is (in effect) describing a "cure" for trauma, as he describes how his grandson (standing in for *every* human infant) "overcame" the originary trauma of maternal separation. The traumatic occurrence needs to be represented and a fiction is invented. That fictional representation of necessity appears where once there was no representation: in the infant's case because it had not previously reached the necessary developmental stage, experiencing the mother not as separate from self but as fused and undifferentiated; in the adult's case because the impact of the trauma has shattered representational capacities, leaving only a flood of terrifying affect, blurring or erasing the boundaries between self and other, subject and object. The nature of the infant's experience of the trauma before the *fort-da* game was invented matches the description of adult traumatic experience in all three of the major contemporary accounts of trauma. That is, an inability to represent the trauma and a consequent inability to make sense (to produce a meaningful account) of the trauma; the shattering of temporal capacities as the trauma repeats only as terrifying and present affect or in so-called veridical memory as if the original traumatic event is happening *now*, in a perpetual experiential present; and a loss of spatial boundaries as the traumatised adult experiences the world as if trapped at the site of the original traumatic occurrence.[11]

Temporality is an essential component of non-traumatic (post-traumatic) experience; for the infant, a sense of time arises from the rhythm of tolerance of displeasure. The successful resolution of this repetition compulsion is the mastering of time and requires a meaningful fictional narrative (narrative is after all simply a representation played out in time) from the very simplest narrative – *fort* then *da* then *fort* then *da,* etc. – to the most complex *construction in analysis*. A fictional narrative becomes the "cure" or at least the catalyst for the "cure". The soothing representation is a *fictive*, or perhaps more accurately in Ernst's case, a *metaphoric* substitution (a wooden reel as mother). Lessening the grip of trauma entails a repetitive return to the traumatic event, although the repetition is more accurately conceptualised as a *spiral*, a form that apparently repeats, but which slowly moves one to a different "place" (a different point in time). This escape from trauma mirrors the process of plunging into trauma as described by Jean Laplanche, where the traumatised individual 'is caught in the repetitions of a spiral of trauma that recapitulates the original wounding' (Ganteau 2015: 58, paraphrasing a passage in Laplanche 2006). For Laplanche, one can spiral into trauma; Freud's description of his grandson's repetitive game (his fictional play) suggests one can also spiral out of trauma given the right conditions. Freud does not use the term 'spiral', so perhaps a better way to conceptualise a repetitive circle/cycle that can eventually lead to change is to think of it as a *Heraclitan circle*, where one goes around the circle but can never return to the same point, as the time dimension makes what is a return to the same point in the spatial dimensions of a circle actually a progression to a different point, time having moved on.[12]

Laplanche's *vicious spiral* into trauma is overcome through the *beneficial spiral* back to psychic health that Freud describes. This is not to give the impression that the process is either painless or a *quick fix*. Freud (1937a) was profoundly aware that an analysis of even neurotic symptoms can be interminable; how much more so when dealing with (arguably) psychotic states. Instead, the psychological damage inflicted by trauma may only be susceptible to amelioration in the most propitious of circumstances. There are no miraculous cures of the sort witnessed by viewers of *The Mystery of the Rocks of Kador* (Perret 1912) where Suzanne, on viewing a recreation (a fictionalised *re*-presentation) of the traumatic event on film, is freed instantaneously from her symptoms (her *démence*) and fully recovers the lost object, her lover d'Erquy. In the real world that Freud is trying to describe, cures are rarely instantaneous and never miraculous.[13] Ernst's "cure" is more accurately described as *a coming to terms with* separation through a fictive, metaphoric representation that constantly returns Ernst to the point of unpleasure (loss) but through its temporal extension, gradually diminishes the terror, turning loss into absence, unpleasure into pleasure.

In his *coming to terms*, Ernst has asserted some control over the terrifying trauma, and so achieves what Guy Maddin (2007) failed to achieve in *My Winnipeg*, the *recovery* (or in Ernst's case perhaps, the *discovery*) of agency. But still, the meaningful representation (the symbolisation) can only be a cure to the extent that it is also the marker of the loss of the preceding state of fusion with his mother. The fictional representation always points towards the lost/absent object and so is always a marker of the original trauma. The separation is irrevocable. Freud's account of his grandson's game is effectively a parable about human representational capacities, which are only called into being in order to contain loss (trauma); representation is a marker of the post-traumatic nature of human experience beyond early infancy. In adults attempting to deal with trauma, representational capacities are not called into being for the first time but need to be recovered, having been shattered by the psychic impact of traumatic events. And a "cure", if it comes (a lessening of the psychological distress associated with the trauma), is never miraculous: it is a coming to terms with trauma not its eradication.

In the acceptance of loss and the process of repetition required to escape the most debilitating effects of that traumatic loss, the *fort-da* vignette mirrors Freud's description of mourning in *Mourning and Melancholia* (1917a). The "cure" for trauma has the temporality of mourning; the passage of time and repetition playing a vital part in the return to psychic health through a constant testing and then an acceptance of reality. For Jean Laplanche, the temporality and the repetitions of the work of mourning are 'the very prototype of analytic endeavour' (Ray 2012: 56): the analytic process itself is a process of mourning.[14] But there is no inevitability to the "cure" as in the same essay (1917a) Freud describes the remarkably similar (atemporal) temporality of melancholia, which repeats and repeats the trauma only to retraumatise or precipitate an escape into mania. The fictions of analysis and documentary can only work within a dynamic temporal context; a context (I will argue in the next section) that is refused in the post-structuralist reading of trauma producing a melancholic account, with the traumatised protagonist perpetually trapped in an unchanging, constantly repeating traumatic present. The trauma remains an open wound[15]: there is no possibility of mastery; there is no possibility of understanding or meaning; the bonus of pleasure is not available. The repetitions of the post-structuralist account of trauma are the melancholic repetitions of the death drive – a deathly compulsion to repeat – 'repeatedly bringing the patient back into the situation of his accident' (1920: 13) as Freud puts it in *Beyond the Pleasure Principle* in the context of the traumatic dreams that beset so many survivors of the First World War. This fits with Laplanche's account of spiralling into trauma. What Freud's account of Ernst's game allows – and what *Beyond the Pleasure Principle* as a whole suggests – is that for some there may be no escape from the deathly repetitions of trauma but that this is not inevitable: certain repetitions of traumatic experience might be in the service of the life drive, allowing a bonus of pleasure, allowing the 'patient' to spiral out of trauma or at least out of its worst excesses.

It is clear from Freud's two accounts of the potential routes to recovery from trauma, a fiction plays a central role, providing a representation that can be worked on and that may in time coalesce into a meaningful and perhaps curative account of the traumatic event. Freud is describing fictional interludes that can have a profound effect on the very real traumatic histories in which these fictions intervene. With Ernst, Freud *shows* us the fiction; in *Constructions in Analysis*, he *tells* us how, in theory, the analyst (and analysand) go about creating the fiction. Both accounts suggest that a 'bait of falsehood' has the potential to take the 'carp of truth' if the bait is set within a temporal and inter-personal process.

The post-structuralist account of trauma: a timeless truth without meaning

In the post-structuralist reading of trauma, there is no place for the imaginative fictions that psychoanalysis sees as the key to unlocking or provoking a meaningful account of traumatic experience. Post-structuralist accounts of trauma – taking the Holocaust as the paradigmatic case – entail epistemological and ontological positions that are incompatible with a belief in the possibility of recovery from trauma. These 'prescriptive epistemologies and ontologies', as Michael Rothberg (2000: 206) calls them, refuse the *middle term*, the signified, where meaning – potentially curative meaning – is created or found. Instead, traumatic experience is seen as fixed and unchanging, one either of aporia and blankness or of veridical flashback memory, with both conceived as non-representational manifestations of a terrible sublime. The place where psychoanalysis deploys its fictions – the place where certain recent documentaries deploy their fictions – where creative play or dreaming can be staged, is closed down. The space of the signified, of meaning-making, is lost between missing or shattered signifiers and the literal return of the referent – the traumatic real.

In this section, I will explore the philosophical underpinnings of post-structuralist trauma theories in the work of Jean-François Lyotard and Cathy Caruth, to help explicate the contrasting philosophical framework in which psychoanalysis operates and which allows it to deploy its fictions. In both Lyotard's and Caruth's accounts, the symptoms of trauma come to mould the theoretical superstructure. The insider's experience of trauma, the symptoms of trauma, are universalised to become the only possible experience of the world, as all of experience is recast as traumatic.[16] Symptomatology becomes ontology. This theoretical account once (or if) accepted is then perfectly consistent in refusing both the emergence of meaning and the possibility of any change in the traumatic condition.

Lyotard and the sublime Event

In a number of works written from the early 1980s,[17] Jean-François Lyotard set out a vision of the post-Holocaust world, a world that escaped representation and refused to coalesce into an account that could make any sense of what had happened at Auschwitz. Lyotard re-worked Kant's long-neglected notion of the sublime and the epoch-changing *Event*, to establish Auschwitz as the terrible *sublime event*, beyond the reach of reason and understanding; an event that could only be experienced directly and unmediated as a shattering encounter with the referent, at once both unthinkable and 'the most real of realities' (1988 [1983]: 58). This shattering encounter came to reform ontology, turning the inability of the traumatised to make sense of their experience into a universal template for human experience of the world. Lyotard discarded each of the mechanisms that allowed the psychoanalytic account of trauma to retain at least the hope that change – amelioration of traumatic experience – might be possible. He stripped away the temporal and the inter-personal and occluded the middle term of the signified where meaning is found or created – a middle term that psychoanalysis seeks in its deployment of fictions – enshrining an implacable *Denkverbot* at the core of his thinking.

The insider's experience of trauma in Lyotard's account is one of either 'silence', the inability to find any representational form for the experience, or of 'insanity', the inability to make any sense of the jumbled, terrifying representations in memory that may remain. But this picture of blankness or confusion, familiar from many other accounts of trauma including the psychoanalytic account, is not confined to the traumatised protagonist – the primary witness to the trauma – but expanded to include all outsiders to the trauma, to all secondary witnesses, who mirror the insider's experience of silence in their 'deafness' and in their inability to make any sense of what has happened.

> [T]he "perfect crime" [which is how Lyotard describes "Auschwitz"] does not consist in killing the victim or the witnesses [...] but rather in obtaining the silence of the witnesses, the deafness of the judges, and the inconsistency (insanity) of the testimony. You neutralize the addresser, the addressee, and the sense of the testimony.
>
> (Lyotard 1988 [1983]: 8)[18]

Those secondary witnesses, who try to construct a temporal or historical account of the trauma, come in for particularly harsh criticism, with history seen as a terrorising and illegitimate meta-narrative. Lyotard demands that the historian

> must break with the monopoly over history granted to the cognitive regime of phrases, and he or she must venture forth by lending his or her ear to what is not presentable under the rules of knowledge. Every reality entails this exigency insofar as it entails possible unknown senses. Auschwitz is the most real of realities in this respect. Its name marks the confines wherein historical knowledge sees its competence impugned.
>
> (1988 [1983]: 58)

For the psychoanalyst or the documentary maker (secondary witnesses of a sort) who try to unravel the psychic and historical aetiology of trauma, the inconsistency and insanity of the testimony – even its absence (silence) – may be a starting point in a process that tries to recover or construct/reconstruct 'the sense of the testimony' and so work back to a meaningful account. But Lyotard sees these efforts as futile and illegitimate as the 'rules of knowledge' cannot encompass the horror of 'Auschwitz', with outsiders to the trauma as afflicted by this state of unknowing as insiders. The 'earthquake' of Auschwitz destroyed all the 'instruments' we thought we once had for understanding and making sense of the world, placing all of us in the same predicament as the traumatised survivor – unable to understand what has happened

> Suppose that an earthquake destroys not only lives, buildings, and objects but also the instruments used to measure earthquakes directly and indirectly. The impossibility of quantitatively measuring it does not prohibit, but rather inspires in the minds of the survivors the idea of a very great seismic force.
>
> (1988 [1983]: 56)

The reality of Auschwitz remains but it is not only unrepresentable but unmeasureable and so, quite literally, unthinkable.

Lyotard reached this extreme anti-rationalist and anti-cognitivist conclusion through his revival and reworking of Kant's notion of the *dynamical sublime* which, for Kant (1951 [1790] *The Critique of Judgment*: section 23), was an overwhelming feeling that strikes the perceiver as a sensation of 'boundlessness' as we are presented with a 'formless object'. The language is mirrored in Lyotard's description of Auschwitz inspiring in 'the minds of the survivors the idea of a very great presentation of the indeterminate' and in his choice of the word 'earthquake' to describe Auschwitz, the same word Kant chose to describe the magnitude of the dynamical sublime, which revealed the failure of sensibility, imagination and understanding (Kant 1951 [1790] *The Critique of Judgment*: section 28).[19] In his description of Auschwitz, Lyotard is here also referencing Kant's ideas about the sublime, apocalyptic, epoch-changing event, which is so momentous it is carried outside of history and beyond understanding. For Kant, 'the event' ('die Begebenheit') was the French Revolution; for Lyotard 'the event' ('l'événement') was 'Auschwitz'.

Lyotard is more or less in agreement with Kant on how we reach the sublime. But Lyotard refused the key Kantian notion, 'Judgement' ('Urteil'), which was crucial to drawing the sublime event back into the realm of 'Understanding' ('Verstand'). In the Kantian scheme, there is no direct *Understanding* of the sublime (only *Reason* can grasp the sublime) but Kant offers a route from *Reason* to *Understanding*; a route that allowed the sublime to be drawn back into the realm of knowledge and meaning through the working of the spontaneous and innate, cognitive capacity of *Judgement* which Kant also calls the 'faculty of thinking' (Kant 1999 [2nd edition 1787]: *The Critique of Pure Reason*). *Judgement* is *the* central cognitive faculty that combines all the other cognitive capacities 'under a single higher-order unity of rational self-consciousness'; a complex meta-cognitive faculty combining conceptualisation, logic, feeling, self-consciousness, intuition, etc. (Hanna 2016).

So, in Kant's account, it is *Judgement* that translates the sublime back from the realm where only *Reason* can operate, to the realm of *Understanding*. But Lyotard absolutely rejects the power of reason (it perished at Auschwitz). With this vital modification, Kant's sublime offered Lyotard exactly the philosophical vehicle he required. Like Kant, Lyotard reaches the sublime by vaulting straight over understanding and meaning (the signified) to a much profounder but formless, unthought, registration of the world we inhabit (the referent). But then, in

Lyotard's account, with *Reason* disabled, *Judgement* cannot act as it does for Kant, as a go-between linking the sublime back to *Understanding*. The journey to this new *post-modern sublime* becomes a one-way ticket; meaning cannot be recovered or constructed. Lyotard refuses the possibility of ever being able to understand the sublime event, leaving 'Auschwitz' permanently beyond understanding, incapable of being translated into a meaningful account and registering only as an inchoate, affective presentation of horror and pain.

In his appropriation of Kant, Lyotard produced an account of Auschwitz – an account of trauma – that was carried outside history, to become a timeless, unchanging description of the human condition. This traumatised, anti-rationalist account then came to reform ontology itself (as is clear in Geoff Bennington's approving gloss of Lyotard's ideas):

> As a sort of emblem, Auschwitz signals the limit of historical competence: but this limit is implied in the structure of "reality" in general.
>
> (Bennington 1987: 148)

Joshua Hirsch (2004: 9) has described this as post-structuralism's tendency 'to universalize trauma as inherent in history, language, or even experience itself'. There is no outside to trauma: experience is traumatic and without remedy.

Lyotard's account certainly reflects the experience of many survivors, like Elie Wiesel (1968: 182) who described the Holocaust as 'a mystery that exceeds and overwhelms us'; a terrible, sublime, unrepresentable, unthinkable event. But it is a traumatised insider's account and one which has refused any outsider's view: we are all co-opted into Wiesel's 'us'. There is therefore no possibility of any inter-personal encounter between the traumatised and the non-traumatised (an outside witness) capable of generating a dialectic that over time might produce some sort of meaningful account. In contemporary psychoanalytic accounts of working with trauma – like that of the Botellas – the process can begin where Lyotard ends. Starting with the analysand's formless, contentless, unrepresented, overwhelming feelings, the analyst acts as "witness" and attempts to provide some form and content (a *regredient dream*, a *construction*, a *fiction*) for the formless, contentless, unrepresented trauma, beginning a process that might ultimately yield some understanding. There seem to be powerful parallels between the Botellas's *regredient* technique – a particular instantiation of the broader notion of the free-floating attention of the analyst – and the complex meta-cognitive faculty combining, conceptualisation, logic, feeling, self-consciousness and intuition that Kant called 'Judgement' ('Urteil'); a form of thinking that allowed Kant to draw the formless sublime back to the middle term where understanding and meaning appear. It is a similar complex, meta-cognitive faculty that allows the analyst to draw the analysand's formless trauma into some sort of representational form (into a fiction produced in the counter-transference) that might catalyse a meaning-generating process. For Lyotard, these techniques and faculties (if they ever existed) were destroyed by the 'earthquake' of Auschwitz.

Caruth and the embodied sublime

In Lyotard's account of Auschwitz, the traumatised flesh and blood survivors of the camps are strangely absent. It is as if the main victim of the Holocaust was thought and philosophy. A more embodied and historically located post-structuralist account of trauma emerged in the United States from the late 1970s, again taking the Holocaust as its archetype, but placing the testimony of survivors centre stage.[20] This has come to be known as 'trauma theory' and was developed by a group of Yale University literary scholars including Shoshana Felman and, most prominently, Cathy Caruth (in her writings from the early 1990s[21]). Caruth combined a variety of practices – post-structuralist literary theory, neurophysiology and a version of psychoanalysis – to articulate her account of trauma. But despite the different theoretical underpinnings of Caruth's trauma theory, it comes to conclusions very similar to those of Lyotard. Once again, trauma is unrepresentable and beyond understanding, registering as an unthinkable, timeless sublime. Lyotard's sublime, unthinkable *Event*, that registered only as a 'negative presentation of the indeterminate' (Lyotard 1988 [1983]: 56), is replaced by a sublime, embodied, traumatised survivor of the work and death camps. Their terrible stories are beyond the comprehension of both themselves and those who witness their testimony.

On understanding, Caruth is unequivocal: 'Traumatic experience suggests a certain paradox: that the most direct seeing of a violent event may occur as an absolute inability to know it' (1996: 91–2). It is, as if, according to Roger Luckhurst, '[t]rauma somehow is seared directly into the psyche, almost like a piece of shrapnel, and is not subject to the distortions of subjective memory' (2008: 4). Trauma registers not as a memory (available to thought and reworking) but as a pristine, unchanging and veridical imprint of the traumatic event, sealed off from other parts of the mind. Caruth describes trauma as 'a symptom of history' and traumatised individuals 'become themselves the symptom of a history that they cannot fully possess' (1991: 4). To substantiate her conjectures, Caruth cites neurophysiological research – especially that of Bessel van der Kolk[22] – to claim that traumatic memory is a 'reality imprint' (Van der Kolk, McFarlane, and Weisæth 1996: 52); or, in Roger Luckhurst's gloss of Van der Kolk, 'the unprocessed fragment of the thing itself' (Luckhurst 2008: 13). Ruth Leys, who holds that memory is always subject to distortions and can never be veridical, suggests that van der Kolk and trauma theorists

> share the same epistemological-ontological commitments. They both think that traumatic flashbacks and nightmares are veridical memories of past traumatic events, and they both believe that those symptoms are literal replicas or reproductions of the trauma that as such stand outside all representation. Van der Kolk believes that the literal nature of the traumatic flashback or memory means that it belongs to a system of traumatic memory different from that of ordinary memory and as such is cut off or dissociated from ordinary recollection, symbolisation, and meaning.
>
> (Leys's spoken comments in: Leys and Goldman 2010: 666)

Without access to explanation and without agency, the victim of traumatic events becomes the embodied, sublime referent, a by-product of a traumatic history, and an unwitting vessel for the literal truth to which they have no access. Survivors' accounts cease to be signifiers or representations of the traumatic event but fragments of the real. And when the trauma does not register as a veridical memory – as a piece of mental shrapnel – it is equally lost to understanding and meaning; it is an impenetrable *aporia*, an "unknown" that is felt only as a painful, affecting absence or nothingness. Neither of these articulations of traumatic memory are representations: one is an embodiment of the referent; the other is a simple absence of representation.

Caruth and other trauma theorists teaching at Yale also drew heavily on the deconstructive theories of Paul de Man to reinforce the idea that trauma is unrepresentable or unreadable and unavailable to understanding. In a recent essay, Stef Craps writes:

> According to Caruth, conjoining a psychoanalytic view of trauma with a deconstructivist vigilance regarding the indeterminacies of representation in the analysis of texts that bear witness to traumatic histories can grant us a paradoxical mode of access to extreme events and experiences that defy understanding and representation. In this account, textual "undecidability" or "unreadability" comes to reflect the inaccessibility of trauma.
>
> (Craps 2014: 45)

Craps's perspicacious observation contradicts a common assumption that trauma theory addresses the real historical world and real survivor's accounts. Trauma theory's "real world" of traumatic experience is the historical world reconfigured either as unreadable "text" or as a remote, noumenal truth to which we have no access. The apparent return to history and the real world by Caruth and others is more accurately an obliteration of history and the temporal. In 1991, Caruth wrote 'a history can be grasped only in the very inaccessibility of its occurrence' (1991: 7) and five years later went on to make the universalising claim: 'I link the notion of trauma to the larger conception of the very "possibility of history"' (1996: 7, footnote 5) – by which Caruth of course means the *impossibility* of history. And this ahistorical, atemporal traumatic world comes to describe all of human experience (conflating, according to Wulf Kansteiner (2004: 194), the traumatic with the non-traumatic and so obliterating 'historical precision'). In trauma theory, a particular version of the inside of the traumatic experience is used to produce an ontology that claims all of human experience as traumatising and beyond understanding. For Pieter Vermeulen (2007: 460), trauma theory can be defined as a 'program of understanding non-understanding'. He substantiates this by quoting Caruth: trauma is not about the 'event itself' but inheres 'solely in the *structure of its experience* or reception'; an experience which in turn is defined as a 'collapse of understanding' (Vermeulen 2007: 459–60, quoting Caruth 1995: 3–12; retaining Caruth's italics). The theory is circular, hermetically sealed, and so in its own terms, invulnerable to challenge.[23] Trauma is everywhere, and *unreadability* and *non-understanding* are everywhere, spilling over the borders of traumatic history to define reality itself.

My position is less hostile than that of Vermeulen and Trezise as I would concur with Caruth that the structure of the experience of trauma is often one of blankness and lack of understanding. But this is not the end point, rather it is the point where the inter-personal (and historicising) practice of psychoanalysis begins its work (as I will argue through the work of Linda Belau below).

Post-structuralism's atemporality and passivation of the secondary witness

It seems that trauma theory closes off all the routes that psychoanalysis pursues in trying to construct or recover a meaningful account of trauma. Where there is some memory of the trauma, even if confused and temporally fractured, the analyst as an outsider to the trauma tries to work with the analysand to piece together a temporal account that reaches behind the screen memories, the nightmares and the hallucinations. But trauma theory excludes both the possibility of recovering a historical account of the trauma and forecloses on the process of working with the insider's account of trauma over time, returning to it again and again, so setting in motion a beneficial spiral (a mournful spiral) away from the initially traumatising account. By claiming that the registration of the trauma is veridical – a fragment of the real – there is no account available to work with. There is nothing for the psychoanalytic process to uncover as we are already in possession of the referent, the truth. Psychoanalysis can work with what we now call traumatic flashback memories but only if these are conceived of as *vivid* not *veridical*; a distinction that retains the notion that 'traumatic memory is always representational, available to memory, and therefore open to constant revision' (Luckhurst 2008: 13). Veridical memory is another facet of the trauma theory's atemporality; like Lyotard's 'Event', it is outside history and not subject to change. I have no doubt that some of those suffering trauma are subject to powerful, terrifyingly real, flashback-"memories" that enter the mind without warning, but this is not proof of the flashback's veridity, only its affective power.

By conceiving the registration of trauma as veridical, non-representational and not available to cognition, the traumatised victim is caught in an unending repetition of the pain of the wounding event. This is the atemporal temporality of melancholia rather than the temporal process of mourning that analysis hopes to set in motion. The temporality of trauma theory is not strictly an experience of time at all but the experience of a perpetual series of traumatic, frozen "presents" (frozen "pasts" if one prefers, constantly repeating in the present), which occlude the possibility of 'working-through'.[24] Without time as an agent of change, melancholia cannot become mourning, and mourning cannot become a process that can lead back to psychic health. Without an active temporal process, Freud's grandson, Ernst, would have remained lost forever in 'nameless and shapeless distress' overwhelmed by the loss of his mother. Instead, through an idea of time as change, and the staging of the fiction with the cotton reel with its repetitions of *fort-da, fort-da,* Ernst is able to reach an accommodation with loss, recasting it as temporary absence. No longer an endless circle of distress but a *spiral* (a *Heraclitan circle*) out of trauma to a more ordinary experience of the world.

And just as the action of time is excluded from Lyotard's and Caruth's accounts, so is the active intervention of the secondary witness; an intervention which (like that of the analyst) could generate a dialectic that might allow an understanding of the traumatic past to emerge. The *witness* (and the act of *witnessing*) plays a central role in trauma theory[25] but it is a passive role. All the witness can do is to passively *receive* the testimony, which the traumatised individual *transmits* to the witness as a kind of bodily or psychic contagion. Just as the primary witness – the traumatised protagonist – experiences the trauma as a nameless, shapeless dread, so the secondary witness plays silent witness to the trauma through a process of vicarious traumatisation. The secondary witness in this account does not have a mind that can try to actively process the experiences that are presented or transmitted.[26] Again, here, post-structuralist trauma theory leaves off where psychoanalysis begins an active process that might lead to understanding. Jean Laplanche, Dominique Scarfone and others (see for example, Laplanche 1999a; Scarfone 2010) write about the analyst passively receiving what is transmitted by the traumatised patient, but the analytic mind (as both inside and outside the trauma) can then begin to actively process the feelings that have been transmitted (feelings that are intuited in the countertransference), transforming them into something new (a *construction*) that can then be offered back to the analysand. Those feelings come with no representational form but the analyst struggles to create that form – to create a fiction – that when offered back to the patient may begin a process that starts to bring understanding to the nameless, shapeless trauma.

Psychoanalysis: working with impossibility

Linda Belau (2001) succinctly characterises the difference between Cathy Caruth and Shoshana Felman's deconstructive approach to trauma (and I would include Lyotard here too) and the approach of psychoanalysis. Deconstructive and post-structuralist accounts begin with the *impossibility* of trauma – its unrepresentability, its incomprehensibility, its perpetual and unchanging repetition (as veridical memory or inchoate horror), its passivation and vicarious traumatisation of the secondary witness – and then raise this experience of impossibility to the level of 'an ideal' (Belau 2001: paragraph 20). The insider's experience of trauma – the symptomatology of trauma – is turned into a new ontology.

Psychoanalysis takes a different approach.[27] As Belau puts it (2001: footnote 32): 'for deconstruction, the subject is impossible, for psychoanalysis, the subject is that very impossibility'. It is at this very moment of 'impossibility' (when post-structuralism *gives up*, turning trauma into a sublime, timeless referent) that psychoanalysis starts its work. Fictions are invented to take the place of lost, missing or never-existing representations. These fictions are generated by the secondary witness (by the analyst or, by extension, by the documentary maker) out of the 'impossibility' – out of the transmission and passive reception of traumatic experience – by using their mind to work actively to give form to the passively received trauma (as Freud advocates in *Constructions in Analysis*, as the Botellas do through their regredient dreaming or as any analyst must do in first feeling and then trying to comprehend what they intuit in the counter-transference). And, in the absence of analyst or third-person documentary maker – in a self-analysis or in an autobiographical documentary – the traumatised protagonist (the primary witness) may be able to produce these fictions or representations intra-personally by conjuring a virtual, secondary witness from within the self (finding a self that is other to the self). These representations or fictions can then work over time within an analysis/self-analysis or a documentary, with time as process and change, rather than post-structuralism's atemporal temporality of perpetual melancholic return to the sublime unchanging event.

There is, of course, no inevitability to time as change leading to amelioration of traumatic experience and no utopian belief that time "heals". For Barbara Johnson (1980: 142), psychoanalysis does not return to the 'knot' of trauma in the belief that a simple interpretation or insight can unknot it, but rather returns again and again to the very impossibility of trauma, with the clinical process being 'an act' or a performance: 'an act of untying the knot in the structure by the repetition of the act of tying it.'[28] In documentary, the filmic return to the knot of trauma and the repetition of the traumatic event (the act of tying the knot) may be the route to untying it. That process of *untying through repeated tying* may begin with a filmic return – perhaps a repeated return – to a representation of the trauma as it apparently happened in its apparent veridity. But by representing the tying of the knot in the film-within, the process of untying may be able to start to play out over time.

The process through which psychoanalysis and documentary may be able to have an ameliorative influence on the structure of traumatic experience demands an ontology at odds with the one post-structuralism offers. But the post-structuralist account of trauma is itself at odds with what I might call the *standard* post-structuralist construction, which Fredric Jameson succinctly summarises:

> [T]he vast majority of structuralist and poststructuralist thinkers wage an implacable war on the "referent" and its supposedly ideological conception of a "real" reality out there (of which truth is the accurate reflection, etc). Yet in this process, in which the old tripartite linguistic scheme is whittled down to the simple opposition of signifier to signified, some of the opprobrium that hitherto attached to the referent now comes to contaminate the second term, the signified, which seems to have more or less taken its place.
>
> (Jameson 2015)

Faced with the *impossibility* of trauma, post-structuralist cultural critics and philosophers have rediscovered the 'referent', the '"real" reality out there', reinventing it in the form of veridical traumatic memory *or* the victim of trauma as the sublime, embodied referent *or* the traumatic *Event* itself as sublime and outside history. What remains in post-structuralist trauma theory from Jameson's description is the opprobrium that contaminates the second term, the signified, where meaning and understanding might coalesce. This contaminated middle term has taken the place once reserved for the referent. The referent, now rehabilitated as the *post-modern* or *traumatic* sublime, then refuses any mechanism that might translate the real out there back to the realm of meaning (as is evident in Lyotard's refusal of the action of *Judgement* that Kant uses to work the inchoate feelings of the dynamic sublime back to *Understanding*).

But this philosophy of impossibility seems to have been erected on a misapprehension of traumatic experience as sublime and "real". What is identified in the work of Lyotard and Caruth seems much closer to what Jameson (1983) calls 'material signifiers' (*schizophrenic* signifiers) rather than the sublime referent. It is very hard to tell the difference between the experience of the sublime victim of trauma theory – an embodiment of the referent – and the experience of schizophrenia as described by Jameson. Jameson's description of schizophrenic experience mirrors very precisely the description of the effects of trauma on those who are in its grip[29]: no sense of 'temporal continuity', a feeling of 'unreality', no ability to make sense of the world, 'the experience of the present becomes powerfully, overwhelmingly vivid and "material"' (or '*literal*'), the schizophrenic living in a world of 'heightened intensity, bearing a mysterious and oppressive charge of affect, glowing with hallucinatory energy'. And Jameson does not mistake this form of experience as an instance of the sublime, instead 'schizophrenic experience is an experience of isolated, disconnected, discontinuous material signifiers which fail to link up into a coherent sequence' (1983; Jameson's italics). The experience of the traumatised is one of shattered signifiers; shattered signifiers masquerading as the traumatic sublime referent.[30] The misrecognition derives from the misrecognition of the schizophrenic or the traumatic signifier. The old construction of *Form – Content – Unform* (for signifier – signified – referent) of "normal" experience has become, under the shattering impact of schizophrenia or trauma, *Unform – Content – Unform.* The referent and the signifier have become very hard to distinguish because the *unform* (the shattered nature) of the signifier feels very like the *unform* of the referent.

In the next section, I will turn my attention back to psychoanalysis and attempt to provide a theoretical account of how fictions fit into the structure representation-meaning-referentiality (which can be mapped on to the structuralist/post-structuralist trilogy of signifier-signified-referent), which will return us by a different route to the question of the fictionality of psychoanalysis's representations and of the fictionality of fictional films-within in documentary. Having argued for the place of these fictions within a non-fictional frame via phenomenology (in Chapter 2), I will attempt to make the same case via psychoanalytic theory.

Psychoanalysis: fictions as representations of unrepresented states

Psychoanalysis as a meaning-seeking enterprise

Post-structuralism's hostility to meaning and understanding – its scotomisation of the middle term, the signified – puts post-structuralist theory fundamentally at odds with the psychoanalytic project (despite its many borrowings from psychoanalysis). Psychoanalysis is at root a clinical practice with its sights set on a "cure"; a cure not conceived simply as the removal of the symptoms of psychic distress but rather presaged upon a belief that psychic pain will only diminish if a meaningful account of psychic history and psychic life can be found.[31] As Terry Eagleton writes

> the aim of the psychoanalyst [...] is to restore the lost signifieds to those who have become stuck in a hard place, and whose discourse has consequently grown rigid and repetitive. To unpick the knot of a neurosis, and unravel a reified piece of signification [...] One of the roles of psychoanalysis is to free us from a fantasy of compulsive repetition on which we have become impaled, converting this stuckness or stumbling-block at the core of one's being into the cornerstone of a new form of life.
>
> (Eagleton 2009: 9)

Psychoanalyst Jacques-Alain Miller (1984: 622) makes a similar assertion:

> The symptom can be attributed to a failure of symbolisation; the cure is an intersubjective process in the course of which the subject reestablishes the continuity of his [*sic*] life history by giving meaning, after the fact, to what has remained opaque in his experience.

or again as Jacques Lacan described the objective of psychoanalysis in a 1967 lecture: 'To restore to the symptoms their meaning, to provide a place to the desires they mask' (Lacan quoted in Patsalides and Patsalides 2001: 207). The centrality of meaning to the psychoanalytic project is not limited to the (essentially) Lacanian thinkers quoted here. Freud wrote of the 'drive to know' (the 'Wissenstrieb') and of an 'epistemophilic instinct' (see for example, Freud 1909: 245; Freud 1917b: 327–8) and at the heart of Wilfred Bion's work, for example, is the notion that human beings are meaning-seeking, driven by an epistemophilic urge to make sense of the world. In conditions of psychic distress, this urge ('K') breaks down and becomes *minus-K* ('-K') as the sufferer fails to link up ideas and impressions and so fails to create meaning: the failure of meaning is a marker of that psychic distress (Bion 1994 [1962]; and see also 1959, 1962).

Trauma and the need to create fictional representations as a route to meaning

But this still begs the question of why, in the case of trauma, there is a need to create fictions within the meaning-seeking enterprise of psychoanalysis. In Eagleton's example of neurotic patients, the process of meaning-making begins with the signified as the analytic pair work to unknot or unravel fixed significations or meanings that are no longer adequate. But in the case of profound trauma, the task cannot begin here but has to begin with representation, with the signifier, as representations have been lost or shattered, or are experienced not as memories or representations at all but as the traumatic event happening in the present (a *re*-presentation of the trauma but experienced as if it were its initial presentation, happening in the here and now). André Green (2005a: 134–5) has described the different forms that unrepresented traumatic experience can take: hallucination (which I take to encompass "veridical" memory), acting out, somatisation (including both "illness" and disturbances to bodily perception) and what he calls 'débordement' or the overflow of intense negative affect, which other psychoanalytic theorists have called 'fear of annihilation' (Melanie Klein), 'nameless anxiety' or 'dread' (Wilfred Bion), 'tormenting anxiety' or 'primitive agony' (Donald Winnicott),[32] 'nameless, shapeless dread' (the Botellas), etc. In the following chapters, when I turn my attention back to documentary films treating traumatic histories, all these manifestations of unrepresented states will be apparent: a filmic representation of a hallucination is central to Ari Folman's *Waltz with Bashir* (2008); whilst Anwar Congo's trauma in Joshua Oppenheimer's *The Act of Killing* (2012) struggles to find representational form, manifesting itself more often as *acting out* or as intense, debilitating somatisation.

The sort of fictions that Freud advocates the analyst should construct in *Constructions in Analysis* or that the analyst must dream in the Botellas's account, are precisely aimed at the particularly acute problem of non-representation in profound trauma (and not Eagleton's neurotic conditions). These fictions provide the representations that have gone missing or been fractured. With profound trauma, analysis cannot begin by reordering or reinterpreting existing representations, but must work at a much more fundamental level (what we might call a more primitive level) and create the representation – that is, produce a fiction that takes the place of the missing representation – a fictional representation that might eventually, if it has some affective traction within the psychic life of the analysand, become the foundation upon which a meaningful account might be built.

Bion addresses this problem directly in *Learning from Experience* through his theorisation of *alpha* and *beta* elements in mental functioning. Beta elements are 'undigested facts' very different from memories. They are pieces of raw experience that have never entered the unconscious through repression – unmetabolised fragments of psychic or somatic or affective experience – which need to be given form by being converted into alpha elements if they are to be made available for thought and allow the construction of a meaningful account (Bion 1994 [1962]:

6–8). These beta elements seem to correspond to the shattered signifiers in Jameson's account of schizophrenia (unsurprising perhaps as Bion's work was much more focused on psychotic states than on the neurotic conditions that absorbed so much of Freud's attention). For the traumatised protagonist, these beta elements are either experienced internally as terror (Green's 'débordement') or are expelled into the external world (to become what Bion calls 'bizarre objects') and lodged in people or things that are then experienced as persecutory and controlling. Those objects, once expelled or projected into other people, allow the traumatised protagonist to *act out* in relation to that person. This *acting* rather than *thinking* can have very troubling consequences in the real world and can also be seen within an analysis as the analysand acts out unprocessed fragments of experience in the present of the analytic encounter.

A generation before Bion, Sándor Ferenczi (1949 [1932]: 225–30) recognised this characteristic of traumatic or psychotic experience and tried to account for it within his clinical practice. The staging of these past traumas within the controlled environment of an analysis and with the help of the analyst's insights (insights that for Ferenczi were reached through feeling or intuiting what he was experiencing in the counter-transference), might just allow the acting out to take representational form; that is to be seen by the analysand to be a representation of something that has gone missing rather than being a concrete "fact" in the present.[33] If this psychic transition can be made by analyst and analysand working together, then this *act* can become an object of thought which might begin a process of change. Repetitious *acting out* in this way can become one of the fictions within the analytic encounter – a play-within-the-play – which might begin a process of psychic change in the life of the analysand. The repetition of the acting out within the analysis is perhaps an example of what Johnson (1980: 142) called 'an act of untying the knot in the structure by the repetition of the act of tying it'.

The insider's experience of these shattered, unformed fragments conforms very closely to the account given in post-structuralist trauma theories of traumatic experience, as a sublime and terrifying encounter with the "real"; with the unchanging noumenal truth. Bion (1994 [1962]: 6) writes that '[i]n contrast with the alpha-elements, the beta-elements are not felt as phenomena, but as things-in-themselves'. But Bion is very careful to say they are *felt* as things-in-themselves and not that they *are* things-in-themselves. Bion, here, remains firmly in the world of phenomena where beta elements can be worked with and given form. This symptom of trauma is not taken as an unchanging and unchangeable ontological fact as it is in trauma theory. Bion works with this apparent impossibility.

Bion's way of working with beta elements is to introduce the creative workings of another mind – an outsider or a secondary witness – who can process the beta fragments and then offer an account back to the traumatised protagonist in the form of alpha elements that are available for thought. Bion's model for this outside mind comes from his observation of the interaction between mother and infant. The infant who has yet to develop a mind capable of thought, experiences lack or need as terrifying, without source, without any temporal notion that it can end, and without meaning. The mother who is attuned to her baby senses the terror, imagines what the problem might be – hunger, separation, cold – and then offers a solution, by feeding the child or holding the child or providing bodily warmth. Bion calls this ability to sense and make sense of the child's experience, maternal 'reverie'. It could also be characterised as the mother intuiting the child's terror in the counter-transference. The mother at first passively and in tune with the child tries to feel what the child may be feeling – the mother tries to experience the feelings the child 'transmits' – and then actively intervenes by imagining a possible solution to whatever it may be that is troubling the child (this switch from passive to active secondary witnessing is absent from the trauma theory account). The solution is a sort of fiction as the mother cannot really know she is offering the "right" solution: if it is right, the child will be soothed; if it is wrong, the first fiction will be discarded and another provided. Like Freud's description of a construction in analysis, if it is productive, the patient (here the baby) is 'touched'; if it is not, the construction will drop out of the analysis and a better one will be sought. The mother's mind does the thinking that infant is not yet capable of, and through their inter-personal exchanges over time, the infant develops a mind capable of thinking for itself and able to make sense of the world for itself. It is a process through which the child enters the world of representation and thought. There are parallels here with Freud's grandson's *fort-da* game, in that the creative fiction of the game is the mechanism through which the child enters the world of representation and learns to contain terrors that were formerly uncontainable.[34] And there are in turn parallels between Ernst's struggle to enter the world of representation and the traumatised protagonist's struggle to recover representational capacities that have been shattered by the impact of trauma.

In adult trauma, these beta elements are again at play. The analyst, taking the place of the mother, must try to passively receive the terrifying and disturbing feelings that are being transmitted. Bion (1970) likened this passivity to Keat's notion of negative capability, describing it as the suspension of memory and desire. The analyst then switches into an active mode and tries, working with the analysand, to find or create a representational form for the formless terror that has been "received". The shattered fragments of the signifier that were received are returned to the analysand having been imaginatively reconstituted into something approaching "whole" signifiers or coherent representations. Again, this is the analyst constructing a fiction – or better, the analytic pair constructing a fiction – that takes the place of shattered or missing signifiers. Beta elements – unmetabolised fragments of psychic or somatic or affective experience – are brought within the representational sphere in these fictional constructions. The fictional constructions themselves can then be reflected on and might allow the analysand to begin to construct a meaningful account of their traumatic history. The fictions bring the analysis to the point where Eagleton began his description of an analysis that deals with neuroses. Having found or created signifiers to replace those lost or shattered, the analysand can then move on to Eagleton's task of developing new signifieds (meanings).

A recent essay by psychoanalyst Howard Levine captures this essential difference between the analysis of neuroses and the analysis of unrepresented trauma, which requires creative fictions:

> In the presence of represented *unconscious*, latent content, the analytic process moves via free association and interpretation from conscious and preconscious surface to unconscious depth. In the analysis of unrepresented and weakly represented mental states, *the elements of mind – conscious, preconscious, and unconscious – must first be created by a work that begins in the analyst's psyche and is then offered to and inscribed in the psyche of the patient as part of an interactive, intersubjective relationship and process*. In other words, the analyst may be required to provide some expressive, catalytic action in order to help precipitate or strengthen the patient's representational capacities.
>
> (2013: 70; Levine's italics)

Levine is one of a number of analysts who have recently (re)turned to the complex issue of the representation of unrepresented states in profoundly traumatised or psychotic patients, and who look back to Freud's *Constructions* essay, to Bion, and to a lesser (but increasing) extent to Ferenczi to find inspiration. The 'catalytic action' that Levine describes is analogous to Freud's 'bait of falsehood' in the *Constructions* essay: the fictional account that takes the place of the missing representation and then acts as a catalyst for the emergence of meaning or in Freud's grander articulation, acts as 'bait' to take the 'carp of truth'. These fictions must always be judged by their impact on the analysis: that is, whether a fiction helps free the analysand to be able to start thinking about the trauma and to find meaning; or, in Bion's terms, whether the fiction helps the analysand to convert unthinkable beta elements into alpha elements – thoughts that can be thought by the thinker.

Meaning as created/found fiction: between Aphrodite and Sleeping Beauty

Levine's recent work goes beyond the description of the clinical interventions that may be required in the face of trauma and its unrepresented states, and places what I am calling *fictions*, and what Freud called *baits of falsehood*, within a broader theory of representation, meaning and referentiality (an epistemological-ontological framework). Levine's ideas, in common with psychoanalysis in general, fall into a broadly Kantian framework.[35] The philosophical system depends on the idea that there are noumenal truths out there somewhere – truths about both the external and the internal world – but that these are inaccessible and unknowable in any direct way. The unknowable, noumenal truth is given various expressions in psychoanalysis from Lacan's 'Real' to Bion's 'O'. Levine turns to Bion for his framework and describes the nature of the representation (the fiction) that is produced by the analyst working with a traumatised patient:

> The representation produced is always to some extent partial and approximate and never a fully complete depiction of the thing-in-itself. […] As Bion put it "(Ultimate Reality) O does not fall into the domain of knowledge or learning save incidentally; it can 'become', but it cannot be 'known'. *It is darkness and formlessness* but it enters the domain K (i.e., the realm of that which can be known)."
>
> (2013: 70–1; Levine's italics)[36]

What Levine is claiming for the co-authored, "invented" representations of the analytic pair is a faint echo – an indirect glimpse – of the *unform* of the referent. The unform of 'O' acquires form and content as a signifier in psychoanalysis's invented, fictional representations. These representations can then become imbued with meaning (that is, form a unified sign where a signifier points to a signified) through further mental activity on the part of the analyst and the analytic pair (and so enter Bion's domain of 'K'). This is the process of symbolisation, which emerges out of reflection on the counter-transferential encounter between analyst and analysand. Post-structuralist accounts of trauma recognise the 'darkness and formlessness' of traumatic reality but refuse all the mechanisms through which the overwhelming and terrifying experience of the traumatic sublime could be drawn into the representational sphere and become objects of thought. Lyotard explicitly rejects the workings of the complex faculty of *Judgement*, the mechanism that Kant defined as the means of drawing the formless sublime back to the realm of *Understanding*. In contrast, psychoanalysis describes a number of mechanisms which perform the function of *Judgement* from regredient dreaming, to reverie, to intuiting in the counter-transference. All these mechanisms seek to provide representational form for the unform of the referent and insist that it is only *through* representation that we might gain 'partial and approximate' access to the referent. It is the 'partial and approximate' nature of these representations, which leads us to see them as fictional.

This brings me back to the nature of the "fictions" deployed in psychoanalysis when dealing with traumatic states. In the previous chapter, I advanced an argument from phenomenology that the fictions of psychoanalysis and the fictions of the film-within-the-film in documentaries seeking to explore traumatic personal histories, might only be fictional to an extent. They may be representations of psychic realities (representations of *factical* events) and so, as I have said, hint that some truth is in play. And, as I have also argued, despite the label fictional, these fictions can sit within the frame of the analysis as a whole or the frame of the documentary as a whole and not compromise the perception of the analysis or the documentary as non-fictional intentional objects (noematic objects). What psychoanalytic meta-theory suggests – drawing on Levine, on Bion and others – is that these fictions may contain fragments of the truth and this brings psychoanalytic theory into line with my earlier argument which was derived phenomenologically. If these "fictions" contain fragments of the truth, calling them fictions seems wide of the mark but the label remains useful as it accords with the commonsense, realist description of these strange, invented, representations and it is the word used (along with its synonyms) by analysts and filmmakers and film viewers to describe these representational forms. They are probably best described as alternative frames of experience that have the appearance of fiction.

But is this an entirely satisfactory theorisation? The radically unknowable nature of the referent or 'O' or the 'Real', means that we cannot know whether these representations contain a faint echo of a psychical truth or whether they really are just fictitious; that is, created out of nothing and so merely delusions. Of course, analysis allows for a pragmatic test. Freud (1937b: 262) believed a false 'construction' would be revealed in its lack of affective impact on the analysand and would 'drop out as if it had never been made' allowing a better one to be created or found (like the mother in her reverie trying various solutions to her infant's terror until one seems to work). Still, perhaps we are deluding ourselves if we construct an ontology that posits noumenal truths that can never be known for certain in this phenomenal world we inhabit.

Winnicott's notion (1990 [1971]a) of the transitional object and potential space[37] seem to offer a viable solution to this conundrum. Potential space is a play space within the analytic frame where ideas can be played with, tried out, discarded, altered, re-made, combined in different ways, as analyst and analysand can go in search of something that seems to be meaningful and has the potential to alter psychic perceptions.[38] Winnicott observed that infants at play occupy a similar potential space, often playing with objects – apparently trivial and everyday objects to the adult mind – which they imbue with deep significance. These play objects, *transitional objects*, appear to help the child negotiate – to transition – between inner experience and the exigencies or brute realities of the external world. The transitional object (a doll, a teddy bear, a piece of cloth) is simultaneously both an imaginative creation of the child and a real object that the child finds in the external world. It is central to Winnicott's account that the child's transitional object is *simultaneously* both created and found; it is brought into being as a creative act of the child's internal, imaginative world and is simultaneously an object that exists in the real external world. To try to separate these two apparently competing ontologies would be to destroy its function as a transitional object.

It is the very ambiguity of the transitional object's ontological status that allows André Green, in his essay on *Potential Space* (1986b), to use it as the basis for a theory of meaning (a slightly more sceptical theory of meaning than the one outlined by Levine). Green is trying to describe the nature of the meanings that arise in the analytic setting (meanings that are prompted into being by the catalyst of fictions akin to those in children's play) but his reflections provide the basis for a more general theory of meaning with universal applicability:

> Meaning does not emerge complete as Aphrodite rising from the waves. It is for us to construct it. Viderman believes that, prior to the analytic situation, the

> meaning that we seek never existed; it is the analytic process which constitutes it *as such* for the first time. Meaning is not discovered, it is created. I prefer to describe it as an absent meaning, a virtual sense which awaits its realization through the cuttings and shapings offered by the analytic space (and time). It is a potential meaning. It would be wrong to think like Sleeping Beauty it merely waits there to be aroused. It is constituted in and by the analytic situation; but if the analytic situation reveals it, it does not create it. It brings it from absence to potentiality, and then makes it actual. To actualize it means to call it into existence, not out of nothing (for there is no spontaneous generation), but out of the meeting of two discourses, and by way of that object which is the analyst, in order to construct the *analytic mind.*
>
> (1986b: 293; Green's italics)[39]

Green's account suggests that the meanings that are attainable in the phenomenal world we inhabit[40] are both created by us and found by us in a real world beyond. They are at once both inventions and discoveries, both subjective and objective, both fiction and truth. With the truth (the referent, 'O', the 'Real') posited as *a priori* unknowable, we cannot know what part of meaning is created and what part found, so the ontological status of meaning must forever be suspended between Aphrodite and Sleeping Beauty. Meanings are both a human creation and a brush with the noumenal, unknowable truth. This places the hard work of analysis (and the hard work of human meaning-making more generally) firmly back in the phenomenal world, in a world structured in time and space, in a world where meanings are tentative and contingent, succumbing neither to a fantasy that we can possess the truth nor to a despairing resignation that there is no meaning (a *fantasy* and a *despair* that trauma theory combines in its positing of a truth that is at once unknowable). Meanings emerge in a potential space that Green describes as 'a ventilated space, a space which is neither that of "this is meaningless" nor that of "this means that" but one of "this may mean that"' (Green 1986c: 42).

In the arena of cultural studies, Annette Kuhn, like Green, co-opts Winnicott's notion of potential space and develops a similar theory of cultural meaning to Green's conception of psychic meaning. Like Green, Kuhn recognises how creative activity in potential space straddles the apparently incompatible, polar opposites of invented ("fictional") representation and noumenal truth: 'Potential space can be understood as a place that contains fantasy and reality, "me" and "not-me", and what in semiotic terms could be characterised as sign and referent' (Kuhn 2013a: 4). I am largely in agreement with Kuhn but side with Green in seeing this straddling as the straddling of signifier and referent (of representation and noumenal truth) rather than a straddling of sign and referent, as 'sign' already contains or presupposes a fusion of signifier and signified (a fusion of representation with meaning). For me, and for Green, the signified (tentative meaning of the 'this may mean that' sort) is the *product* of the straddling of signifier and referent. Kuhn's use of the notion of potential space has exerted an influence on film theory, introducing Winnicottian ideas and conceptions of meaning into the field (a subject I will return to in the next section).

In the light of Green's theory of meaning, the construction in analysis *or* the regredient dream *or* the analyst inventing solutions like Bion's mother in her reverie *or* the quasi-historical reconstruction of events – all of psychoanalysis's fictions – are the baits of falsehood that tempt meanings into existence; meanings that in turn have the same ambiguous ontological status as Winnicott's transitional object, suspended somewhere between fiction and truth.[41] Likewise, the "fictional" films within the non-fictional frame of documentary open up a potential space within documentary: a play space where ideas (meanings) of ambiguous ontological status are provoked into existence. In the end, perhaps we should heed Adam Phillips's observation (1988: 118) that the child is not concerned with what the transitional object *is* but what it *does*. It is an observation that validates psychoanalysis's pragmatic test of its "fictions": if they work keep them; if they don't work let them 'drop out' and try others. We are left with a functional account of meaning. If the fictions provoke meanings that have an ameliorative or curative impact on the traumatised protagonist's current psychic experience, the job is done.

In developing this functional account of meaning, I am not suggesting that it is only applicable to psychic meanings: I am *not* advocating a lower threshold for the achievement meaning in relation to the psychic, quite the contrary. The notion of meaning that I derive from Green is universally applicable across all of human meaning-making activity whether in relation to psychic phenomena or those of natural science. Like psychoanalysis, natural science has its meaningful fictions – that is, its tested and as yet unfalsified hypotheses often backed up with empirical data – that function to advance further scientific discoveries. But it would be a mistake to think of these theories as the noumenal truth: they are functional theories of which we can at least say 'this may mean that' and contain elements of both the created and the found. Whilst these theories continue to "function" science will keep them; when they fail (as aspects of Newtonian physics did in the face of Einstein's speculations of 1905), they will drop out of the frame.

Of more immediate impact on the conduct of an analysis or on the making of a documentary are the creative possibilities that are opened up by the notion of potential space. The idea of potential space grants the analyst or filmmaker permission to bring the freedoms and unbounded imaginative potential of children's play into the serious business of analysis or filmmaking. This freedom is particularly needed in the case of traumatic histories where representations must be conjured up to take the place of those that have been fractured, have gone missing or have never achieved representational form. Green pays Winnicott the highest compliment for placing the notion of play at the heart of analysis. He rejects Freud's suggestion that the analytic situation can be compared to a game of chess with its fixed and rigid rules, preferring Winnicott's games:

> If Winnicott is the master player of psychoanalysis, it is surely not chess that he plays with his patient. It is a game with a cotton reel, with a piece of string, with the doll or a teddy bear.
>
> (Green 1986b: 293)

The essence of an analysis is to provide a setting, which enables the patient to play these games:

> Analytic technique is directed toward bringing about the capacity for play with transitional objects. The essential feature is no longer interpreting, but enabling the subject to live out creative *experiences* of a new category of objects.
> (1986b: 285; Green's italics)

Games 'with a cotton reel, with a piece of string, with the doll or a teddy bear' perhaps best captures the spirit of the imaginative strategies deployed in the fictional films-within in the documentaries that form the core of this study. The films-within are transitional objects that sit within the potential space of the documentary, just as the games Winnicott encourages sit within the potential space of the analysis. For Green 'Winnicott has [...] described not so much an object as a space lending itself to the creation of objects'; a 'playground of transitional phenomena' (Green 1986b: 285). It is the frame of the documentary and the frame of the analysis that define the potential space where meaning might emerge through the playing of games (through the exploration of fictions).

And although articulated in a very different idiom, Green's speculations about the nature of the meanings that become available through the analytic process seem to be very similar to the sort of "truths" that Linda Williams sees as becoming available through a documentary-making process that deploys fictions. Williams argues that 'documentary can and should use all the strategies of fictional construction to get at truths' (1993: 20); truths which she describes as 'postmodern' truths; relative and contingent truths (or the fragmented and 'receding horizon' of the truth if we figure the truth as absolute) (1993: 11). These post-modern truths (like Green's meanings) are never stable and are subject to change – 'never absolute and never fixed' but always 'under construction' as Williams describes them – so 'the truth figured by documentary cannot be a simple unmasking or reflection. It is a careful construction' (1993: 20).

The Winnicottian viewer watching the Winnicottian viewer: the emergence of meaning for both extra- and intra-diegetic audience

Over the last thirty years or so, a few cultural critics have applied Winnicott's idea of potential space to the space of the fictional feature film. Ira Konigsberg (1996: 887) describes the 'transitional' filmic space of fictional cinema, as a 'world of shadows half-way [...] between signifier and reality'. Phyllis Creme, in her 1994 PhD thesis,[42] invented the idea of a *Winnicottian viewer*, a viewer who enters the film on the screen and plays an active role.

> Film and spectator interact in a mutual, overlapping potential space as the apparently uncrossable offscreen/onscreen barrier appears to be crossed. As I engage with it, the film that is given me out there on screen becomes my own creation, like a found object.
>
> (Creme 2013: 41)

For Creme (2013: 48), we (as viewers) 'both "find" and "create" this film as it unfolds before us, with us as willing participants', whilst Konigsberg (1996: 885) sees the on-screen characters as transitional objects, part oneself (as viewer) part other. And for Creme, this playful, creative activity (like the play Winnicott observed in his child patients) is a meaning-making and a therapeutic activity: 'For Winnicott, play is everyone's birthright. It is a mark of psychic health and the major aim of therapy – not just to cure "illness" but as a way of experiencing a sense of meaning and of self in life' (2013: 39). Play takes place in the potential space of the film just as it did in the potential space of the therapeutic setting of Winnicott's consulting room.

The entanglement between the viewer and the viewed – between spectator and film – that Konigsberg and Creme describe through Winnicott, seems to fit very closely with the entanglement between spectator and film that Sobchack (1999) describes through phenomenology, where viewer and film are not a separate subject and object but mutually implicated as an experiencing-subject perceives an experienced-object.

And just as Sobchack took the insights of a film phenomenology developed to interpret fictional films and then applied them to non-fiction films (documentary), so I want to take Konigsberg's and Creme's psychoanalytic insights about fictional film and apply them to documentary. I also want to shift the frame of reference to allow me to sustain my contention that the film-within can make meanings available to the traumatised protagonist who exists *within* the documentary. The frame of reference used by Creme and Konigsberg is that of the cinema goer (their Winnicottian viewer) entering the potential space of the film on the cinema screen, who both finds and creates meaning through their active, playful spectatorship. In the documentaries that concern me, the films-within are viewed (sometimes repeatedly) by the traumatised protagonist within the documentary. This traumatised diegetic spectator becomes my primary Winnicottian viewer. Creme's and Konigsberg's extra-diegetic Winnicottian viewer (you or I watching the documentary) therefore witnesses another Winnicottian viewer (an inner Winnicottian viewer) within the diegesis who, like us, reacts to and enters into the film that they are watching. We watch the documentary, and within that documentary we see this inner Winnicottian viewer watching the film within the documentary. It is the meanings (*intra-diegetic* meanings) that may become available to this inner Winnicottian viewer, that are my primary focus.

Even these two frames of reference cannot capture the complexities of some documentaries (Albertina Carri's *The Blonds* (2003) has frames within frames within frames) or the complexity of the analytic encounter as described by André

Green. Taking the theatre rather than cinema as his model (a common metaphor in "French" psychoanalysis), Green (1979: 3–4) builds a picture of frames of reference nesting one within the other like *Matryoshka* ("Russian") dolls. There is the outside world that contains the theatre (a theatre that I take to be the analysis sitting within the frame of the everyday life of the analysand); inside the theatre there is the auditorium and the stage (which marks the divide between the analysand's outer and inner selves); and then there is the stage itself, where the analysand might try to put on a performance of their inner life. But this on-stage space contains another frame, a hidden frame – off-stage space – which remains forever off limits. In Green's metaphor, off-stage is the unconscious, the unseen part of the stage where the truth hides.[43] Linking this notion of frames back to ideas put forward in the previous section, the stage is the place where Terry Eagleton's neurotic patient puts on a performance of existing representations of their inner life as they search for new signifieds (new meanings) which it is hoped will be in close proximity to the truth that sits just out of reach, off-stage. It is also the place where the analyst (as theatre director) might have to stage a fiction (a *construction*) for a traumatised analysand as the traumatised patient may have no play of their own to stage, trauma having fractured or obliterated those representations which might have formed a play.

In the next chapter, I will turn my attention away from psychoanalytic metatheory and towards documentary film and ask if parallels can be drawn between psychoanalytic practice and documentary practice where fictions are deployed in pursuit of a traumatic personal history.

Notes

1 The role of memory was already clear in Freud's early work with Breuer treating hysterics (where the hysteria was viewed as a symptom of a buried trauma) and is captured in the famous epigram of 1893, 'Hysterics suffer mainly from reminiscences' (Freud and Breuer 1893 [1955]: 6).
2 Freud frequently draws on literary fiction to describe trauma, from E.T.A. Hoffmann (2004 [1816]; 2012 [1819]) to Shakespeare.
3 For the visual nature of these dreamt or imagined fictions, see Birksted-Breen (2016: 227).
4 Nichols's comments appear in chapter 8 (pp. 99–110) of his *Speaking Truths with Film* where he endorses the thoughts Werner Herzog expressed in an NPR (National Public Radio) interview (Herzog 2005).
5 Hamlet in *Hamlet* Act II Scene II: 'I have heard / That guilty creatures sitting at a play / Have by the very cunning of the scene / Been struck so to the soul that presently / They have proclaim'd their malefactions'.
6 Although, of course, it is a description of an extended dialogue between an infant and the infant's internal idea of his mother. This could be described as an intra-personal (rather than inter-personal) encounter; an encounter that is at the heart of self-analysis and the autobiographical film (which will be explored in Chapter 4); an encounter between the self and aspects of the self that are other to the self.
7 *Beyond the Pleasure Principle* as a whole is steeped in trauma. Whilst Freud was working on the text, he was mourning the untimely death of his daughter (Ernst's mother), Sophie Halberstadt-Freud (Chaplin 2027).

8 Donald Winnicott further developed this pioneering work of Klein's with children: see, for example, *The Piggle* (1989 [1977]).

9 That said, some analysts – notably André Green – believe play (if not specifically toys) is vital in the process of coming to terms with trauma. Green wrote 'it is in the presence of horror that we understand the necessity of play in making it bearable' (2005b: 8).

10 Panh has said he was working on *The Missing Picture* for eighteen months before he stumbled on the idea of recreating his memories through the use of clay figurines. 'The first moment they start to sculpt, it was like a miracle. There was something very pure in the gesture – something linked to your childhood.' Panh revealed that he himself had made clay figurines as a child. Panh's comments come from a filmed interview with Deirdre Boyle (Panh and Boyle 2015). There is a fuller discussion of *The Missing Picture* in Chapter 4.

11 The spatial component of traumatic experience is perhaps less well-appreciated than the temporal component but it is recognised in the frequent use of place names as the markers of traumatic events: Auschwitz for the Holocaust; the references to the principal traumatised protagonists in Alain Resnais's *Hiroshima mon amour* (1959), as 'Nevers' and 'Hiroshima', after the sites of their traumas.

12 My coinage *Heraclitan circle* is a reference to Heraclitus's famous epigram: 'You could not step twice into the same river' (recorded by Plato in *Cratylus*).

13 Although of course Freud and Breuer did point to the immediacy of abreaction in the treatment of hysteria in the 1890s.

14 This is the same temporal rhythm required to *work through* an analysand's resistances, described by Freud in his essay *Remembering, Repeating and Working Through* (1914a).

15 As Freud wrote: 'melancholia behaves like an open wound' – a perpetually 'open' trauma (1917a: 252–3).

16 This contrasts with the Freudian account which casts all of human experience (beyond very early childhood) as *post*-traumatic as we enter the world of representation and thought, having worked through the originary, ontogentic trauma of separation (loss).

17 Especially *The Differend: Phrases in Dispute* (1988 [1983]) and also *Lessons on the Analytic of the Sublime* (1994 [1991]) where Lyotard reworks Kant's (1951 [1790]) ideas as set out in sections 23 to 29 of *The Critique of Judgement.*

18 Thomas Trezise (2013) provides a powerful theoretical and ethical critique of the notion of 'silence' in Lyotard and in the later theoretical work of Cathy Caruth, Dori Laub, Berel Lang and Giorgio Agamben (see for example, Agamben 2000). For Trezise, Lyotard and other trauma theorists fail to listen to the countless, articulate survivors' accounts, seeking instead to theorise away (to be deaf to) the content of these testimonies in pursuit of a preconceived notion of the unrepresentability of trauma and the Holocaust. Trezise describes this as 'a pronounced listening impairment' (2013: 3).

19 Romantic writers who followed Kant (although not Kant himself) also commonly described the French Revolution as an earthquake (Salmi et al. 2016: 24).

20 Caruth's colleague Dori Laub has listened to and recorded hundreds of hours of Holocaust survivors' testimony.

21 Beginning with Caruth's essay of 1991, 'Introduction to Psychoanalysis, Trauma and Culture'.

22 See, for example, Van der Kolk and Van der Hart (1989: 1530–40).

23 Thomas Trezise (2013: 47) recasts trauma theory's self-defined invulnerability to challenge as *fatally vulnerable to challenge*, writing 'the inaccessibility of traumatic experience to knowledge undermines the very foundation of the theory that asserts it'.

24 Referring to Freud's essay *Remembering, Repeating and Working-Through* (1914a).

25 See, for example, Shoshana Felman and Dori Laub. 1991. *Testimony: Crises of Witnessing in Literature, Psychoanalysis, and History.*

26 The notion of 'transmission' is a key term in trauma theory and is used frequently by Shoshana Felman, Dori Laub and others. See, for example, their essays in Caruth, ed. 1995. *Trauma: Explorations in Memory*, e.g. Felman on page 56; Laub on page 68, etc.

27 And it is not just psychoanalysis that challenges a post-structuralist ontology that universalises the experience of the traumatised. Film theorist, Joshua Hirsch, writing about the representation of the Holocaust in film argues that the post-structuralist position is actually one of ethics and aesthetics and not ontology (symptomatology is *not* ontology): 'The discourse of trauma [...] transforms the inherent limit of the witness's private memory into a moral limit of public memory; it transforms an involuntary psychological symptom into a voluntary aesthetic' (Hirsch 2004: 20).

28 Jean Laplanche also describes (at least the first part of) the analytic process as one of untying knots (deconstruction) or unweaving. Laplanche writes: 'the very model of psychoanalysis [is] unweaving so that a new fabric can be woven, disentangling to *allow* the formation of new knots' (1999b: 253–4; Laplanche's italics). The etymology of *analysis* itself suggests unknotting: *ana* meaning back/again/anew/towards; *lysis* meaning to unfasten/loosen/set free/untie, etc.

29 A description that the psychoanalytic account, trauma-theory account and PTSD account share.

30 Freud makes a parallel point in his essay on *The Unconscious* (1915b) where he writes that the schizophrenic mistakes *words* for *things*; words become concrete, real, literal. Here post-structuralist accounts of trauma mistake fractured, broken or absent memories (signifiers) for the concrete, real and unchanging truth (the referent), producing what could be described as a traumatised account of trauma. These shattered signifiers seem to equate to André Green's list of heterogeneous signifiers (as described in Chapter 1).

31 For Paul Ricœur, the aim of psychoanalysis is to discover a new, meaningful, narrative identity for the analysand with the desire for meaning expressing itself as a desire for narrative (for exploring 'untold or virtual stories'). See David Wood's Introduction to: *On Paul Ricœur: Narrative and Interpretation* (Wood 1991: 1–19; especially 11–14).

32 The foregoing list of other theorists' terms is taken from Green (2005a: 134–5).

33 According to Green, Freud was only able to account fully for acting out after he developed the so-called *second topography* and introduced the notion of the 'id' which is non-representational (and non-linguistic) unlike the unconscious of the first topography (Green 2005a: 155–6).

34 The profound difference between Freud's and Bion's account is that Ernst is *apparently* author of his own meaning and his own "cure" whilst for Bion the intervention of another mind is critical. That said, it is not worth making too much of this difference, as Freud's description of his grandson's game is short and unelaborated and there is even a hint that another mind might have been involved in inventing the game, when Freud writes: 'It is of course a matter of indifference from the point of view of judging the effective nature of the game whether the child invented it himself or took it over on some outside suggestion' (1920: 15). What is certain is that in *Constructions in Analysis* (1937b), Freud is fully aware that another mind is a necessary condition for change to occur.

35 In one of his rare explicit references to the Kantian framework of his thought, Freud wrote in his 1915 essay on *The Unconscious*: 'Just as Kant warned us not to overlook the fact that our perceptions are subjectively conditioned and must not be regarded as identical with what is perceived though unknowable, so psycho-analysis warns us not to equate perceptions by means of consciousness with the unconscious mental processes which are their object. Like the physical, the psychical is not necessarily in reality what it appears to us to be' (1915b: 171). Here Freud seems to chime with Kant's statement in *The Critique of Pure Reason*: 'I [...] know myself, like other phenomena, only as I appear to myself, not as I am [...] So far as inner intuition is concerned, we know our

own subject only as appearance, not as it is in itself' (Kant 1999 [2nd edition 1787]: B152–6). For an overview of the influence of Kant on Freud's thought, see Brook (2003).

36 Levine is referring to Bion's ideas in *Attention and Interpretation* (1970) where he develops the idea of 'O'.

37 Winnicott always used the term 'potential space' but it is frequently referred to by commentators as *transitional space* to emphasise its link to the transitional object.

38 Play is always central to analysis for Winnicott: '*Psychotherapy takes place in the overlap of two areas of playing, that of the patient and that of the therapist. Psychotherapy has to do with two people playing together*' (1990 [1971]c: 38; Winnicott's italics) or '[P]sychoanalysis has been developed as a highly specialised form of playing in the service of communication with oneself and others' (1990 [1971]c: 41).

39 Note: Viderman, who Green mentions, is Serge Viderman (1916–91) the Romanian-born psychoanalyst who practised in Paris and whose work profoundly influenced César and Sara Botella. See Viderman *La construction de l 'espace analytique* (1970).

40 Meanings that are unified signs combining signifier and signified that are the outcome of what Alain Gibeault (2005: 1712–4) describes as the 'process of symbolization'.

41 Green (1986b: 293) describes the transitional object as 'constructed within the space of illusion never violated by the question, Was the object created or found?'.

42 Ideas she reprises in Creme (2013).

43 And that off-stage unconscious is not restricted to the represented but hidden, repressed unconscious of the neurotic but includes the idea of the psychotic and traumatised, unstructured, unrepresented unconscious (inchoate and ineffable) which Bion and others have hypothesised.

Chapter 4

Cinéma vérité as filmo-therapy and autobiographical filmmaking as self-analysis

In Chapter 2, I briefly surveyed the gradually expanding boundaries of documentary as audiences and filmmakers came to adopt a more permissive attitude towards such practices as the deployment of fictions in documentary and to accept more subjective modes of address, especially the autobiographical.

In this chapter, in pursuing my argument that documentary is capable of producing meaning in the wake of trauma, I want first to make a case for *cinéma vérité* – and specifically Jean Rouch and Edgar Morin's 1961 documentary *Chronique d'un été* – as having pioneered many of the practices that are central to contemporary documentaries that use fictions to explore traumatic histories.[1] Rouch and Morin theorised their filmmaking and its ability to produce "truths" in both phenomenological and psychoanalytic terms; and they did this thirty years before film scholars began to apply the insights of these bodies of theory to the interpretation of documentary film.

But one practice that *cinéma vérité* and *Chronique* did not pioneer but which is common in documentaries today treating traumatic histories, is the autobiographical mode of address. And so, in the second part of this chapter, I want to look more closely at how autobiographical documentaries produce meaning when the key, meaning-generating, interpersonal relationship of conventional documentary – between the director and the principal protagonist – is missing.

Cinéma vérité

Chronique d'un été: *documentary as 'filmo-therapy'*

Chronique d'un été was conceived as an anthropological study of contemporary Parisian life, which both Rouch and Morin treated as an experiment in phenomenological filmmaking; truths would be revealed in the intensity of the encounters between ordinary Parisians in the filmmaking present. *Chronique* was made at the high point of Bazinian phenomenological realism and, more generally, whilst French intellectual life was still heavily influenced by Jean-Paul Sartre's existential phenomenology. Rouch and Morin, like Sartre, sought an immediate, authentic engagement with the world. Truth was to be grasped through direct experience

DOI: 10.4324/9781003657187-6

of the world and was to be found in the impressions of the individual. Truth was revealed in the encounter with the world not in withdrawn contemplation and this encounter could be captured on film and sound tape. For Sam Di Iorio (2007: 30), 'Rouch and Morin shared a Bazinian faith in cinema's power to uncover fundamental truths: in showing appearances (things as they seem) they hoped to reveal essences (things as they are)'.

And those essences were understood by Rouch and Morin to conform to a psychoanalytic model of the production of meaning or "truth". Rouch described the *cinéma-vérité* approach to filmmaking pioneered in *Chronique d'un été* as 'filmo-therapy' (said on film in Dauman 2011)[2] and believed that the documentary camera actively creates and records something new and transformative in the filmic present.

> Yes, the camera deforms, but not from the moment that it becomes an accomplice. At that point it has the possibility of doing something I couldn't do if the camera wasn't there: it becomes a kind of psychoanalytic stimulant which lets people do things they wouldn't otherwise do.
>
> (Rouch quoted in: Renov 2004: 197)

Morin (2003 [1960]: 232) made a parallel point when he described the encounters to be filmed in *Chronique* as a 'sociodrama' or a 'game [that] has the value of psychoanalytic truth, that is to say, precisely that which is hidden or repressed comes to the surface in these roles'. The truth is seen as emerging from an examination of the structure of experience in the present just as it is in the analytic encounter.

Edgar Morin's two interviews with 'Mary Lou'[3] (a young Italian woman who had recently moved to Paris) are examples of the revelatory and creative power of the camera in *Chronique*. The combination of Morin's searching questions about Mary Lou's personal happiness and the close camera work focusing on Mary Lou's face, capture her troubled state. She is agitated and close to tears, her speech is hesitant and broken. However we might interpret Mary Lou's state of mind, it is clear that the conversation in the presence of the camera was very exposing. Morin and Mary Lou generated an encounter that had not been seen in documentary before; a moment of highly charged "reality". Towards the end of *Chronique*, Mary Lou is filmed commenting on her experience:

> I feel that to obtain even the tiniest grain of truth, the subject has to be alone and on the verge of hysteria – that is if it is to talk of anything intimate.

The *tiny grains of truth* are not revealed simply in the intensity of the moment of filming, they emerge from the interpersonal relationship between filmmaker and protagonist (despite Mary Lou's feeling of being 'alone'). It is encounters like that between Morin and Mary Lou which prompted Emanuel Berman many years later to describe documentary contributors becoming 'invested in their relationship with the filmmaker in a way that evokes what goes on in psychoanalysis or psychotherapy' (Berman's comments reproduced in Chanan 2007: 216). The revolutionary interviewing techniques and the open group discussions pioneered in *Chronique* transformed subsequent documentary practice to such an extent, that in 2006 Kevin MacDonald could write:

> It may be a truism to liken the interviewing process to that of psychoanalysis, but in my experience that is very much the case. People will say things to you in front of the camera and a film crew that they might not have said ever before.
> (Macdonald in: Cousins and Macdonald 2006: 392)

Macdonald's observation is echoed by another British documentary maker, Richard McKerrow, in an interview in 2012: 'Documentary made in the right way, is a form of docutherapy' if the documentary makers are 'brave enough to go forward, and ask questions that are psychologically exploratory' (Lennon-Patience and Røkeberg 2014: 141).

In *Chronique*, the mechanics of the filmmaking process and the interpersonal relationships that this process entails are fully visible. It is a Brechtian mode of filmmaking, where the director, film crew and filming equipment are not hidden; it is a mode Allan Casebier (1991: 157–8) describes as 'reflexive' as it unmasks the mechanics of the filmmaking process in documenting a subject. The camera is not seen as a transparent window on the world – rather the filmmaking process actively creates what it then records.

And the *cinéma-vérité* mode of filmmaking was not simply reflexive but self-reflexive, allowing protagonists to reflect back on their own performances and perhaps to find something meaningful in what they witness. Morin certainly knew that self-reflexivity was a necessary part of the process of revealing the truth, as he wrote about it before the filming of *Chronique* had even started:

> We will show them [the participants] what has been filmed so far (at a stage in the editing that has not yet been determined) and in doing so attempt the ultimate psychodrama, the ultimate explication.
> (Morin 2003 [1960]: 233)

This psychodrama was played out towards the end of the filmmaking process, in a scene where a partly edited version of the film is shown in a small movie theatre to all the protagonists, with Rouch and Morin present. The protagonists are encouraged to comment on their own performance and on the performances of others. This scene was filmed and the sometimes heated exchanges that ensued were then cut into the final version of *Chronique* to create the film that was released to the world. Casebier (1991: 157–8) describes this self-reflexive process as the process of mediation involved in the reception of the documentary playing out within the documentary itself. It is a highly self-conscious mode of filmmaking, where the documentary itself becomes a subject of the documentary. It allows for an examination of the processes through which the truth is produced – and a questioning of the validity of those processes – to form an aspect of the completed film as cut and presented to the audience.

In making the documentary itself a subject of the documentary, *Chronique* suggested an approach to filmmaking where isolated moments of insight or revelation in the filmic present can become an evolving series of successive "presents" that play out over the screen time of the film. It is not unlike analyst and analysand in later sessions, revisiting interpretations and constructions from earlier sessions which are then re-considered, re-made, abandoned, seen in a different light, as perhaps profounder insights become available. In structural terms, it provides the space within documentary where the fictional film-within-the-film finds it place. It is here that the outer Winnicottian viewer (us as extra-diegetic audience) watch an inner Winnicottian viewer (an intra-diegetic audience member) being acted on and affected by and perhaps changed by the film and the filmmaking process and by their own performance within the film.

Chronique d'un été *and the fictional film-within: 'walking through' trauma*

One scene in particular opened up these possibilities, moving documentary beyond the talking-head encounter towards the performative, offering the potential to harness the creative power of the fictional film within the frame of documentary. It was a scene that shifted the focus of *Chronique* from the present of life in Paris to the past and to the traumatic past.

Rouch had experimented with fictions before making *Chronique*, placing his documentary protagonists into entirely made-up scenarios and having them improvise in front of the camera. Whether these scenarios were devised by Rouch or by the protagonists themselves, Rouch believed that these fictions would reveal a deeper truth that was not otherwise available.[4] In *La pyramide humaine* (1959), Rouch brought together black pupils and white pupils from a high school in Abidjan on the Ivory Coast who usually kept apart from each other and had fairly distant, even hostile, relations. He arbitrarily assigned the students character traits (racist, non-racist) and had the pupils play out everyday scenarios (meeting at the beach, falling in love). The fictional scenarios dramatised often previously unspoken racial tensions and prompted the students to reflect on their attitudes, which had formerly been concealed (perhaps even from themselves). Rouch was putting into practice his belief that 'fiction is the only way to penetrate reality' (Rouch 2003: 6). At the close of the film, we see a friendship has developed between a white and black pupil, leading Rouch to tell the audience: 'This small film accomplished in its daily improvisations what years of being in the same classroom could not.' Although some critics have questioned Rouch's claim that the film really shifted entrenched racist attitudes (see for example, Margulies 2007: 125–33), if we take Rouch's optimistic summation at face value, the improvisations, the fictional interlude within the documentary frame, had a transformatory impact on the real lives of the participants. A 'truth', to use Rouch's term, a social truth about the here-and-now, had emerged from the filmmaking process: a truth that facilitated the transformation.

When making *Chronique*, Rouch again experimented with a fiction. Keen to test the potential of the new light-weight cameras and synchronised recording equipment that were just becoming available in France in 1960, Rouch and Morin designed a scene in which one of the film's researchers, Marceline,[5] would walk through *La place de la Concorde* and *Les Halles* whilst delivering a monologue. The light-weight camera allowed her to be filmed at a distance whilst on the move, with her words picked up on the portable sound-recording equipment. Marceline, who was an Auschwitz-Birkenau survivor, talked about her wartime experiences.

Marceline performed a "dialogue" (or more accurately a monologue) between herself and her father who died in Auschwitz. On her lonely walk, Marceline refers to her father as 'you', as if he were there alongside her. We hear Marceline saying: 'Here I am now in the *Place de la Concorde*. I came back, you stayed.' She tells her "father": 'I was almost happy to be deported, I loved you so much' (her father having been deported to Auschwitz six months before her own deportation). Late in the scene Marceline says: 'Papa, papa, I wish you were here now'. Her last word is: 'Papa', followed by a heavy sigh. The experience is laden with affect for Marceline. The scene could be described as fictional as it involves a protagonist engaging in dialogue with someone who is dead. This is not to suggest a temporal confusion; Marceline uses the past tense and knows very well that the father she addresses is dead. But the scene has an intensity that comes from the performance happening in the present and, in an emotional sense, Marceline *is* accompanied by her father on her long, lonely walk across *La place de la Concorde*.

What resulted was a sequence in which the film's phenomenological method was applied to the past. The past was evoked through memory and not by recourse to an account that made any claim to historical objectivity. Marceline's words remained an examination of the structure of present experience but the structure of a present experience of a remembered and reimagined past. The past is not *out there* somewhere, to be looked at as an object: it only exists in the embodied form in which it is being recounted; it only appears as perceived by a consciousness (an indivisible subject-object phenomenon). This opens up a space in documentary for fantasy, imagination and fictionalisation.

It was a very different approach to documentary to the contemporaneous North-American practice of *direct cinema* (with which *cinéma vérité* is frequently equated). Direct cinema purports to capture truths about the world *out there* as if the camera and crew did not exist; the camera is a transparent window on reality. Joshua Oppenheimer, who sees himself working in the *cinéma-vérité* tradition pioneered by Rouch, draws a stark distinction between the two filmmaking practices:

> It's a great pity that in the Anglophone world we conflate *cinéma vérité* and Direct Cinema. *Cinéma vérité* was all about giving people the space to perform on camera, to imagine, to stage themselves as a way of documenting how they

> see themselves and make sense of their world. It's trying to do something fundamentally more profound. Direct Cinema tries to be insightful by looking at reality in a very close way, while in fact much more is staged than we like to think. In *cinéma vérité* it's about trying to make something visible – the role of fantasy and imagination in everyday life.
>
> (Oppenheimer quoted in: Bradshaw 2013: 38)

Rouch was not trying to capture an objective reality directly on film but using the interfering presence of the camera to create a space for fantasy and imagination as this, he believed, was the route to a deeper truth (a deeper reality). Alisa Lebow (2006: 235) makes a similar point when she notes 'documentary realism can be said to disavow its fantasy, and [...] it is precisely fantasy that is necessary to achieve a glimpse of the Real.'[6] And Peter Loizos (1993: 46; 50), writing about Rouch's ethnofictions more generally (not specifically *Chronique*), sees Rouch's 'use of improvisation and fantasy as projective methods in the exploration of people's lives' which 'convey something fundamental about real lives'.

Rouch's *phenomenological-historical* method, pioneered in Marceline's scene in *Chronique*, was an approach uniquely suited to trauma as trauma exists only in the present and is manifest in a variety of disruptions of memory and physical symptoms. It is an approach to the traumatic past that Claude Lanzmann deployed to devastating effect in his 1985 documentary, *Shoah*; a film made in the "present" through memory and without the usual paraphernalia of old photographs and film footage, authoritative voice-over narration, linear historical chronology or extra-diegetic sound or music. Shoshana Felman (1991: 51), writing about *Shoah,* has called it 'the story of the past in the present of the telling'. For Felman, this 'telling' includes what is not said and unconscious enactments of aspects of the past that evade memory.

> What is not available in words, what is denied, what cannot and what will not be remembered or articulated, nonetheless gets realized. What takes place in the film, what materially and unexpectedly occurs and what returns like a ghost is reference itself, the very object – and the very content – of historical erasure.
>
> (Felman 1991: 68)

Felman's words capture the potential of documentaries like *Shoah* to bring to light things that were hidden (erased), but I question the idea that what returns is reference in the strong sense of the veridical, the truth, the thing-in-itself, and instead take what is articulated to be an embodied representation (a signifier) of a missing traumatic past which might allow meaning to emerge.

For this phenomenological-historical method of documentary making, Joshua Hirsch (2004: 69) coined the term *historical vérité*, making explicit its debt to the *cinéma vérité* of Rouch and Morin and Marceline's famous scene. Through Marceline, because of her personal history, *Chronique d'un été* had opened up the possibility of using a traumatised individual to represent a trauma with deep historical roots directly to the viewer and also to themselves.[7] Rouch and Morin's innovation was to give us not just the words of the traumatised protagonist but also their body, allowing us to hear and see the past performed in the present through memory (and its distortions and aporias) and to witness that memory performed in the body of the protagonist. Joshua Oppenheimer acknowledges his debt to Lanzmann and *Shoah* and the potential of *historical vérité* to reveal meanings about the traumatic past.

> The now of the film is the time that it's made and that becomes the present. I think what that also does is that it somehow makes the film fundamentally about that now. It's about how that traumatic past is alive in the present. For me it becomes about how these real time moments of people remembering and working through layers of resistance to their memory has become for me how people struggle to make meaning of the unimaginable in the present and how the present is traumatized by the past. People are literally becoming coherent in the face of such a traumatic history.
>
> (Oppenheimer interviewed in: Oppenheimer and Hoberman 2015)[8]

Beyond offering documentary makers a way to explore trauma through the memories, bodies, silences, and identifications of protagonists, *Chronique* opened up the possibility of the documentary-making process itself intervening in the life of the protagonist (the life as it is seen within the diegesis). Through its self-reflexive structure, *Chronique* allowed Marceline to review her performed, embodied monologue when she watched it back and reacted to it in the movie theatre alongside the other protagonists. At first, she doubted its veracity. She felt her performance had been forced and unnatural. She worried that she had been 'acting' whilst being filmed; *acting* here being a synonym for *untruthful* (fictitious). But she also said:

> They were very personal, intimate memories. Maybe when I was saying the words, I was reliving the past, feeling it.

In *Chronique*, Rouch and Morin gave documentary its first, traumatised inner Winnicottian viewer in the character of Marceline. Marceline walked and talked through her traumatic past and was later able to watch back and comment on her own performance and so, potentially, reach a new understanding of that past. But Marceline's scene remains a largely unexplored potential in *Chronique* as it was neither a film about Marceline nor about her traumatic past and the scene in which she reflects on her performance is short, with no subsequent or evolving elaboration of her responses to her performance. But the scene is suggestive of a number of possibilities for documentary.

Marceline's *walk* moved *Chronique* beyond *talk* towards an enacted, embodied and fictionalised dramatisation of the traumatic past. Stella Bruzzi, in writing about re-enactment in much more recent documentaries, emphasises the 'emotive' power of these fantasised, dramatised, constructions/reconstructions:

> [T]he permanent now of the documentary re-enactment [...] remains an emotive form of revisiting history, especially because it muddies the documentary waters by incorporating drama, fantasy and personalization. In this sense, it becomes a logical extension of the psychotherapeutic 'talking cure'. Enacting – or *walking* through, not merely *talking* through – pain or trauma, renders it even more immediate and palpable, as the audience is invited to identify and empathize with the re-evoked past event, to become engrossed with it.
>
> (2015a: 94; Bruzzi's italics)

Bruzzi's observation recognises not just the emotive or affective forces to which documentary re-enactment gives us access but, in giving us access to the bodies of the protagonists, it can offer clues (somatic clues) to the protagonist's psychic state that are not necessarily captured in the web of words of a psychotherapy narrowly conceived as a talking cure. And as viewers, we may ourselves experience the re-enacted trauma at a bodily level before we can translate that experience into words: it is 'an overtly visceral, physical viewing experience that conveys the trauma of the events being re-enacted in a literal way, a transference that makes our bodies *feel* the impact of the emotional impact [*sic*] of the film' (2015a: 95; Bruzzi's italics).

Bruzzi's account adopts the viewpoint of those who watch the documentary (the extra-diegetic audience member). But in documentaries that fully exploit the self-reflexive potential suggested by *Chronique*, the protagonist within the diegesis also becomes an audience member (an intra-diegetic audience member) watching back their own performance, responding somatically and affectively, forming identifications and empathetic attachments within the diegesis. In watching their own *walking through* of their own traumatic past, the protagonist is actively caught up in a series of intra-diegetic identifications that play out within the frame of the documentary film. Marceline's short walk and talk revealed an intense transferential encounter between Marceline and a fictional object (her dead father). The scene is an embodied performance or dramatisation of Marceline's encounter with one of her own internal objects and the identifications that this encounter entails, as she *works through* (bodily *walks through*) her traumatic past. It defines a form of 'post-traumatic cinema' that 'not only represents traumatic historical events but also attempts to embody and reproduce the trauma for the spectator' (Hirsch 2004: x–xi).

Rithy Panh's *S21*: the embodied past in the historical-*vérité* tradition

Rithy Panh's *S21: The Khmer Rouge Killing Machine* (2003) is just such an attempt to explore the embodied nature of trauma in documentary. Two of the survivors of the Khmer Rouge's notorious Tuol Sleng prison (known as S21) – Van Nath and Chum Mey – return to the prison where they were tortured and beaten and are brought back together with the perpetrators of the murder, violence and cruelty that took place there in the 1970s. Rithy Panh's film presents both victims *and* perpetrators as traumatised by their past experience. In S21's now empty cells, former prison guards are asked to recreate their daily routines and interactions with the prisoners, but with no one playing the part of the prisoners. They shackle and unshackle, beat and verbally abuse these unseen, reimagined victims and seem to readily fall back into the rhythm of their daily routines of more than twenty-five years earlier. The manner in which the actions are performed suggests that memories of the 1970s are as much *body memories* as they are the product of conscious recall. For Jacques Rancière (2011: 101), the scene 'reactivates the machine' (the impersonal killing machine of the film's title) with the re-enactors in a trance-like or 'hallucinatory' state, a contention confirmed by Panh himself when he described how he directed this scene: 'I [...] simply said "so show me your work, show me how you worked." And that's what opened up the bodily memory' (Panh quoted in Oppenheimer 2012: 245). The imagined prisoners seem to be very real to the guards in their re-enactments and the performance of this fictional scenario makes the prisoners very real for us as viewers of the film; the story of the past returning in the present of its embodied re-enactment.

In self-reflexive mode, the film stages confrontations between the guard-re-enactors and "victim" Vann Nath, and between one of the guards, Houy Him, and his parents. Houy Him revisits the experience of the re-enactment in these inter-personal encounters. In Van Nath's meeting with the guards, he makes it clear what he hopes for from the experience:

> I don't really want to come to these meetings, because we're not here to tell pleasant stories. We only talk about this unbearable past, which we can't escape. I can't anyway. I'm trying to understand what happened, to make sense out of it. I want to understand it.

But the potential of this self-reflexive process to bring understanding seems to be unavailable to Houy Him. He is unable to engage in any meaningful way with the fictional recreations of the past. When talking to Van Nath, he hides behind the justification that he was following orders and so he is not responsible. And with his parents, he attempts to stop them talking about his role at S21, exclaiming: 'Stop it. I have a headache. I'm sick all day long. I can't eat a thing' and so rather than the embodied traumatic past becoming available for a meaningful reworking, it re-emerges only in a different bodily form; in its return as a psychosomatic symptom. The traumatic past may become available for the viewer to work with and develop a deeper understanding (through a reflection on the *re*-presentation of the past in the *hallucinatory*, dramatic re-enactments) but it is not available to Houy Him. The extent to which *historical verité's* embodied, self-reflexive approach to filmmaking can reveal new meanings to the protagonist is always limited by the protagonist's psychic capacity to confront these meanings.[9]

Cinéma vérité *as a partial model for contemporary "trauma" documentaries*

The *cinéma vérité* of Rouch and Morin – in its self-consciously reflexive and self-reflexive form, in its phenomenological approach to meaning-making (producing something new and transformative in the filmmaking present), in its belief that documentary gives access to embodied meanings, and in its deployment of fictions as a means of getting at psychological "truths" on a psychoanalytic model – can be viewed as a precursor of recent documentaries that try to *coax out* a meaningful account of a traumatic past through the deployment of a fictional-film-within-the-documentary.

But this statement needs some qualification. Several contemporary films that explore trauma through fictions do not present the body of the traumatised protagonist directly to the audience. In animated documentary, for example, the body is represented graphically and we are reliant on the voice of the traumatised protagonist to tell us (to talk us through) how they responded physically and affectively to the unfolding filmmaking process and to the fictional interludes within the documentary. And sometimes, the body of the traumatised protagonist is not available as it is substituted by the body of a double who takes the protagonist's place (for example in Albertina Carri's *The Blonds* (2003)). But *cinéma vérité* – and *cinéma vérité* in its evolution into *historical vérité* – delineated a range of filmmaking practices and techniques that were capable of engaging with the complexities of psychological trauma, even if not all the contemporary documentaries conform precisely to the *cinéma/historical-vérité* model.

But perhaps the most marked difference between contemporary films exploring trauma and *vérité* is that the autobiographical mode address has become so common in recent films. Rouch may appear in a number of his films, but none could be described as autobiographical. In the second section of this chapter, I turn my attention to autobiographical explorations of trauma to tease out the mechanisms through which meaning emerges in the absence of the key interpersonal relationship between director and protagonist: the very interpersonal relationship that has led several documentary theorists (from Berman to Piotrowska) to make an equation between the documentary encounter (director-protagonist) and the analytic encounter (analyst-analysand).

Autobiographical documentary-making as a self-analytic process

Michael Renov credits the emergence of the autobiographical mode of address with reinventing the very idea of documentary (2008: 41). The films at the core of this study – documentaries that deploy fictions as part of a process of working through a "real" traumatic history – are frequently autobiographical: Carri's *The Blonds* (2003); Maddin's *My Winnipeg* (2007); Folman's *Waltz with Bashir*

(2008); Panh's *The Missing Picture* (2013). And even when in third-person mode, like Oppenheimer's *The Act of Killing* (2012), there is a strong autobiographical element, as it was the traumatised, principal protagonist who conceived, scripted and directed the film's fictional interludes (the films-within-the-film).

In Chapter 3, I likened the fictions that are deployed in documentary to the fictions the analyst constructs (Freud) or dreams (the Botellas) when attempting to represent otherwise unrepresented traumas. But in documentaries where it is the traumatised protagonist who constructs or dreams the fictions, and where the director and principal protagonist are one and the same, it might be better to think of these films as exercises in self-analysis rather than in terms of a conventional, two-person, analyst-analysand model. This raises the question of whether self-analysis is even possible and if it is, who performs the critical role of the secondary witness in a self-analysis and by extension in an autobiographical film?

Freud's self-analysis

Didier Anzieu's detailed account, *Freud's Self-Analysis*, establishes beyond question that not only is self-analysis possible but that 'the basic corpus of psychoanalytic notions' emerged from Freud's self-analysis rather than from the analysis of his patients (Anzieu 1986 [1959 & 1975]: 232).[10] James Barron (1993: xix) echoes this view arguing that 'psychoanalytic theory and practice are the intellectual children of Freud's self-analytic efforts.' In the subsequent history of psychoanalysis, Freud's reliance on his own unconscious and his own dreams as objects of research has been under-acknowledged. Freud himself rarely mentioned his self-analysis in his public presentations of psychoanalysis, perhaps out of fear that the practice would be seen as lacking the objectivity required of a "science" (Mitchell 1993: xiv).

But the psychoanalytic model that is most familiar is that of analysis taking place in the dynamic, inter-personal encounter between analyst and analysand: the "other" of the analyst is a crucial (perhaps *the* crucial) element in a transactional process from which meaning may emerge. How can autobiographical documentaries on the one hand, or the isolated practice of examining one's own psychic mechanisms, hope to unearth psychological meanings or insights without that creative – sometimes traumatic – encounter between a "self" and an "other"? In his foreword to a collection of essays on self-analysis by practising psychoanalysts, Stephen A. Mitchell acknowledges the problem:

> Self-analysis, as it turns out, is very hard to do […] [T]here is an omnipresent danger of self-absorption, self-indulgence, self-deception.
>
> (Mitchell 1993: xvii)

Documentary theorist Alisa Lebow (2012: 1) points to similar dangers confronting documentary practice when she notes the widespread perception of autobiographical or *first-person* documentaries as 'self-absorbed, myopic, ego-driven films that only a mother could love'.[11]

Away from the public stage in Freud's private correspondence, a picture of self-analysis emerges that belies the assumption that self-analysis is a solitary and solipsistic endeavour. Freud's self-analytic practice *was* dependent on others; both "real", external others and others Freud conjured from within himself. In a letter to Wilhelm Fliess, Freud hints at the internal other:

> My self-analysis remains interrupted. I have realized why I can analyze myself only with the help of self-knowledge obtained objectively (like an outsider). True self-analysis is impossible; otherwise there would be no [neurotic] illness.
> (Freud and Masson 1985: letter dated 24 November 1897)

In this highly ambivalent statement, Freud at first describes the condition that makes a self-analysis possible and then seems to retreat, and to doubt the very possibility of *true* self-analysis.[12] But to focus on the positive part of the statement, the other in self-analysis must be conjured from within the observing self; a part of the self that can observe another part of the self, 'like an outsider'.[13] Freud's internal other was joined by external others; trusted colleagues and family members who Freud used as sounding boards for ideas and insights that emerged from his self-analysis. So important were these external others to Freud's self-analysis that Anzieu (1986 [1959 & 1975]: 569) claims '[t]here can be no proper self-analysis unless it is communicated to someone else.'[14]

Self-analysis in documentary

In documentary, a number of others are generated by the very mechanics of the filmmaking process itself. The director even of an autobiographical film is never alone. The film is made with the participation of others: camera and sound crew, producer, editor, who act as external others. In reflexive films that unmask the mechanics of the filmmaking process, these external others are not simply assumed to exist by the film's viewers but appear in the diegesis and can be seen to perform their role of other to the director. In Albertina Carri's autobiographical documentary *The Blonds* (2003), Carri appears to reach a profounder understanding of her traumatic past in part through her continual dialogue with her film crew.

The nature of the filmmaking process also produces a very present and tangible internal other in the images and words of the autobiographical director captured on film. In the editing process especially, the director of an autobiographical film is confronted by an alien self – a filmic *Doppelgänger* in sound and vision – who it is hard to hear and view in any other way than 'like an outsider'. This *Doppelgänger*-effect is given more play in *self-reflexive* documentaries as the encounter between the director and his or her *Doppelgänger* is brought within the diegesis, as the encounter is filmed and then this new material is cut into the final version of the film (the film-within-the-film is witnessed within the diegesis). In being confronted by a filmic other in the midst of making the film, the direction the final film will take is almost certainly altered. Meanings are likely to emerge for the director/protagonist from this confrontation with their *other self*.

Finally, there is the prospect of a future external other that constantly plays in the imagination of the director throughout the making of a film; the film's eventual audience. At the end of Rithy Panh's *The Missing Picture* (2013), he says he is handing over his film to his audience so he can be rid of it and so rid, he hopes, of the painful recollections it contains. This fictional transaction with a fictional (that is imagined) audience provides Panh with a profoundly important external witness to his self-analytic efforts. The audience is, even though only in prospect, that 'someone else' that Anzieu says is essential to any 'proper self-analysis'. The filmmaker's prospective audience acts on the filmmaker in much the same way as the prospect of an eventual reader acted on psychoanalyst, Rivka Eifermann, in her self-analytic writing:

> My audience, fantasized and real, took form and gradually became a constant presence. Indeed, unanticipated discoveries concerning the unconscious role the audience played, or served, in the course of writing, turned out again and again to be integral to the subject of the paper I was writing.
>
> (Eifermann 1993: 173)

The same 'unanticipated discoveries' are available in autobiographical film.

Both Alisa Lebow (2012) and Michael Renov (2008) have written about the emergence of the autobiographical documentary[15] and its transformatory impact on our perception of the nature of documentary. Both see the autobiographical form as carrying within it its own others; others which are inevitably in dialogue with the autobiographical filmmaker. In *The Cinema of Me*, Lebow takes Jean Luc Nancy's formulation of the *singular plural*, where the "I" is always ontologically a "we", and argues that in documentary articulations of the self, others are always inferred, indeed are constitutive of the self (Lebow 2012: 2; referencing Nancy 2000). There is no Cartesian singular-self – the self as an island – but instead a social "I" whose language and culture both precede the "I" and form the "I". She extends this *singular plural* (the "I" that contains the other of "we") through Emmanuel Levinas's formulation of subjectivity as created in and through our subjection to the other, and Judith Butler's formulation of the subject as always in a social relation, in dialogue, with the norms defined by a wider community (Lebow 2012; referencing Levinas 1998, and Butler 2005). I am entirely sympathetic to this notion of a culturally and linguistically constituted "I" and would even expand the domain of the "we" in the "I" that Lebow defines, to memory and the unconscious both of which are central to my way of approaching autobiographical and non-autobiographical documentaries that deal with trauma. I am thinking here of Maurice Halbwachs's notion of 'la mémoire collective' (Halbwachs 1992) and Jean Laplanche's formulation of the unconscious as a receptacle for untranslatable remnants of other people's unconscious (Laplanche 1999a).

For Lebow (2012: 3), 'the speaking, and in this case filming, subject is neither solipsistic nor monologic, but always already in dialogue or as Nancy would have it, always already "speaking with"'. Michael Renov (2004 [1989]: 112) makes a similar argument. The structure of autobiographical documentary, with its dual focus on the self and the self in relation to a real outside world, inevitably produces the outside perspective of an other through 'a practice of inscription in which the domain of the subject and the enveloping world are mutually constitutive: self and other/self through other'.

The presence of others in the filmmaking process, the threat or the promise of an eventual audience and the 'dialogic splitting of subjectivity' (Lebow 2012: 3) entailed in the act of autobiographical filmmaking are all instances of others entering the process. But for those filmmakers trying to explore their traumatic past, something more seems to be required, often involving the deployment of elaborate fictions which the filmmaker invents (constructs or dreams) and in which internal others and alternative versions of the self are brought to life in animation, in clay models, in the bodies of actors, etc. Fictions are required as the primary internal other that is sought in these self-analytic films is the unconscious, which by definition is unrepresented and can only be known through its derivatives. By fictionalising the self and being able to view this fictionalised self in relation to others, a picture of unconscious structures may emerge. It puts on the filmic stage, structures of identification and object relating that might otherwise remain obscure. The task is further complicated as this internal other is one we are 'not constitutionally inclined' to look for (as Freud put it in his paper *The Unconscious* (Freud 1915b: 169)). And in filmic explorations, as in life, when we do seek the unconscious, it is not "simply" a case of trying to find ways of lifting repressions that block our access to painful and difficult memories that have undergone repression by the dynamic unconscious. In the wake of trauma, these memories might survive only as vestiges without representation, as a *blank* 'that has no history and is incapable of taking the form of represented memories' (Botella and Botella 2013: 108). Albertina Carri faced precisely this problem in her autobiographical documentary *The Blonds* (2003) where the traumatic loss of her parents was not remembered but felt as an aching absence. By fictionalising herself in the body of an actor, she was able to represent (reconstruct) the emotional *form* of her connection to her parents even if the *content* remained blank.

The fictions and fictionalisations of the self in autobiographical documentary are attempts to both represent the self and gain the necessary critical distance to view the self like an outsider; to gain the distance that Freud and Anzieu see as crucial to a successful self-analysis. Jordana Blejmar describes these documentaries with their elaborate fictions as 'docu-fantasy'[16] and points to what she calls an 'autofictional turn' in documentary (Blejmar 2016).[17] Blejmar is borrowing a term coined by Serge Doubrovsky to describe his form of literary autobiography that saw fictions and fictionalisations of the self as the route to forms of self-knowledge (or 'truth' in Doubrovsky's language). For Doubrovsky (1989), these fictions were 'fiction[s] of strictly real events or facts'; fictions that are a route to the 'truth' not to its downfall. The fictionalised self becomes an object for the author of the autofiction that can be viewed as if from the outside. It is a self that autofiction writer,

Camille Laurens (quoted in Cusset 2012) describes as decentred, at once 'I, it's not me'; an exteriorised and fictionalised self that can be viewed like an outsider, so that the truth of past emotion can emerge.[18]

Rithy Panh's The Missing Picture*: an exercise in self-analysis*

Fictional and fantasised internal and external others play a crucial role in Rithy Panh's autobiographical documentary *The Missing Picture* (2013). We do not have access to the body and the somatic responses of the traumatised protagonist on screen in the way that a film made in the *vérité* mode would allow; Panh "appears" in the film represented by a clay manikin. Instead, the affective and subjective voice of the director (Panh's words voiced by actor Randal Douc)[19] guides the viewer through the evolving process that was the making of *The Missing Picture*. Rithy Panh had spent four years of his childhood as a slave labourer in Khmer Rouge camps where most members of his immediate and extended family met their deaths. In his subsequent career as a filmmaker, Panh explored the history and traumatic aftermath of the Khmer Rouge's period in power in Cambodia in documentary and docudrama, in feature film and through film biography. With the project that became *The Missing Picture* (2013), Panh tells us that the past finally caught up with him, compelling him to confront his personal trauma directly through autobiography, and to try to lay it to rest.

> I seek my childhood like a lost picture
> or rather it seeks me.
> Is it because I am fifty?
> Because I've seen troubled times
> When fear alternates with hope?
> The memory is there [pause] now
> Pounding at my temples.
> I'd like to be rid of it.[20]

The film describes Panh's attempts to find the *lost* or *missing picture:* some way to represent his traumatic past to himself that might bring him some peace. As the film progresses, Panh's understanding of the nature of that missing picture gradually shifts. In the film's trailer, Panh tells us that he began the filmmaking process thinking that the key to his past would be found in the artefacts and objects that are the focus of the historian and the realist documentary maker. He sets out to find the picture that will somehow *reveal* the truth; the indexical object that will *be* the truth.

> For many years I have been looking for a missing picture. A photograph taken between 1975 and 1979 by the Khmer Rouge. [...] I searched vainly for it in archives, in old papers, in country villages across Cambodia. Today I know this image must be missing – I was not really looking for it – would it not be obscene and insignificant? So I created it.[21]

What Panh creates is a film that he calls *The Missing Picture.* It is a realisation that the key to the past lies inside himself – in his memory and fantasies – and not in some external piece of documentary evidence. Panh recreates his memories and the *factical* (fantasy) world that played in his head as a child, in clay scenes populated with clay figurines.

As the film progresses, the fictions that Panh deploys with his clay models are increasingly not fictionalised recreations of past events or even the representation in clay of childhood fantasies but entirely fictional present encounters between people; intersubjective encounters of the sort that psychoanalysis brings into play in the transference and the counter-transference and that self-analysis brings into play as the self confronts alien selves. The dialogues happen internally, inside Panh, between the middle-aged Panh and a variety of internal others – his dead parents, his lost childhood self – in an intra-personal dialogue between Panh and his own internal objects. Panh gives voice to both "himself" and these other aspects of himself in the voice-over narration. He both speaks and ventriloquises.

Panh's main internal interlocutor is his former self, the boy Rithy Panh. As Panh tells us late in the film, 'Now, it is the boy who seeks me out'. It is a dramatisation with clay models of Joyce McDougall's evocative description of what happens in analysis: 'Whether we will it or not, our inner characters are constantly seeking a stage on which to play out their tragedies and comedies' (McDougall 1986: 3); a stage she saw, following Winnicott, as a *potential space* 'that lies between fantasy and reality' where we can try out or stage productions (1986: 10). Like a character in Pirandello's *Six Characters in Search of an Author* (1995 [1921]), the boy marches into the theatre and demands to put on his show for the director.

If we were in any doubt that *The Missing Picture* is an exercise in self-analysis, these doubts are dispelled in a wonderfully comic and moving scene late in the film. A clay manikin of the middle-aged Panh lies on a model couch beneath a huge portrait of Sigmund Freud. A clay-manikin analyst sits by Panh. It is soon apparent that the "analyst" is also the middle-aged Rithy Panh.[22] The two Panhs, analyst and analysand, sit and lie under the stern gaze of Freud. The voice-over begins with the words: 'Sometimes I picture a child. Let's say it's me', and the clay analysand on the couch morphs into the child Rithy Panh in a mix lasting a couple of seconds. Now the adult analyst-Panh is analysing the child analysand-Panh. As the scene progresses, the model set of the analytic consulting room fills up with more and more characters from Panh's past (parents, siblings, friends). Panh, as his own analyst, has produced a facilitating set or stage that might cast light on his traumatic past, as Joyce McDougall (1986: 10) describes:

> The analyst might be likened to the stage manager of Luigi Pirandello's celebrated *Six Characters in Search of an Author*, in that he or she seeks to maintain a space that is ready to welcome all the internal inhabitants of each analysand's secret theater.

But the self-analysis appears to fail. Panh tells us that the boy 'wants to speak to me. But words are hard to find.' And Panh admits that he does not really want to hear what the boy has to say anyway: 'I want to leave it all, leave my language, my country in vain and my childhood returns'. Panh seems to be struggling to avoid that other we are not constitutionally inclined to 'hear'; our own unconscious. There is a missing picture locked up inside the fifty-year-old Panh and it seems the picture is destined to remain missing as he cannot bear to look for it.

Towards the end of the film, Panh explains that he is trapped in perpetual melancholia unable to mourn, identified with the dead ('Their flesh is my flesh'), and himself perhaps already *psychically killed* by his past ('It is me they will kill. Or maybe they already have'). Mourning has failed. Panh is caught in an unending repetition of his painful past (both within this film and in all the other films he has directed about his and Cambodia's past (Boyle 2014b: 32)[23]): attached to the unmourned, *lost object* of dead parents, siblings, family and friends and to the *lost object* of his former self whose childhood was murdered by the Khmer Rouge; feeling 'guilty for not having helped the destitute'; and unable to understand or to make sense of what has happened to him.[24]

Panh's sense of loss is felt at a bodily level ('I want to touch them. Their voice is missing, so I won't tell'). It is a sense of bodily disconnection and loss that precedes representation and cannot be represented. It is the overwhelming sense of loss and separation that we assume Freud's grandson Ernst felt before he was able to find a soothing fiction – a missing picture – and to bridge the gap of loss with his *fort-da* game. For Panh, the sense of bodily disconnection is presented as an insuperable melancholic fact and for all the inventive fictions he deploys, he cannot bridge the gap. After a second visit to the analytic consulting room, Panh concludes: 'Of course, I haven't found the missing picture. I looked for it, in vain.'[25]

But in the film's trailer, made after the film was completed, Panh reaches a different conclusion. The missing picture is actually hiding in plain sight. It is the film Panh creates and calls *The Missing Picture*. He is only able to see it when the film is finished. It is in the trailer that Panh tells us of his giving up on the search for the unique, missing photograph taken at some time between 1975 and 1979 that somehow would *be* the truth and explain everything:

> Today I know this image must be missing – I was not really looking for it – would it not be obscene and insignificant?

But he immediately goes on to say:

> So I created it. What I give you today is neither the picture nor the search for a unique picture, but the picture of a quest, a quest that cinema allows.

Panh's words suggest that it is the autobiographical documentary-making process itself that *allows* the possibility of reaching an understanding of a traumatic past. It is the filmmaking process conceived as Rouch conceived it, not as a transparent window on reality, but as an active intervention in the world, a provocation and a catalyst for the emergence of truth or meaning that would not otherwise be available. This active process plays out in intra-personal encounters with internal others or alien selves. The fictions that Panh stages – the films-within-the-film of *The Missing Picture* – are attempts to give representational form to the contents of his own post-traumatic consciousness as it manifests itself in memory and fantasy, and in imagined encounters and identifications with internal objects. These fictional representations in themselves do not bring understanding. The process involves self-conscious reflection; a questioning of the adequacy of the representations that have been produced. It is perhaps ironic that in a film that contains a fictional representation of a failed self-analysis that the documentary-making process can be seen to echo most closely the strategies and the possibilities made available by the analytic process as it attempts to find meaning in a traumatic past. But the irony is perhaps explained in Barbara Johnson's perception of the analytic process. The knot of trauma is not untied in a sudden revelatory interpretation or insight. If the knot can be untied or at least loosened, it is through a temporally evolving process that involves constant failure and constant painful repetitions (re-knottings) of the "unresolvable" trauma until in the end the knot might be untied through the very repetition of failure: 'an act of untying the knot in the structure by the repetition of the act of tying it' (Johnson 1980: 142).[26] If understanding can be reached in analysis, it is reached through a process and in *The Missing Picture*, Panh provides himself and us with a picture of a quest, a picture of a process; an unfolding process of self-examination made possible through film ('a quest that cinema allows').

The filmmaking process can open up a space – a Winnicottian play space – where trauma can be explored experimentally in all its manifestations including those we might conventionally call fictions. The analytic space is a space for fantasy, memory, dreams (even hallucinations), free associations, acting out, transference, counter-transference. The filmic space in documentary, in the hands a director such as Panh, is a similar space. The film-within-the-film in documentary is a way of importing fictional representations – psychically *real* fictions, fantasies, imagined intra-personal encounters – into the arguably factual frame of documentary. There is then a secondary part of the process – both in analysis and documentary – which was encapsulated by Jean Laplanche when he described Freud's analytic method as having a patient go step by step from one representation to another and 'reminding him of those steps' (quoted in Fletcher and Stanton 1992: 87–8). The being *reminded of the steps* is made possible in self-reflexive documentaries where the protagonist views and reviews their own fictional creations as an intra-diegetic audience member (an inner Winnicottian viewer) watching their own fictions. The self-reflexivity of both certain documentaries and analysis is what turns the process into a truly dynamic process; a process that might be able to loosen the knot of trauma. Panh said in an interview (IDFA 2013): 'Personally I don't know where I am going [...] if you know before, it is not documentary film'[27] confirming Stella Bruzzi's contention about performative documentary that 'documentary is an unpredictable act' (Bruzzi 2006: 214). Panh reminds us of that unpredictability by telling us about the failures of the process; telling us and reminding himself of the steps that have been taken.

But for all its representational ingenuity and its deployment of fictions within the frame of the documentary, did the process bring any greater understanding for Panh? Was the process cathartic? Panh's final piece of voice-over suggests that it is the transaction with us – the external other of the imagined audience – that has cathartic potential.

> Of course I haven't found the missing picture. I looked for it, in vain. [...] And so I make this picture. I look at it. I cherish it. I hold it in my hand like a belovèd face. This missing picture I now hand over to you, so that it never cease [*sic*] to seek us out.

This is an ambiguous statement. Is the handing over of the film to the secondary witness – us as audience who have witnessed the filmic representations of Panh's traumatic past – a perpetuation of the trauma which is now transmitted to us and seeks us out and haunts us too, or is there some relief for Panh in the inter-personal exchange with this imagined other of the audience? My feeling is that if we read this closing statement both in conjunction with the upbeat images and music that accompany and follow the closing credits *and* in conjunction with Panh's statement that opens the film, there might be at least a glimmer of optimism to be found. Panh opens the film explaining why he must make the film:

> The memory is there [pause] now
> Pounding at my temples.
> I'd like to be rid of it.

And he ends the film handing over the picture he has created out of his memories, fantasies and encounters with internal objects. He is rid of something to the extent that he hands over this picture of a process of psychic self-exploration. As in the analytic process, there is a hope of catharsis in the handing over or the sharing of the traumatic past with a secondary witness.[28] And if there is some sort of catharsis – some sort of therapeutic benefit – through filmmaking or analysis it emerges from the process as a whole, not in an isolated moment of epiphany or in a single interpretation. It is a process or a quest; a quest that Panh tells us 'cinema allows'; the process of making a film.

If this is Panh's own verdict on his making of an autobiographical film, then it seems to echo Ari Folman's experience of the autobiographical, self-exploratory process of making *Waltz with Bashir*, which he described, in retrospect, as 'four years of therapy' (Folman in interview quoted in Schäuble 2011: 210). And it was not just in retrospect that Folman pointed to the therapeutic potential (the self-analytic potential) of autobiographical filmmaking. He explores it *within* the diegesis of *Waltz with Bashir*. At the start of the film – when Folman's friend Boaz Rein recounts his nightmare vision of ferocious dogs rampaging through Tel Aviv – Folman asks Rein why he has not tried 'therapy, psychiatry, shiatsu, anything...' but has instead contacted Folman about his nightmares. 'I'm just a filmmaker', opines Folman. Rein replies 'Can't films be therapeutic?'. Both *Waltz with Bashir* and *The Missing Picture* seem to be filmic experiments that attempt to answer Rein's question in self-analytic form.

Notes

1 Joshua Oppenheimer, for example, explicitly acknowledges his debt to Rouch, declaring 'I'm absolutely standing on his shoulders' (interview with Oppenheimer in Spiessens 2014: 69). That said, associations between *Chronique* and current practice are not offered in the spirit of a genealogy – a continuous teleological progression from then to now – but more to indicate points of connection.

2 Rouch says this in a piece of footage from 1960–61 that did not make the final cut of *Chronique* but which is included in Florence Dauman's 2011 documentary *Un été +50* (in which *Chronique*'s original participants, fifty years after its release, reflect on their experience of making the film).

3 Credited as 'Mary Lou' in the film but in life, Marilù Parolini.

4 In *Moi, un noir* (1958), Rouch employed this tactic by having his economic-migrant protagonists portray themselves as the Hollywood stars they most admired: it was a way to unearth the hopes and fears and disappointments in the lives of migrant workers in a foreign country. There are powerful echoes of *Moi, un noir* in *The Act of Killing* (2012) where director Joshua Oppenheimer provides a stage for his protagonists to act out scenes from their murderous past in the style of the Hollywood movies they loved.

5 Marceline Loridan (later Loridan-Ivens) who was born Marceline Rozenberg of Polish Jewish parents living in France.

6 Lebow is referencing Slavoj Žižek's ideas on fantasy and the "Real".

7 I should note that *Shoah* lacks the self-reflexive element of *Chronique*, where the traumatised protagonist within the diegesis represents the traumatic past not just to the audience but also to themselves through the medium of the film-within-the-film (as they watch back their own performance).

8 In Oppenheimer's appropriation of Lanzmann's *historical-vérité* method, he makes claims for its meaning-generating potential which Lanzmann explicitly rejected. In conformity with the trauma-theory paradigm, Lanzmann utterly rejected the idea that we can reach a meaningful account of trauma (a meaningful account of the insider's experience of the Holocaust): 'There is indeed an absolute obscenity in the project of understanding. Not to understand was my ironclad rule during all the years *Shoah* was in the making' (Lanzmann in Liebman 2007: 51–2). Oppenheimer rejects Lanzmann's view very directly in an interview with Irene Lusztig: 'Lanzmann famously said that it's obscene to ask that question "why". I utterly disagree' (Lusztig 2013: 52).

9 Similarly, in Oppenheimer's *The Act of Killing* (2012), some of what Anwar Congo witnesses in his own films-within proves too difficult for Congo to comprehend and what results is not understanding but somatisation (see Chapter 5).

10 Anzieu is not alone in seeing Freud's self-analysis as central to the development of psychoanalysis. See, for example, Gay (1988).

11 This is not Lebow's view but her recognition of a widespread perception.

12 Doubts as to the objectivity of self-analysis dogged Freud throughout his life. In the late essay *The Subtleties of a Faulty Action* (1935: 234) he wrote: 'in self-analysis the danger of incompleteness is particularly great. One is too soon satisfied with a part explanation, behind which resistance may easily be keeping back something that is more important perhaps'.

13 From the perspective of the subsequent genesis of psychoanalysis, this tentative statement about how self-analysis might work is perhaps the first glimmering of an idea that

would develop into object relations, with different parts of the self in communication with each other. The ambivalence of Freud's comment in his letter to Fliess, perhaps reflects Freud's lack of an *internal objects* model at that time. It was only with the publication of *On Narcissism* (1914b) and *Mourning and Melancholia* (1917a) that Freud developed a theoretical construct capable of explaining how one could take oneself as an object (a self-observing self).

14 Freud's principal external others were (according to Anzieu) first Wilhelm Fliess, then sister-in-law Minna Bernays and finally daughter Anna Freud.

15 Lebow prefers the term 'first-person documentary' (to the more common 'autobiographical documentary' used by Renov and others) as films can be highly personal and subjective without being strictly autobiographical (Lebow 2012: 1–2).

16 A similar term, 'docu-fantasia', is used by Guy Maddin to describe his autobiographical documentary *My Winnipeg* (2007), which deploys fictions, and a fictionalised version of himself played by actor Darcy Fehr, to explore his traumatic past. See Ebiri (2008).

17 Blejmar's 2016 book, *Playful Memories: The Autofictional Turn in Post-Dictatorship Argentina*, cites Albertina Carri's *The Blonds* (2003) as an early and important exemplar of this 'turn'.

18 The quarry for Laurens is 'past emotion' but the construction of a fictionalised self is equally valuable when the quarry is traumatic experience. Note: in this paragraph (for references to Doubrovsky and Laurens), I am indebted to a conference paper delivered by autofiction writer Catherine Cusset (2012).

19 Strictly speaking, the narration was co-written by Panh and novelist Christophe Bataille (printed version available in Panh and Bataille 2013).

20 This is the film's opening voice-over.

21 The trailer is included on the DVD of the film issued by New Wave Films (2013).

22 Jennifer Cazenave (2018: 44–5) writes about this scene as an *analysis* not a *self-analysis*, apparently not equating the middle-aged analyst with Panh. I am unable to argue definitively that the middle-aged analyst is in fact Panh as clay manikins closely resemble each other (even though the two manikins that represent the middle-aged analyst and the middle-aged analysand look identical and are dressed identically). Nevertheless, even if this scene is of a conventional two-person analysis (where only the analysand is Panh), the film as a whole remains an autobiographical exercise in psychic self-examination (and so is, in effect, an exercise in self-analysis).

23 Deirdre Boyle quotes Panh as saying he has been making 'one film' throughout his adult life even though, in 2014 when he made the statement, he had actually made thirteen documentaries and five fiction films. Since 2014, Panh has made seven more films. Most are about his or Cambodia's troubled past.

24 These are all aspects of failed mourning (melancholia) as described by Freud in *Mourning and Melancholia* (1917a).

25 All quotations in this paragraph and the preceding two are taken from Panh's voice-over.

26 The apparent paradox of untying through tying is the paradox of mourning: constant painful repetition and failure over time being the route back to psychic health (the untying of the knot). As Jean Laplanche asserts, the process of mourning (knotting and unknotting) is 'the very prototype of analytic endeavor' (see Ray 2012: 56).

27 Panh made these comments just after completing *The Missing Picture*. In the same interview, he also re-emphasised the theme of unpredicability, saying: 'You can't order reality to go to your script' (IDFA 2013).

28 The process we see in *The Missing Picture* (Panh's creation of fictions where he encounters internal and external others) seems to closely mirror the analytic process as described by André Green (1986b: 296): 'the essence of analytic action concerns the representation of intrasubjective and intersubjective psychic processes'.

Chapter 5

Joshua Oppenheimer's *The Act of Killing* (2012) 'the play's the thing'

Third-person documentary or documentary-making as analytic encounter

'… I have heard
That guilty creatures sitting at a play
Have by the very cunning of the scene
Been struck so to the soul that presently
They have proclaim'd their malefactions;
For murder, though it have no tongue, will speak
With most miraculous organ. I'll have these players
Play something like the murder of my father
Before mine uncle: I'll observe his looks;
I'll tent him to the quick: if he blench,
I know my course. The spirit I have seen
May be the devil: and the devil hath power
To assume a pleasing shape; yea, and perhaps
Out of my weakness and my melancholy,
As he is very potent with such spirits,
Abuses me to damn me: I'll have grounds
More relative than this: the play's the thing
Wherein I'll catch the conscience of the king.'

Hamlet in Act II, Scene II of William Shakespeare's
The Tragedy of Hamlet,
Prince of Denmark

The Act of Killing: its structure and central conceit

The final scene: the rooftop re-enactment and how to read it

In the extraordinary closing scene of Joshua Oppenheimer's 2012 documentary *The Act of Killing,*[1] Anwar Congo returns to the rooftop above what is now a handbag shop in Medan in North Sumatra where half a century before he had murdered

DOI: 10.4324/9781003657187-7

scores, perhaps hundreds of people. As he tries to re-enact the methods he used to kill his victims for Oppenheimer's camera, he is convulsed, he retches, he doubles up, he sits and breathes deeply, he leaks tears and nasal mucus, he emits strange, guttural noises. Gradually Congo recovers his composure and carries on with his re-enactment only for his body to rebel again. It seems Anwar Congo, the thinking, conscious "I", has been completely upstaged by his body; a body that although it 'speaks no known language' has forced its way centre stage and provided 'a framework for communicating the psychic scenes of the internal theatre' (McDougall 1986: 53) through a series of extreme, observable bodily *blenches*. Congo struggles on to the end of his re-enactment after several attempts, and then quietly leaves the rooftop stage and heads off into the city night. The film ends.

What are we to make of this bizarre, climactic scene? I felt I was witnessing something terrible, something agonising, something primitive.[2] It made deeply disturbing viewing; a disturbance I struggled to understand. What was going on inside Congo that made this attempt to replay a memory so difficult? Could Congo make sense of it and did that sense bring any relief from the pain of traumatic memory?[3]

My reading of *The Act of Killing* and the character Anwar Congo emerge from my experience of disturbance and the struggle to understand what unfolds on screen. My theoretical justification for this reading begins with Vivian Sobchack's thoughts about the *act matter* (the noematic content of film) and the nature of the phenomenological experience of a viewer watching a film that is perceived to be non-fictional and concerns non-fictional characters. It returns to documentary the referentiality it claims in its self-declaration as non-fictional. For Sobchack, the non-fictional filmic object opens up a space through or behind the screen that allows the viewer to speculate about the life – and that must include the psychic life – of an on-screen protagonist. But Sobchack also describes the *act quality* (the noesis); the viewer's act of perceiving and speculating about the life of the on-screen protagonist. The *act matter* cannot be separated out from the *act quality* and so my speculations about the internal psychic life of Anwar Congo cannot be separated off from my own subjective, unconscious and embodied responses to the film that unfolds before me. Phyllis Creme, in a different idiom, construes this entanglement through Winnicott's transitional object and the impossibility of separating the found (the referential) from the created (the invention of the perceiving subject). Rather than treating this *inseparability* as invalidating the attempt to understand the psychic life of an on-screen character,[4] I conceive of it as the route to that understanding through the notion of a counter-transferential reading, where meaning (symbolisation) emerges in a 'system of intra- and intersubjective exchanges' (Gibeault 2005: 1712–4) between viewing subject and viewed subject. The disturbance I felt on first encountering Anwar Congo might be taken to be a bodily and affective contagion, an entanglement, a psychic identification with Congo who – although I only encounter him as a filmic avatar – I know to have a real life beyond the screen. My feeling of disturbance, if it can become an object of reflection, might offer me a glimpse into the internal psychic life of Congo but it begins with my subjective, non-cognitive, unconscious, affective responses to what I see and hear on screen.

The fictional film-within-the-documentary-frame

To begin to understand this closing scene, which graphically enacts both the impossibility and the possibility of representing trauma, we need to spool back to the start of the film. Over the opening shots of Medan city, we are provided with a series of "cards" (on-screen texts) which situate us in the context of Indonesian politics and history, asserting the film's "facticity" and describing the film's central conceit:

> In 1965, the Indonesian government was overthrown by the military.
>
> Anybody opposed to the military dictatorship could be accused of being a communist: union members, landless farmers, intellectuals, and the ethnic Chinese.
>
> In less than a year, and with the direct aid of western governments, over one million "communists" were murdered.
>
> The army used paramilitaries and gangsters to carry out the killings.
>
> These men have been in power – and have persecuted their opponents – ever since.
>
> When we met the killers, they proudly told us stories about what they did.
>
> To understand why, we asked them to create scenes about the killings in whatever ways they wished.
>
> This film follows that process, and documents its consequences.

With Indonesia's troubling history and the film's central conceit explained in a few words,[5] the viewer enters the main body of the documentary, which takes place in a dynamic and evolving present driven in part by the scenes the killers create; scenes that were shot to produce what the killers thought would be a feature film about the events of 1965 and which appear as short interstitial scenes (short films within the Oppenheimer documentary). These scenes take many forms from historical re-enactments of events from the killing years of the mid-1960s, through fictionalised re-enactments often in the style of the Hollywood movies so loved by the killers, to fantasy sequences that bear no relation to anything that ever happened. These films-within sit within the frame of Oppenheimer's documentary which follows the killers over several years: he films them talking to each other; he films them answering questions that he poses from behind his camera; he films them talking to survivors of the 1965–66 massacres and to the children of victims of those massacres; he films them making their feature film; he films them reflecting on what they have shot as they watch their rushes – and rough and fine cuts of their film – on a monitor. This last technique gives the film a self-reflexive quality like *Chronique d'un été* but Oppenheimer deploys the technique much more extensively, in a cycle of 'shooting-screening, shooting-screening, shooting-screening' (Oppenheimer 2016).[6] We are not simply presented with the final version of the killers' film (in fact we never see their film in its entirety nor was it ever finished) but we hear the killers reflecting on the process of making the film, reflecting on scenes they have shot, as their initial intentions are modified and recast in the light of their own production, experienced as an external object. The killers form an intra-diegetic audience for their own film. We as documentary viewers (as extra-diegetic audience) see the film-within, see the intra-diegetic audience watching and responding to scenes from the film-within and see the documentary frame in which Oppenheimer places this material. Just as in *Hamlet*, we as extra-diegetic audience watch an intra-diegetic audience (the 'guilty creatures sitting at a play') but with the added twist that the 'cunning' scenes we watch are of the killers' own devising and they take roles in their own "play". We witness the consequences of this process: the process and the consequences of this process as seen within the diegesis are the subject of this chapter.

Errol Morris, who became Joshua Oppenheimer's executive producer on *The Act of Killing* after the film had been shot and editing had begun, identified a parallel between Oppenheimer's film with its films-within and *Hamlet* with its plays-within, calling his 2013 essay on *The Act of Killing* – 'The Murders of Gonzago'. Morris describes the film's disquieting nature and its deployment of fictional scenes and quasi-fictional re-enactments to unearth hidden truths:

> *The Act of Killing* is truly unlike any other documentary film. A good thing in my opinion. One of the extraordinary things about documentary is that you get to continually reinvent the form, reinvent what it means to make a documentary – and Oppenheimer did just that. He identified several of the killers from 1965 and convinced them to make a movie about the killings. But the film is even weirder than that. Oppenheimer convinced these killers to act in a movie about the making of a movie about the killings. There would be re-enactments of the murders by the actual perpetrators. There would be singing, and there would be dancing. A perverted hall of mirrors.
>
> But there is method to Oppenheimer's madness – the idea that by re-enacting the murders, *he, the viewers of the movie, and the various perpetrators* recruited to participate could become reconnected to a history that had nearly vanished into a crepuscular past. Oppenheimer has the optimistic thought that the past is inside us and can be brought back to life.
>
> (Morris 2013; my italics)

Morris claims '*The Act of Killing* is truly unlike any other documentary film'. It is. But *The Act of Killing* is also heir to all the possibilities for documentary opened up by the work of Rouch and Morin, later pursued by Ari Folman, Guy Maddin and others[7]: the use of fictions, the re-enactment of the past in a dynamic present, the exploration of trauma through fantasy and hallucination, the implication and complicity of the director in the filmmaking process, the director acting as an active secondary witness, the inclusion of the film's protagonists in a potentially meaning-making exercise through their exposure to a film-within which they respond to and are affected by in an evolving temporal process.

I want to ask whether the complex structure of the documentary with its film-within-the film ('a movie about the making of a movie about the killings') can generate the possibility of meaning emerging (what Morris calls becoming 'reconnected to a history') in all the frames Morris describes: for the director who exists within the diegesis (the director as he appears in the film)[8]; for the 'various perpetrators' who exist within the diegesis; and for us as 'viewers of the movie' (the film's extra-diegetic audience)? Of these three frames, it is the frame of the perpetrator-protagonist which is my central concern: the protagonist I call in Chapter 3 the *inner* Winnicottian viewer who can be witnessed by us (the audience or *outer* Winnicottian viewer) creating and responding to their own or the director's filmic fictions. Can the creation of and the reflection on fictional constructions – here filmed fictional scenes – help to bring understanding of a real, non-fictional traumatic past and can that understanding have a material impact on the psychic life of the traumatised protagonist? Behind this question lies a second question: are there parallels between the filmmaking process and the analytic process where fictions are deployed to represent traumatic histories that have all but 'vanished into a crepuscular past'?

The Act of Killing is not a historical film; it is, in Oppenheimer's words (2016), about 'now'. It is firmly in the *vérité* tradition of Rouch and its evolution into the phenomenological-historical (*historical vérité*) tradition of Lanzmann. We do not see the world as it was in 1965–66. This is a re-articulation of the traumatic past as it is experienced, re-enacted, *acted-out*, lied about and fantasised about, in the present.[9] For Milo Sweedler (2014): 'Oppenheimer's strikingly original approach to filmmaking dilates the category of testimonial documentary to include what the filmmaker evocatively calls "documentary of the imagination," in which truth emerges in and as a fiction'. Through fictions – and responses to these present (here-and-now), imaginative fictions – Oppenheimer explores both the political and the psychological ramifications of the past in present-day Indonesia. I am concerned here particularly with the psychological or psychic ramifications for those filmic protagonists who had been perpetrators of violence in 1965–66.

But if the film is not historical, it has its own temporality. Major scenes are edited together in more or less the chronological order in which they were shot and so the viewer is confronted by a series of successive experiential "presents" that reveal changes in the protagonists' relation to the past as the documentary's chronological structure plays out. The viewer is able to gauge changes in the protagonists that have occurred over the production period of the film and so we can speculate as to whether the filmmaking process itself has altered perceptions of, and psychic responses to, a traumatic history as those present perceptions of the past change over filmic time. Can it bring about changes in the traumatised protagonists' relation to the traumatic past as psychoanalysis claims to be able to do? Is it possible to use film and the filmmaking process to reach a less painful accommodation with a traumatic past as Guy Maddin hoped to do when he began to make *My Winnipeg* (2007) and expressed the desire to 'film my way out of here'.

At the heart of the film is an evolving relationship between the director and Anwar Congo, one of the killers (or gangsters) of 1965–66 and the one who appears the most troubled by his past. He emerges as the film's central character. The relationship between Oppenheimer and Congo develops over filmic time with the chronological construction of the documentary leading the viewer to assume that the development of this filmic relationship mirrors the development over time of the "real" relationship between Oppenheimer and Congo.[10] The temporal component of this documentary allows the viewer to witness Congo's increasing reliance on Oppenheimer and his powerful need to gain *something* from Oppenheimer (his support, his sympathy, his approbation, his absolution perhaps) as Congo apparently spirals deeper *into* trauma rather than *out of* trauma. The film's linear, chronological structure is also circular as the film is bookended with two re-enactments by Congo of his killing methods on the roof of the handbag shop in Medan city. The final bizarre and climatic scene where Congo seems to lose control of his body repeats a visit to that same roof and repeats a re-enactment by Congo of the same killing methods, shot early on in the filmmaking process. The contrast between these two visits affords us a yardstick by which to measure changes in Congo's psychic state and his relation to his traumatic past; changes which we can perhaps attribute (at least in part) to Congo's engagement in the filmmaking process playing out over time.[11]

An early scene: the initial rooftop re-enactment

On Anwar Congo's first visit to the rooftop site of his murders he is accompanied by a neighbour who plays the part of a murder victim. Congo places a garrote around the neighbour's neck and explains how he developed this method of killing in order to dispatch his victims without spilling too much blood. Garroting was efficient and clean. Through most of the scene Congo is calm and matter-of-fact and apparently untroubled by the past and the horrors he is describing. But there are some signs of a more troubled relation to his past. There are physical gestures which suggest disquiet – frequent massaging of his forehead as he recounts the story of his murders – and his admission that '[t]here's so many ghosts here; because many people were killed here.' And towards the end of the scene, Congo confesses: 'I've tried to forget all this with good music…Dancing…Feeling happy…A little alcohol…A little marijuana…a little…Ecstasy…Once I'd get drunk, I'd fly and feel happy.' The scene ends with Congo demonstrating his dancing and his neighbour opining, in a spectacular act of misrecognition, 'He's a happy man'.

The Congo who we meet at the start of the film appears at his happiest when discussing the film project that Oppenheimer has facilitated; the making of the film about his murderous past. 'Whether this ends up on the big screen – or only on TV, it doesn't matter' a broadly smiling Congo tells his friend and fellow gangster

Herman Koto, 'we have to show, that this is the history. This is who we are.' The making of the film seems to provide a substitute for alcohol and drugs as Congo's chosen route to 'feeling happy'. Somehow, the making of the film will bring him absolution and justify what he did. But the 'consequences' of making a film about that traumatic past that for years Congo had been trying so desperately to obliterate with alcohol and drugs, are not those Congo expects or hopes for. They lead him back to the same rooftop to once again demonstrate his killing method, and his near physical collapse.

The play-within-the-play: the truth uncovered or 'miching malicho'?

Scenes from the film-within: the Apotheosis of Anwar Congo

The sort of film Anwar Congo is imagining, we see as an edited actuality near the end of *The Act of Killing*. In a scene Congo has designed and scripted we see him, arms aloft, standing in a sunlit landscape, surrounded by women in long white skirts and elaborate headdresses, dancing slowly, a vast waterfall tumbling behind them; it is Congo's vision of heaven and elicits something close to joy in Congo as he watches it back on a monitor in his living room. He tells an off-screen Oppenheimer: 'This is great Joshua. This is very good. I never imagined I could make something so great. One thing that makes me so proud is how the waterfall expresses such deep feelings'. In flowing gown, he is approached by actors playing the "communists" he murdered in 1965–66, the wire garrotes Congo had used to kill them still around their necks. One by one, they thank Congo for killing them and present him with a gold medal – which they hang around his neck – whilst Congo "graciously" bows.

Murdered "communist": For executing me and sending me to heaven
I thank you a thousand times, for everything.

This utterly bizarre scene, perhaps the strangest and most perverse I have ever watched in a documentary – a dark and unintended parody of the post-modern sublime perhaps – is played out to a music track of a version of Matt Monro's upbeat, popular, 1960s song, *Born Free*. But this scene of the beatific Congo, coming so close to the end of *The Act of Killing*, rings hollow. By this stage, we have already witnessed Anwar Congo's progressive traumatisation and psychological collapse. He may know that he was *born* free, but his past actions leave him haunted, suffering a traumatic reaction which cannot be expunged by a piece of cinematic fiction however 'great' the depiction of his apotheosis may be. This quasi-religious, fictional attempt to be forgiven his sins by the victims of his murderous violence echoes a scene that only appears in the longer, director's cut of the documentary. Here Congo – who is suffering with recurrent, nightmare dream-visions of his victims – confides that when he was little and had bad dreams, his mother would tell him he had the dreams because he had not washed his feet before he went to bed. Although not stated explicitly, Congo, the elderly, haunted killer, seems desperate to find a way to *wash his feet*; to wash away his sins. To try to achieve it he constructs an elaborate filmic fantasy. The scene of the apotheosis of Anwar Congo appears to be a conscious attempt by Congo to produce a self-protective screen memory or screen fantasy. In an interview, Oppenheimer described Congo in this scene as 'trying to run away from his pain, to build up a cinematic psychic scar tissue around his trauma' (Oppenheimer quoted in Barnes 2013). Is this fiction as a shield against the "truth" rather than a route to it?

So how should we think about the film-within-the-film in *The Act of Killing*? Is it a vehicle for hiding unpalatable truths, where former killers indulge in elaborate fantasies that seek to hide guilt and wash away sins[12] or is it a more dangerous and unpredictable vehicle that cannot be controlled by the killers, as Congo's second trip to the rooftop suggests?

Claudius and Congo compared: The Murder of Gonzago *and the films within* The Act of Killing

In its presentation of quasi-historical reconstructions and out-and-out fictions, *The Act of Killing* seems to be deploying the techniques of both reconstruction and construction that Freud proposed in his attempts to find or create representations of a traumatic past, and the two models that *Hamlet* offers of the fictional play-within-the-play (a form of re-enactment and a forgery) with both acting as catalysts to provoke the emergence of the "truth". But given the persistent criticism that in *The Act of Killing* the killers use their fictional films to justify their past actions, to evade guilt and to imply that the murders were necessary, even ethical, it is important to explore the counter-argument that the fictions might obscure the truth.

Hamlet is aware of the possibility that the story he reproduces in *The Murder of Gonzago* might have been suggested to him by a malevolent spirt that 'Abuses me to damn me' (*Hamlet*: Act II Scene II). And on two other occasions, Hamlet suggests that his plays might be 'false' in the sense of malicious, obscuring or misleading. First, on seeing the dumb show, Ophelia enquires of Hamlet: 'What means this, my lord?' and Hamlet replies: 'Marry, this is miching malicho. It means mischief' (*Hamlet*: Act III Scene II). Secondly, later, in the middle of the staging of *The Murder of Gonzago* – as the King rises from his seat ready to storm out of the production – Hamlet comments: 'What, frighted with false fire?' (*Hamlet*: Act III Scene II). Is the entire project of staging a fictional production, the 'false fire', or is it only false in Polonius's much more limited sense; a falsity but a falsity with the power to provoke the emergence of truth?

Hamlet, and Freud in *Constructions in Analysis* (1937b), both suggest that there is a lurking danger that the play or construction might be merely false and misleading. But both also suggest the potential to provoke the truth. For both Hamlet and Freud, the play's or the construction's truth-provoking credentials are established in the reactions elicited and in how those reactions come to be understood by the diegetic play-goer or by the analysand. Freud (1937b: 260–1) argues that a valid or productive construction will *touch* the patient and that a false construction will leave the analysand 'untouched' and fade out of the analysis. Hamlet describes his parallel strategy in a speech in Act II Scene II (reproduced at the front of this chapter), where he defines both what he hopes the theatrical production might reveal and the manner in which that revelation will become apparent. The play-within-the-play, if it is a *cunningly* constructed conceit, has the power to force the guilty to feel their guilt ('the play's the thing / Wherein I'll catch the conscience of the king') and they will publicly proclaim 'their malefactions'; that is, confess to their crimes. This confession – this public proclamation – will take a particular form. The malefactors will be 'struck [...] to the soul', a condition that reveals itself to the eye ('I'll observe his looks') with the visual evidence of the guilt apparent in a bodily response (a 'blench'). It is in this bodily response that the crime will speak (it will 'speak / With most miraculous organ'), as actual speech – a verbal confession – is not the expected response (the malefaction – 'murder' – has 'no tongue'). In staging his play, Hamlet seeks a bodily reaction that cannot be suppressed and will reveal something hitherto unseen; specifically, evidence of the Queen's, and especially the King's, as-yet-unseen guilt for the murder of Hamlet's father, old King Hamlet. The new king, Claudius, Hamlet hopes will be *soul struck,* precipitating an affective, involuntary, bodily response. That this response is to be seen rather than confessed in words is amplified in Hamlet's instruction to his accomplice Horatio in Act III Scene II, to keep his gaze fixed on Claudius as the play is staged. Hamlet tells Horatio to 'Observe mine uncle' and undertakes to do the same himself ('I mine eyes will rivet to his face') hoping to observe his uncle's 'occulted guilt', which will 'unkennel' itself. And when the plays are staged before King Claudius, his reaction is indeed bodily and observable; he rushes from the scene in anger, shouting, 'Give me some light: away!' (Act III Scene II).

But final confirmation of the King's guilt only comes later, in the period immediately after he has watched the play (in Act III Scene III). In an act of personal reflection on what he has just seen and heard in the play, Claudius confesses his guilt in a soliloquy that is overheard by Hamlet.

> O, my offence is rank, it smells to heaven;
> It hath the primal eldest curse upon't –
> A brother's murder.

Only then is Claudius able to symbolise into words what had been a purely bodily response (an *acting out*) when he watched the theatrical production. And it is only at this point that it becomes more certain that Hamlet's play is not a mere devilish trick, or miching malicho, or false fire. I have followed the same approach in judging the fictional films within *The Act of Killing*: looking for involuntary, visible, physical blenches from Anwar Congo as he witnesses his various filmic fictions and then waiting to see if these somatic and affective responses can be reflected on by Congo and can coalesce into words; into an account that is meaningful to Congo.

There are striking similarities between Claudius and Congo. Both are murderers traumatised by their past actions, neither seems able to confess their guilt before being precipitated into doing so by watching a play-/ film-within, and both are desperate to wash away the stain of their crimes. Congo (as we have seen) is troubled by his inability to *wash his feet*, to wash away his sins as his mother had advised; whilst Claudius, in his soliloquy, reveals a similar desire to be cleansed:

> What if this cursed hand
> Were thicker than itself with brother's blood,
> Is there not rain enough in the sweet heavens
> To wash it white as snow?[13]

And both men are still in possession of the fruits of their crimes which neither wishes to give up. Congo enjoys being a hero and minor celebrity in his hometown, fêted as one of the men who rid the country of the "communist menace" in the 1960s; whilst Claudius revels in the power his crime has brought him (and is unwilling to relinquish it):

> O, what form of prayer
> Can serve my turn? "Forgive me my foul murder?"
> That cannot be, since I am still possess'd
> Of those effects for which I did murder –
> My crown, mine own ambition, and my queen.
> (*Hamlet*: Act III Scene III)

Where *The Act of Killing* does part company from *Hamlet* is in the casting of the malefactors as the players. It is as if Hamlet had cast King Claudius and Queen Gertrude in his play and asked them to re-enact their own malefactions 'in whatever ways they wished'.[14] This is, perhaps, Oppenheimer's unique bit of mischief – his bit of miching malicho. But, and once again in conformity with *Hamlet*, the Oppenheimer we hear within the diegesis plays a role similar to that of the character Hamlet. He appears as a character (as a voice and an off-screen presence) in the play-without, talking to the killers whilst they make or watch-back the film-within and, like Hamlet, he keeps a close eye – a focused camera lens – trained on them to see how they will react to witnessing the fictional production to see if they will *blench*.

Scenes from the film-within: the Kampung Kolam massacre

In a major scene in *The Act of Killing*, Anwar Congo directs his friends and local extras – many of them children – in re-enacting the destruction of Kampung Kolam (a so-called "communist" village in the 1960s) and the rape and massacre of its inhabitants. Like Hamlet's staging of a play that is 'something like the murder of my father', this scene is Congo's attempt to recreate a historical event for the camera. Congo himself (like Hamlet) does not take an acting role but observes as the action is filmed. He is an intra-diegetic audience member watching the live performance of his own "play".

During the filming of the scene, Congo speaks to Oppenheimer's documentary camera.

Congo: What I regret … [long pause and cannot finish his sentence] … Honestly, I never expected it would look this awful.

Congo then tries to gather his thoughts, looking troubled:

Congo: Imagine those children's future. They've been tortured. Now their houses will be burned down. What future do they have? They will curse us for the rest of their lives. This was so, very, very, very … [Congo tails off into silence].

Congo seems to be taken by surprise by his emotional and affective response to witnessing his own reconstruction even though it re-enacts an event he clearly remembers. His response is largely affective and has 'no tongue'; he is scarcely able to articulate – to represent in words – what is so 'awful'. But what does struggle into words is his fear of being cursed (a fear Claudius also voices in his soliloquy in Act III Scene III of *Hamlet*) and a confusion of past and present in his use of the future tense for something that happened long ago (their houses *will be* burned down and they *will* curse us). The film-within – despite it being of Congo's own 'cunning' design – has unexpectedly revivified the past in the present, blurring the distinction between them and exposing a temporal confusion: the past bursting into the present or past and present overlaid, inter-mixed and inseparable, revealing in Congo a facet of traumatic experience that is recognised in all the major accounts of trauma.

What also emerges, again apparently unexpectedly for Congo, is that he is brought into an empathetic encounter with the victims of his violence ('Imagine those children's future'). The intermingling of self and other implied by the notion of empathy is only one of a number of interminglings or *identifications* that psychoanalysis recognises, including imitation, sympathy, mental contagion, introjection, projection, etc., which will be explored later in this chapter. Part of the mischievous force of the play- or film-within is to activate these identifications and reveal their workings in the traumatised diegetic protagonist as they witness the re-creations and forgeries of the play or film. For André Green, bringing identifications into representational form (making the analysand aware of their own identifications) is at the heart of the analytic process: '[T]he essence of analytic action concerns the representation of intrasubjective and intersubjective psychic processes' (Green quoted in Delourmel 2013: 133). Congo's filmic representation of a massacre has opened him up to these processes. Meaning or understanding of the past might become available to Congo if these identifications can be understood rather than simply being experienced as troubling, largely inarticulate, affect.

Scenes from the film-within: Congo as "communist" victim

As I have suggested, the film-within in *The Act of Killing* has a radical twist that makes it more mischievous than Hamlet's *The Murder of Gonzago.* The malefactors do not merely watch re-enactments of their "pasts" played by actors, they are also the players. Often they play their own past selves but they also engage in role reversal when they choose to play their own past victims. This role reversal is a second, radical, mischievous twist on the play-within-the-play model provided by *Hamlet.* This device – despite being of the killers' own choosing – is highly revealing, generating the possibility of meanings emerging that might otherwise have remained hidden both from the killers themselves and from the cinema audience. The device forces the perpetrators to embody and perform – to imaginatively enter – the experience of the victim. Those perpetrator-actors who are open to this process, find themselves forced into an empathetic engagement with their victims' experience at the very moment of their torture and imminent death. This is perhaps the most devious and mischievous of all the 'indirections' in *The Act of Killing* by which 'we find directions out'.[15] Congo again and again places himself in the most difficult and potentially revealing circumstances. It is as if Congo understands and deliberately adopts the methods of psychodrama for uncovering hidden truths about a traumatic past, rather than proceeding evasively like a guilty man trying to cover his tracks. The lack of a social imperative for him to examine his past actions (Congo, like the other killers, is still celebrated as a hero by many in Indonesia) suggests that Congo is driven by psychic imperatives. One suspects he is driven by a powerful desire to confess or perhaps by an epistemophilic urge to understand his past in the hope that this will be cathartic.

A scene in the film-within has Anwar Congo reversing roles and playing a "communist" who has been brought in for interrogation. We do not find out why Congo chose to play a victim but it clearly has physical and psychological consequences for him.

Congo is seated at a table, bloodied and bowed, being interrogated by three men; the principal interrogator role being taken by Congo's friend, Herman Koto. After playing this scene for a little while, there is a call of 'cut' from someone off-camera but the camera keeps running, focused on Congo who looks troubled. He takes deep breaths and blows the air out slowly, apparently trying to calm himself. He drinks water from a plastic bottle with his eyes closed. Koto crouches next to him, looking concerned, his arm on the small of Congo's back as if to comfort him. Eventually Congo manages to say, breathily and quietly, 'OK, let's do it'. Congo is blindfolded and Koto winds a wire around his neck ready to garrote him, saying 'I place this medal around your neck' in a perverse reference to the apotheosis scene in which the murdered "communist" places a medal around Congo's neck.

Congo is strangely still during all this activity. Koto then tightens the wire and Congo twitches, making a strange, gurgling, snorting noise; a noise Congo has already demonstrated in the documentary both as the sound he remembers being made by someone who is being garroted and as the sound that was made by the severed neck of a man Congo had murdered by decapitation. It is a sound that Congo has told us haunts him in his dreams. As I watched Congo apparently close to bodily collapse, I was struck by the raw, bodily nature of the scene; guttural noises issued from somewhere apparently deep inside Congo.

Congo begins to make small, agitated gestures with his right hand. It appears Congo is trying, wordlessly, to stop proceedings. Koto stares at the stricken Congo and then looks anxiously in the direction of the camera, seemingly asking someone off-camera (Oppenheimer perhaps) – *what's happening? – what's wrong with Anwar?*

Congo is now utterly still again. Eventually he manages to pull off the blindfold. Koto asks, 'Are you alright?' and Congo replies, 'I can't do that again.' The camera again keeps running, although now of course the camera is recording the reactions of the "players" to having played a scene and is no longer recording a scene from the film-within itself. This is a seamless switch of frames from the *film-within* to the frame of the *documentary-without*. Congo remains seated: head bowed, eyes closed, arms limp. After a while Koto says, 'Get him some water' but Congo cannot grasp the water bottle placed in his hand and so Koto pours water into his mouth, before Congo pushes the bottle away and returns to sitting limply, breathing deeply, lost in some inexpressible, inner awfulness.

In the director's cut we are shown a different take of this same scene. Congo is, if anything, even more physically afflicted, Koto having to lift Congo's "lifeless" arms from where they dangle by his side and place them on his knees. After a while Congo says, 'I feel like I was dead for a moment'. Koto stares at Congo and then responds, 'Don't get so into it … Don't think too much about it', aware, as the cinema audience is aware, that playing the part has physically overwhelmed Congo. The playing of a part – a role reversal – in the film-within has had a profound impact on Congo; an impact that registers bodily and scarcely registers in words beyond 'I can't do that again' or 'I feel like I was dead for a moment'.

How these physical and affective reactions – these blenches – might be read is fraught with uncertainty. Interpreting affective and somatic responses is a hugely challenging task. As André Green wrote of affect: 'Affect constitutes a challenge to thought' as it 'is difficult to speak of something which is, in essence, only partially communicable as affects often are' (Green 1977: 129). Any interpretation is liable to misrecognitions, as affects can easily become attached to the *wrong* 'ideational representative' in the mind of the person who is affected, let alone in the minds of others (outsiders) who witness the affected body (Green 2005a; especially Chapter 9: 125–64). But what is clear is that wherever the film-within-the-film sits in a spectrum running from historical re-enactment to elaborate fantasies set in no time (like the apotheosis scene), it has the power to precipitate powerful, affective, bodily responses. That the killers had total control over what was represented and how it was to be represented, brought no concomitant power to control their affective responses to playing a role or to watching back their own fictions. One imagines that Congo did not anticipate his own almost-total collapse and his inability to carry on playing the part when he designed the scene in which he reversed roles with one of his victims. The power of the film-within in documentary is in its potential to generate unexpected and unanticipated responses; this is its miching malicho. Like so many sorcerers' apprentices, the killers of 1965–66 produced a film-within that made them the unwitting playthings of their own creation; a creation which acted back upon them in ways they did not anticipate.[16]

Scenes from the film-without: Congo watches himself playing the victim

Some time after the shooting of the scene in which Congo plays a victim of interrogation, torture and garroting – how long we are not told – we meet Congo again.[17] In a deft piece of structural editing, Oppenheimer places this scene immediately after the scene in which we see his apotheosis. We move from Congo's bizarre fantasy of absolution to his much more troubled reaction to inhabiting the body of a victim. The cinema audience sees most of the apotheosis scene unframed but towards its end, we cut to a wide shot and see that Congo is watching the scene on a monitor in his house (again a seamless move from film-within to film-without, and a seamless move from the filmic present of the apotheosis scene to the later filmic present of reviewing that scene). Having pronounced the apotheosis scene to be 'great', Congo asks an unseen Oppenheimer to put the interrogation scene on the monitor. That Congo moves directly from the apotheosis scene to the interrogation scene may suggest that he is not convinced by the self-protective fantasy of being forgiven by his victims and that something more meaningful might be available in reviewing the other scene.

As the scene progresses, Congo begins to look troubled. He stares intently, frowns, blinks repeatedly.

Congo: Did the people I tortured feel the way I do here?
I can feel what the people I tortured felt.
Because here my dignity has been destroyed and then fear comes, right there and then.
All the terror suddenly possessed my body.
It surrounded me, and possessed me.

It seems that Congo is now able to articulate – to represent in words – his affective responses to playing a part in the film-within. He describes how he felt, providing a meaningful account of his bodily, *tongueless*, reactions on set. In the gap of time between the shooting of the scene and the "present" of recording his reflections, Congo has found a way to represent his experience. This later present in his house is also a dynamic present like the present when he was on set in character.

His reflective comments at home come not as recollections in memory alone but through a new affective confrontation with the past as represented by the images and sounds of himself on the monitor; a confrontation generated by a self-reflexive engagement in a filmmaking process playing out over real (and filmic) time. In front of the monitor, Congo is no longer the actor or the "player" but a member of the intra-diegetic audience.

But the glimmerings of understanding, soon dissipate. The experience of watching himself rendered still and almost lifeless in the film-within seems to retraumatise Congo. By the end of the scene in front of the monitor, Congo *the-intra-diegetic-audience-member* closely mirrors Congo *the-player-of-a-victim-of-interrogation* in the film-within. Oppenheimer's intercutting between film-within and film-without reveals both "Congos" to be absolutely still, silent and seemingly 'struck […] to the soul'. The twitching hand of the *player*-Congo is replaced by the twitching jaw muscles of the *viewer*-Congo. In both frames, Congo blenches. In both frames he is physically overwhelmed by the playing/witnessing of traumatic events. As a member of the extra-diegetic audience, I am able to 'observe his looks' and to see him 'blench'.

If Congo's own attempt to interpret his blenches is brief and soon dissolves back into overwhelming affect and bodily ticks, are we as members of the extra-diegetic audience able to read these *blenches*? Let us accept Congo's own account of what he experienced: 'I can feel what the people I tortured felt. […] All the terror suddenly possessed my body.' Congo is overwhelmed bodily, undone to the point of near lifelessness. Congo is telling us that he is experiencing what his victims experienced. This is not a conscious, cognitive recognition of how he *thinks* they might have felt but a far more "primitive", body-to-body encounter that comes entirely unbidden. In fact, encounter is too distancing a word, implying a separation between Congo and his victims. He *is* the victim at the moment the terror arrives or, to use Congo's own word, he is 'possessed'. And 'possessed' has far more affective resonance in Indonesian culture than in the West. For some social groups within Indonesian society – predominantly the uneducated like Congo – possession is a live, real and terrifying notion and not a term of purely historic interest (Lusztig 2013: 53).

Thomas Wartenberg, writing recently about the role-reversing interrogation scene from a philosophical and ethical perspective, reaches conclusions similar to my psychological reading of this same scene (and indeed of the later scene with Congo watching his interrogation at home in front of the monitor). Playing the part of one of his own victims precipitates what Wartenberg (2017) calls an ontological collapse in Congo; a collapse of the gap between self and other with profound consequences.

> Two dichotomies are necessary to characterise this ontological situation: that of an actor playing a role, thereby creating a distinction between reality and fiction, and another within the reenactment between the roles of perpetrator and victim. So, Congo is a real perpetrator acting in the fictional role of one of his

> own victims. What transpires is an *ontological collapse* of this structure, for the actor playing a character actually becomes that character, at least briefly in his own imagination, and a perpetrator of torture and murder becomes his own victim albeit only imaginatively. As a result of this double collapse of roles and reality – in which the actor *becomes* the character he is supposed to simply be playing, experiencing himself as a victim of his own crimes – Congo is no longer able to repress an ethical assessment of his own actions.
>
> (2017; Wartenberg's italics)

The ontological collapse that Wartenberg describes precipitates a profound ethical crisis for Congo. My reading of this double collapse is cognisant of its ethical dimension (it is ethical to the extent that in reviewing himself playing this part, Congo acknowledges his own guilt) but I am more interested in the psychological dimension of the collapse(s). The difference between my reading and Wartenberg's is that Wartenberg is asking ethical questions framed within the grander question: *can documentaries do philosophy?* I am asking psychological questions framed within the grander question: *can documentaries do psychoanalysis?* Wartenberg answers his own grand question with a *yes*: 'My discussion of *The Act of Killing* presents the film as an important example of cinematic philosophy because it provides better support for Arendt's banality of evil thesis than Arendt was able to by means of her own account of Eichmann' (Wartenberg 2017, with reference to Arendt 2006 [1963]). I also hope (in what follows) to be able to answer my grand question with a *yes* – even if tentatively.

My reading of this scene is that playing the part undermines Congo's *ego ideal*; his heavily defended sense of himself that he has for so long sought to bolster (for example in the apotheosis scene). In the heightened, phenomenological present instant of the *playing*, distinctions between reality and fiction, between self and other, collapse, precipitating a psychological crisis (and perhaps creating the conditions for a meaningful or "truthful" account to emerge).

Slavoj Žižek reaches a very different conclusion about this scene. He argues that despite Congo showing the glimmerings of guilt and remorse, this does not lead on to an ethical or psychological collapse. As Žižek puts it, it

> does not lead to a deeper crisis of conscience – [as] his heroic pride immediately takes over again. The protective screen that prevented a deeper moral crisis was the cinematic screen: as in their real killings and torture, the men experienced their role play as a re-enactment of cinematic models: they experienced reality itself as a fiction.
>
> (Žižek 2013)

What Wartenberg and I see as the catalyst for the collapse (the playing of a part in a fiction in the style of a Hollywood movie), Žižek sees as Congo's defence against collapse, protecting him from having to face his traumatic past and his culpability. And Žižek goes further. Not only do Congo and the other killers not experience their re-enactments in *The Act of Killing* as real, but they did not experience the actual killings in 1965–66 as real because (as Congo has told us) at that time, they imagined themselves to be film stars acting in violent Hollywood movies. For Žižek, filmic fictions are a screen *against* truth and reality – both in 1965–66 and now – and not a *bait of falsehood* capable of taking *the carp of truth.*

Whilst wanting to acknowledge Žižek's powerful reading, I do not share it. My reading of the scene is that playing the victim prompts a powerful identification that precipitates a *collapse*. For Wartenberg (2017), this identification is empathy: 'The reenactment process employed by *The Act of Killing* forces empathy upon Congo by making his own experience of victimisation the bridge to his understanding of what his victims experienced.' In the rest of this chapter, I will consider empathy alongside other forms of identification as the potential motive force behind the collapse.

Congo possessed: empathy, affect, identification and meaning in the counter-transference

The nature of Congo's possession

Congo describes his collapse as *possession*. But what is the nature of this possession? The word certainly implies that Congo believes something alien to himself, something other to himself, has entered him and changed him. But what is it, and crucially, does Congo *understand* what it is?

For Wartenberg (2017), the possession is *empathy* which, extrapolating from his text, is a sharing, real or imagined, of the psychic or emotional state of another human being that *also* has a cognitive component ('understanding'). This entails a theory of mind, a conscious, cognitive ability to place oneself in "someone else's shoes": what Shannon Spaulding (2017: 13) calls 'the capacity to understand another person's state of mind from her perspective' which (in Karsten Stueber's words (2017: 138)) 'presupposes an awareness of the difference between self and other'. Wartenberg may be right, but there is no stable definition of empathy and the balance between its "felt" and its cognitive components. It is a much-contested term that has attracted a vast and expanding literature in recent years. Dan Zahavi, writing recently in *The Routledge Handbook of Philosophy of Empathy* (Maibom, ed., 2017), surveys current conceptions of empathy and finds a range of definitions from 'contagion' – a sharing of mental states that comes with no understanding ('empathy does not involve knowledge') – through 'both sharing and knowing' – an account which 'requires some cognitive grasp and some self-other differentiation' – to 'knowing' – an account by 'those who emphasize the cognitive dimension and argue that empathy doesn't require sharing, but that it simply refers to any process by means of which one comes to know the other's mental state' (Zahavi 2017: 33–43). Elsewhere in this same Routledge volume, editor Heidi Maibom suggests that the categories Zahavi defines represent not competing definitions of empathy but delineate different forms of empathy: broadly (in the order Zahavi describes them), emotional contagion/personal distress, 'affective empathy' and 'cognitive empathy' (Maibom 2017: 1–10; 22–32). But there is no consensus and within philosophy the term remains a 'conceptual quagmire' (Stueber 2017: 138).

Psychoanalysis is equally unable to provide a stable definition of the term. The first of Freud's many references to empathy ('Einfühlung' in German) was in his essay on *Jokes and Their Relation to the Unconscious* (1905b: 186, 195; etc.). Analyst, George W. Pigman, has argued that throughout his career, Freud deployed it most frequently in the context of *understanding* (a meaning-making activity akin to Maibom's category of 'cognitive empathy'): 'Perhaps the most striking aspect of Freud's conception of empathy is his emphasis on its intellectual features and his relative neglect, even suspicion, of its affective ones' (Pigman 1995: 251–2). But there is little consensus within psychoanalysis and Freud never attempted a formal definition. If I were to venture a consensus view, empathy (in both philosophy and psychoanalysis) is a form of sharing of mental states that has both affective and cognitive components: what Zahavi calls 'both sharing and knowing'; a definition that accords with Wartenberg's deployment of the term.

But empathy – conceived as an appreciation of the other's predicament that operates *with* understanding – seems inadequate as an explanatory tool when attempting to interpret Congo's blenches in the scene where he plays the "communist" interrogation victim. Whatever Congo is experiencing, it expresses itself as a bodily reaction. What we witness is in part *mental anguish* but also clearly *bodily anguish* that apparently bypasses his cognitive faculties and manifests itself as a temporary paralysis.

Perhaps, instead of a collapse induced by empathy, we could think of Congo as being overwhelmed by an intense surge of negative affect that comes without understanding. Unrepresented trauma may in fact be best described as registering as overwhelming affect as Freud implies his grandson experienced before he found/created his fictive narrative of the cotton reel and the piece of string or Bion's generic infant experienced before the intervention of the mother in her reverie interpreting the child's distress. Congo's near paralysis may imply a hysterical conversion of some of that negative affect into a purely bodily symptom. And, if Congo is experiencing an intense surge of negative affect, this is not to suggest the absence of an interpersonal (or perhaps intersubjective, inter-psychic, intercorporeal) encounter with someone or something that is other to himself. Affect can be experienced by a body alone ("autochthonic" affect) but many accounts of affect highlight its transmission, its capacity to move from one body to another: a characteristic often described as resonance or contagion. Melissa Gregg and Gregory Seigworth (2010a: 2) describe affect as 'swells of intensities that pass between "bodies"' and Félix Guattari (1996: 158) writes about the 'transitivist character of affect' where there is a confusion or an intermixing of self and other, with one body apparently mimicking the affect expressed in another body.[18]

As with empathy, affect has generated a vast and expanding literature in recent years[19] and little consensus as to a definition. But within the multitude of different constructions of affect, it is clear, at least, that a cognitive component is far less prevalent than in definitions of empathy and many commentators *specifically* exclude cognition. In my use of affect, I concur with this exclusion as without it there is a blurring and overlapping of terms, such as *affect* and *empathy*, which then lose precision. In philosophy, cultural/critical theory and psychoanalysis, affect is generally considered as a bodily phenomenon, as transmittable between bodies and as non-cognitive, non-representational and unsymbolised. André Green (1977: 129), for example, writes that '[a]ffect constitutes a challenge to thought' and Lawrence Grossberg (lamenting the imprecision with which the term is currently used) confirms that, at the very least, it is 'non-representational' and 'non-semantic' (interview with Grossberg in: Gregg and Seigworth 2010b: 316).

Post-structuralist "affect theory" has often stressed the embodied, non-representational, pre-/non-cognitive, pre-/non-personal nature of affect and so offers a way of thinking about Congo that stands in stark contrast to empathy, certainly as it is conceptualised by Wartenberg with a cognitive component.[20] Congo seems to display the symptoms of what Eric Shouse (2005)[21] calls a body overwhelmed by 'a non-conscious experience of intensity' (2005: paragraph 5) as 'affect is transmitted between bodies' (2005: paragraph 12) breaking down the barriers between inside and outside, between self and what's beyond the self. For Shouse, the 'transmission of affect is about the way that bodies affect one another' and occurs '[w]hen your body infolds a context and another body (real or virtual) is expressing intensity in that context, one intensity is infolded into another' (2005: paragraph 14). Shouse distinguishes the impact of empathy (when 'one person's feelings become another's' consciously or not (2005: paragraph 14)) from affect, and gives a gloss that is key to my appropriation of this theoretical construction, in making it clear that 'another' body can be 'real or virtual'. In Congo's case, that body is *both* 'virtual', as he is inhabiting a long-dead body suffering torture, *and* 'real', as Congo *is* the torture victim in the affective, phenomenological present of the film-within. The idea of a 'real or virtual' body is key to my understanding of how the viewer of documentary constructs meaning through a process that often *begins* with the non-cognitive, affective force of the filmic object and the filmic characters on the viewer (before the viewer attempts to interpret what that experienced affect might *mean*). Here, the other body which affects the viewer is necessarily 'virtual' as the film and its protagonists exist only on screen.

But the overarching theoretical construction I want to propose to describe Congo's physical collapse as he plays victim is the notion of *identification*: an umbrella term denoting the various ways in which bodies and especially psyches affect each other and become *like* each other – or, more accurately, the *same* as each other – encompassing the notion of empathy (when the feelings of one are shared or exchanged and become another's and are understood to a greater or lesser extent by another) and the transmission of affect (when the bodily state of one becomes another's). Identification includes these ideas but is broader, taking in the exchange of unconscious material and even of material that has never properly entered the dynamic unconscious. All identifications entail – to a greater or lesser extent – the collapse of the gap between self and other (a collapse Wartenberg sees happening to Congo in his re-enactments and describes as empathy). Jean Laplanche and Jean-Bertrand Pontalis (1988 [1967]: 205–8), borrowing the words of André Lalande, describe identification both as the notion of one idea being substitutable by another (as in dream-work) and as an 'act whereby an individual becomes identical with another or two beings become identical with each other (whether in thought or in fact, completely or *secundum quid*)'. It is this second articulation I want to pursue. It contains, in Laplanche and Pontalis's words, 'a whole group of psychological concepts – e.g. imitation, *Einfühlung* (empathy), sympathy, mental contagion, projection, etc.'

In what follows, I explore various identifications including projection and projective identifications but also (and in particular) projection's counterpart, introjection and introjective identifications. The formal omission of introjection from Laplanche and Pontalis's list (its ghostly presence marked by the 'etc') is symptomatic of introjection's lack of prominence (until recently) in much psychoanalytic writing about clinical practice, where along with projection it is a facet of the transference/counter-transference. Outside of the clinical context, though, introjection has played a key role in meta-psychological theory (and continues to do so)[22] and it is central to Bion's theory of infantile development.

Projection and introjection both describe interactions between the inner and outer worlds. In projection, an aspect of one's inner world is projected – excreted – into an external object (often a person), who is then experienced as the incarnation or embodiment of the expelled psychic material but with no sense, no understanding, that what is then experienced originated in the self. Often the expelled material (in the language of object relations) is a *bad object* that the projecting psyche wishes to be rid of. By contrast, introjection rests on the unconscious fantasy of ingestion – an oral fantasy – where the characteristics of an external object (often a person) are taken into the self which then acquires those characteristics (and again with no sense or understanding that this psychic transaction has taken place). Often the introjected object is a *good object* that acts, say, as a defence mechanism in the case of introjecting the attributes of strength in another to help bolster a self that is felt to be weak and vulnerable. But Karl Abraham's and Sándor Ferenczi's work suggests that the logic of projecting bad objects and introjecting good ones is not always the case. In 1924, Karl Abraham (1927 [1924]: 418–79) wrote about the projection outside the self of good objects, impoverishing the ego with psychotic consequences. And in 1932, Sándor Ferenczi (1949 [1932]: 228) explored the notion of the introjection of bad objects, and specifically the child's 'introjection of the guilt feelings of the adult' in the case of a child that has been maltreated or sexually abused by an adult.[23]

Returning now to Congo, the notions of introjection and projection seem to offer ways to read Congo's *blenches*. In the scene from the film-within where Congo plays the victim of the sort of torture that Congo himself in "real" life meted out to countless victims, he is a very complex object to observe. Is he victim? Is he perpetrator? It also makes any conjectures about projection and introjection very difficult to distinguish. We are presented with a single body that is both perpetrator and victim and projections and introjections are taking place, not between separate bodies, but within this already-complex body. Nevertheless, I am going to attempt a reading that suggests a toxic introjection – an introjective identification – that leaves Congo physically (and psychically) undone.

That he is physically undone seems incontrovertible. Congo says of playing the part of a victim: 'I can't do that again' and 'I feel like I was dead for a moment', and he ends the scene utterly immobile *as if in* (or *in*) a state of paralysis. His very stillness suggests that something very bad is happening inside Congo. My only direct evidence of introjection, of taking in something from outside – taking something in "orally" – is the negative evidence of Congo pushing away the water bottle proffered to him by his concerned friend, Herman Koto. It is as if he can take nothing else inside. The enormous effort of rousing himself from near torpor to push the bottle away suggests the power of his urge either not to ingest anything more or perhaps to refuse something being forced into him from outside.

Scenes from the film-within: the cannibal forces Congo to cannibalise himself

Another scene from *The Act of Killing*'s film-within invites this specifically *introjective* interpretation. Congo and Herman Koto appear in a jungle setting, with Koto in extravagant drag playing the part of Aminah, a female, communist activist. He (she) sits next to a decapitated Congo. Again, Congo is playing a victim of murder and torture, but this time (in another of the bewildering twists of the film-within) he is playing himself, a perpetrator, who has fallen victim to a cruel communist woman, so turning the objective historical record on its head. It is a paranoid, persecutory fantasy in which the killers have re-invented themselves as victims of the communists.

In reading Congo in this scene, we must bear in mind that this inversion is not simply a private fantasy (delusion) but is supported in wider Indonesian society. The scene is explicitly making reference to the docudrama feature film, *Pengkhianatan G30S/PKI [The Treachery of the 30th September Movement of the Communist Party of Indonesia]* (Noer 1984), made with Indonesian government sponsorship, which purports to retell the events of 1965 and the rise to power of General Suharto. It was a piece of propaganda that shifted the blame for the bloodbath of 1965 from Suharto and his supporters to the communists, who are falsely portrayed as the violent aggressors in an attempt to justify the government-sponsored mass killings that followed. The film particularly demonises women of the leftist Gerwani Movement – an activist women's organisation with links to the Communist Party of Indonesia – who in *Pengkhianatan* kidnap and murder loyal army generals. The reference to *Pengkhianatan* would be clear to an Indonesian audience as the film was, for more than twenty years, compulsory viewing in Indonesian schools and was shown annually on national television. Herman Koto's character Aminah would be immediately identifiable as one of these merciless, violent Gerwani women.[24] But what is so striking about Congo's re-articulation of this myth is his decision to portray Aminah as a cannibal. Aminah does not simply kill and mutilate her victim, she eats him and forces him to eat himself.

Congo-the-victim has already been decapitated in an earlier scene shot in studio. Congo's headless body (a ghoulish manikin that has been made by the props department) lies on the jungle floor. Congo's apparently decapitated head (his real head) rests upright on a fake rock, the illusion of decapitation sustained through the concealment of his real body behind the rock so only his head is visible to us. Congo's decapitated head speaks to Koto. We are still in the framing documentary at this point, as Oppenheimer's camera captures Congo's preparations for the shooting of the Aminah scene for his film-within. Congo is giving Koto some last-minute directorial instructions.

Congo: You should be furious, but also sad.
You should be angry, sad. Sadistic.[25]

Filming the film-within now begins. Koto (playing Aminah) speaks to Congo's decapitated head:

Koto [Aminah]: Look at your blood.

Koto smears blood over Congo's face and laughs manically.

Koto [Aminah]: Look what I found in your stomach.
Look at this! Your liver.

Koto picks up a huge piece of raw offal – probably a cow's liver – and puts it in his own mouth.

Koto [Aminah]: Look, I'm eating you.

Then Koto dangles the raw liver near Congo's mouth and Congo gags. Koto tries to make Congo eat the offal. Congo gags again, coughs, retches (a more violent reaction this time). One expects him to throw up but the retching produces nothing. Congo cannot resist what is being done to him as his body is concealed (trapped) by the fake rock and so his arms are not free to push the offal away.

Koto [Aminah]: It's rotten!

Koto spits out some of the liver that is in his mouth. Congo continues to gag and retch, on the verge of vomiting.

Koto [Aminah]: Look at this. Look, your penis! I'll stuff it in your mouth.

Koto holds up a bloody, penis-shaped piece of offal, and rubs it over Congo's face. Congo's physical discomfort increases.

As Koto attempts to force-feed Congo, the actor Congo seems to be genuinely disturbed. As a spectator, I read Congo's responses not as those of an actor skillfully playing a part but as signs of viscerally real disgust and horror. As Koto pushes the raw liver into Congo's face and mouth, Congo's reactions appear to be involuntary and unrehearsed. There could hardly be a more literal depiction of the taking-in (or here the attempt to refuse the taking-in) of something bad from outside.

That Congo chose to stage this encounter as an act of cannibalism resonates with psychoanalytic accounts of introjection. In psychoanalytic theory and metapsychology, the taking in of both bad and good objects from outside the self is invariably an oral and ingestive act but frequently also, in metaphor and sometimes literally, a cannibalistic act. Metapsychology might offer some clues as to what is happening in this scene – it might help us to read Congo's blenches – even if we don't know what impelled him to give a cannibalistic twist to the popular myth of the violent Gerwani women.

The metaphor of cannibalism is mentioned by Freud as early as his *Three Essays on the Theory of Sexuality*, where it is linked specifically to the 'aggressive element of the sexual instinct' (1905a: 159) and to early oral, pre-genital sexual organisation (1905a: 198). There are echoes of this in Karl Abraham's (1927 [1924]: 418–79) description of what he called the second or oral stage of child development – the 'oral-sadistic phase' – as one of biting or sadistic 'cannibalism' in which the infant incorporates objects in order to destroy them. Abraham referred to this as the 'cannibalistic stage'. Freud returns to cannibalism in 1913 in *Totem and Taboo*. Here cannibalism is pursued not as a metaphor but as a historical-anthropological speculation about early human societies where the act of eating another (who is ritually sacrificed and consumed in the 'totem meal') is an attempt to gain their powers: 'By incorporating parts of a person's body through the act of eating, one at the same time acquires the qualities possessed by him' (1913: 82).

Whatever credence we place on Freud's historical-anthropological speculations, he is describing the fantasy that *I become you by eating you.* In section seven of *Group Psychology and the Analysis of the Ego* (1921) on 'Identification', Freud pursues this same theme of (what we now call) *introjective identification*:

> the object that we long for and prize is assimilated by eating and is in that way annihilated as such. The cannibal, as we know, has remained at this standpoint; he has a devouring affection for his enemies and only devours people of whom he is fond.
>
> (1921: 105)

Freud is clear that we should not mistake the cannibal's 'devouring affection' simply as an act of loving identification; it also involves destructive theft and the desire to annihilate the other:

> Identification, in fact, is ambivalent from the very first; it can turn into an expression of tenderness as easily as into a wish for someone's removal.
>
> (1921: 105)

The ambivalent nature of 'devouring affection' brings both love and hate into play (a theme Freud had already pursued in *Instincts and their Vicissitudes* (1915a)). Freud again makes reference to cannibalism in *Mourning and Melancholia* (1917a) where in both the successful process of mourning and in the failure of this process in melancholia, the dead love object is taken in psychically by the bereaved in an incorporative act he equates to cannibalism.

> The ego wants to incorporate this object into itself, and, in accordance with the oral or cannibalistic phase of libidinal development in which it is, it wants to do so by devouring it.
>
> (1917a: 248–9)

But in *Mourning and Melancholia* the process of mourning is seen not simply to restructure the ego but also the super-ego, which is described in this essay as 'the critical activity of the ego' (1917a: 249).[26] By 1923, in *The Ego and the Id*, under the aegis of the new tripartite division of the psyche, a fully formed theory of the structuring of the super-ego through incorporations from outside the self has emerged:

> this ego ideal or super-ego [is] the representative of our relation to our parents. When we were little children we knew these higher natures, we admired them and feared them; and later we took them into ourselves.
>
> (1923: 36)

In thinking about Congo and his cannibalistic film-within, which of these articulations of cannibalistic incorporation in psychoanalytic theory might offer a key? Incorporation to gain qualities from beyond the self *or* to annihilate those qualities (in sadistic incorporation) *or* in incorporation as an aspect of mourning (or melancholia)? And where might the effects be felt: in the ego, or in the super-ego as punishing guilt? My reading of Congo's blenches in both the cannibalism film and in his other performances in *The Act of Killing* will encompass all these elements.

Guilt unkennelled or the introjection of failed projections: first incorporative/introjective reading

I have described Congo watching the interrogation scene on the monitor at his home up to the point where he says:

Congo: Did the people I tortured feel the way I do here?
I can feel what the people I tortured felt.
Because here my dignity has been destroyed and then fear comes, right there and then.
All the terror suddenly possessed my body.
It surrounded me, and possessed me.

But the scene continues with an intervention from Oppenheimer (a disembodied voice from off-screen):

Oppenheimer: Actually, the people you tortured felt far worse
because you know it's only a film.
They knew they were being killed.

Congo looks surprised at Oppenheimer's comment and he replies:

Congo: But I can feel it, Josh. Really, I feel it.
Or have I sinned?

Congo's eyes well up, he bites his lip, and then he continues with his voice cracking.

Congo: I did this to so many people, Josh.

Now Congo is in tears.

Congo: Is it all coming back to me?
I really hope it won't. I don't want it to, Josh.

Congo puts his hand over his face as the crying increases, he shakes his head and seems to search for more words but none are forthcoming. The camera stays on his face.

Here Congo in the film-without (as a member of the intra-diegetic audience watching his own performance and his own bodily blenches in the film-within) offers two interpretations of the effect on him of performing a role reversal with one of his victims. At first, he describes a bodily and affective identification felt as terror and possession. But in his intervention, Oppenheimer confronts Congo with his own responsibility as the source of this terror[27] and this elicits his second interpretation – 'Or have I sinned?' – which he immediately seems to confirm in the next sentence: 'I did this to so many people, Josh'. Congo's empathetic and affective encounter with his victims has, with Oppenheimer's prompting, unleashed something perhaps even more terrifying for Congo; a confrontation with his own guilt. Hamlet hoped that showing Claudius his own murderous acts in the form of a performed fiction, a play, would 'unkennel' his uncle's 'occulted guilt'.[28] It did. Congo seems to have suffered the same fate. Congo's encounter with his victims in a performed fiction, a film, seems to have unkennelled his super-ego to punish him.

But we can also read this moment of crippling confrontation with guilt as a return of guilt that Congo had been projecting out. In the apotheosis scene, the guilt was projected and then magically abolished in the fantasy of his victims forgiving him and even thanking him. In the cannibalism scene, Congo projects his guilt into Aminah and she is recast as the monstrous one. Aminah, like Ferenczi's abused child, must carry the guilt that properly belongs to the abuser. It is a psychic projection that is supported and exploited by Indonesian state propaganda (as exemplified in the film *Pengkhianatan*) where the "communist" victims of murder and torture are recast as the perpetrators. As Congo says to Oppenheimer in an earlier scene: 'For me, that film [*Pengkhianatan*] is the one thing that makes me feel not guilty'. But in the cannibalistic exchange that takes place in the film-within between Congo and Aminah, that projection is reversed or rather returned. In forcing Congo's own internal organs into his face and mouth, Aminah enacts in the most graphic and concrete way, Congo's forced introjection of the toxic bad object (the guilt) that had been projected out and into the other (into Aminah). Congo experiences crippling guilt as his projections begin to fail and so return. There is even a hint that Congo has an intuitive understanding of the process of introjecting *failed projections* in his exchange with Oppenheimer in front of the monitor, where a desperate Congo says 'Is it all coming back to me? I really hope it won't. I don't want it to, Josh.' The projection has returned; it has *all come back*. It is an argument that runs in parallel with Freud's metapsychological speculations, where the things the infant "self" ingests from the outside play a vital role in structuring the super-ego. The affective present moment of the role-reversal interrogation scene in the film-within – a moment repeated and re-experienced as it is watched on a monitor in the film-without – precipitates the collapse of projections and the introjection of failed projections into the super-ego (the 'critical activity' of the self),[29] radically challenging the self-image to which Congo had desperately clung for fifty years. This reading brings the ontological collapse that Wartenberg (2017) sees as empathetic and ethical into conformity with my reading that sees it as introjective and psychological. The two readings are not in competition but are facets of the same ontological collapse.

In this psychological reading, unconscious processes taking place within Congo seem, rather miraculously, to have been able to find expression in the fictional vehicle of the film-within. But perhaps it is no more miraculous than Winnicott's child patients revealing unconscious processes in their drawings and games. Meaning – certainly for the patient – emerges not directly in the game itself but when the game is reflected on by the mind of the analyst in dialogue with the patient. Congo's game – his film-within – seems to yield some meaning (albeit a very uncomfortable and dangerous meaning) in the reflective space of the dialogue between Oppenheimer and Congo.

In a conference paper, Julian Koch (2019) has pointed to the crucial role Oppenheimer plays within the diegesis (never in shot but appearing as a voice or as someone out-of-shot who the protagonists address). Oppenheimer's presence acts as the guarantor of the non-fictionality of what we see in *The Act of Killing;* as the guarantor of the "truth" or reality of the documentary. Koch says 'Oppenheimer pursues two metaleptic strategies in his film, the first of which deliberately merges fact and fiction, yet the second enables the viewer to tell them apart.'[30] It is only this first metaleptic strategy that most of Oppenheimer's critics see, where Oppenheimer "allows" the perpetrators to play fast and loose with fact and fiction in the making of their films.[31] But '[t]he second metalepsis [Oppenheimer's intra-diegetic interventions] creates a distance to the first, betraying the fictionalised history, and asserts the film's own factual stance' (Koch 2019). It is in these interpersonal encounters of the second metalepsis that what might be called "truth" – what Koch calls the 'factual' and what I call meaning – is able to emerge.

Shame unkennelled or the breaking open of the crypt: second incorporative/introjective reading

I want to suggest a second introjective reading of Congo's blenches. It emerges from beneath the first reading in the final, climactic scene on the rooftop above the handbag shop (Congo's second visit to the rooftop to demonstrate his killing methods). From the very start of this final scene, Congo looks deeply troubled. The *faux*-jollity that has characterised so many of Congo's appearances in the film-without has gone; its only trace is perhaps the loud, bright-yellow, double-breasted suit that he is wearing. He begins to speak quietly.

Congo: This is where we tortured and killed the people we captured.
I know it was wrong but I had to do it.

Out of the blue, and with no signs or warnings the viewer can see, Congo begins to gag very loudly. Each time, it convulses his body. He paces slowly around the rooftop, hands in pockets. The gagging increases in ferocity and the noises that emanate from Congo increase in volume. It is the sound we have already heard Congo making in the interrogation scene where he reproduces the sound his victims made as they were garroted or decapitated. It is also a noise Congo has told us he hears in his nightmares when the ghosts of his victims haunt his dreams.[32] He eventually walks to the railings that run around the edge of the rooftop and he doubles up, resting his hands on a low perimeter wall beneath the safety railings. The noises coming from Congo are now very loud. He retches several times, then spits, coughs, still bending forward, supporting himself with both hands on the wall. Even as the ferocity of the retching increases, nothing is thrown up; he is dry-heaving. Eventually he stands straight again, snorts loudly, trying to clear the phlegm obstructing his nose and throat. The camera stays on him for quite a while in a medium-wide shot and then there is a cut.

We next see Congo (evidently very shortly after the last shot ended) sitting on the wall, quietly trying to compose himself. He glances to his left, and seeing a length of wire, he picks it up.

Congo: This is…

Congo pauses and breathes deeply, puffing out air.

This is one of the easiest ways to take a human life.
And this …

He holds up a hemp sack.

> This was used to take away…

His voice cracks at this point. He is struggling to speak.

> …the human beings…

He can now barely speak.

> …we killed…
> because without this maybe people would know.

Congo throws the sack down, sits quietly for two or three seconds, and then begins to dry retch again. The noises Congo makes are deep and guttural, and now even louder. The convulsions come closer and closer together. Eventually, Congo sits stock still, breathing deeply, not looking at the camera but off into some private, middle-distance.

The camera cuts to Congo leaving the rooftop by the stairs, supporting himself on the bannister, and descending the steps very unsteadily. The next shot (the film's finale[33]) is a wide shot of the back view of Congo leaving the shop through the open door and out into the night. The shot of the open door, with the night-time city and traffic visible beyond, is held still for a long time (twenty-eight seconds), Congo having departed. The film then cuts to black. The credits roll. The manner in which the film closes – its metaphoric message – strongly suggests that the filmmaker can see little hope for Congo and that whatever demons he has confronted on that rooftop will continue to haunt him.

Before embarking on my detailed reading of this scene, it is necessary to confront an issue that has divided critics. Is Congo *acting* (in the sense of dissembling) in order, perhaps, to gain sympathy or to try to convince himself or an audience that he is a "decent" man, *or* are his actions involuntary and out of his conscious control as he remembers and relives his past? I take Congo's bodily contortions and the guttural noises that emanate from him in this scene (and in other scenes in the film) to be involuntary and "genuine" – *blenches* in Hamlet's sense – and not a performance that he puts on for the camera. This is a judgement about authenticity which I accept is highly subjective. Those critics (for example Nick Fraser (2013)), who have profound moral objections to the film, see Congo's bodily actions as being manipulative, dissembling and disingenuous and consider those of us who think his actions are "genuine" to be credulous. But neither of these positions can be substantiated as neither Fraser nor I can really know. So instead, having made my personal position clear, I will proceed from the more sceptical position set out by Janet Walker (2013: 16–8). Walker cites an exchange between Errol Morris (the film's executive producer and a powerful advocate of the film) and Oppenheimer over Congo's retching in this final scene (an exchange reproduced in Morris's 'The Murders of Gonzago' (2013: 24)).

Morris: Yes. The vomiting – whether the vomiting is one more performance for himself and for us, or if it is the result of something real. Can we ever know?

At first, Oppenheimer is taken aback by Morris's scepticism, calling it 'a very, very scary thought'. But, on reflection, Oppenheimer manages a more measured reply:

Oppenheimer: It's both – in the same sense that an actor can tap into a real emotion through acting or we can make ourselves sad by choosing to remember something and talking about it in a way that makes us sad. It's definitely both. He's performing for my camera. He's certainly aware of the camera and he's thinking about that. At the same time, he's performing in such a way that he allows the past to hit him with an unexpected force in that moment.

Walker (following Oppenheimer's recalibration of his views in the wake of Morris's scepticism) writes: 'I would resist the opposition between "performance" and "something real" and concur with Oppenheimer that it's both at once.' Walker's point is that whether Congo is acting or not, his performances nevertheless *make meaning*. The therapeutic practice of psychodrama proceeds on this same basis as does my reading of this scene that follows.

If one tracks the sequence of events in the final rooftop scene very closely, the precise trigger for each of Congo's most violent bodily *blenches* is something Congo says about guilt, responsibility, or culpability for his past actions. The first retching seems to come *out of the blue*, after he utters the words: 'This is where we tortured and killed the people we captured. I know it was wrong but I had to do it.' And, to be very precise, the trigger is 'I had to do it'. It is something in that lie – in that self-deception – that precipitates the violent reaction in Congo's body. It is a self-deception that Congo has maintained ever since 1965–66; a self-deception supported in wider Indonesian culture by the power of state propaganda. His only alternative over the years has been the oblivion of alcohol and drugs. In the director's cut, which provides a slightly extended version of the scene, there is a further clue. A little before the second bout of retching, as Congo sits on the low wall at the roof edge, he says

Congo: Why did I have to kill them?
I had to kill…[*pause*]
My conscience told me they had to be killed.

This response to his own question seems more perverse. Although Congo attempts to link 'conscience' to the imperative to murder, it is a piece of self-deceiving psychic-gymnastics too far. Each of Congo's conscious, verbal attempts to disown and project out his guilt seem increasingly desperate, precipitating violent bodily reactions. These reactions appear to be signs of what Raya Morag (in the context of perpetrator guilt in Israeli documentary) calls the 'somatic conditions of guilt' (2012: 98). Or, as Janet Walker puts it, Congo's 'body testifies' (2013: 16)[34] even as his words dissemble. Or, again, as Elizabeth Cowie writes of documentary moments that are like this one on the rooftop:

> In documentary film, sights as well as sounds of reality are seen and heard that are a record of their occurrence in time and space independently of specific statements by the film-makers, or interviewees. For we make sense of the uncontrolled, the polysemic, in documentary as well as the organized and narrated.
>
> (Cowie 2011: 28)

One bout of spasms comes in response to a slightly different trigger. When Congo shows us the sort of hemp sack used to dispose of the bodies of his victims, he says the sack was necessary, 'because without this maybe people would know'. This is not the moral language of guilt and conscience but a statement about shame. Of course, the desire to prevent people from knowing what was happening on the rooftop in Medan might have been out of fear of being caught but as the murders were state-sanctioned and there were no legal consequences, this seems unlikely. One of Congo's fellow killers, Adi Zulkadry, made it very clear earlier in the film that he, Congo and the others, killed openly and with impunity.[35] So if this is a statement about shame – and shame that precipitates as violent a bodily response in Congo as his statements about conscience and guilt – what is Congo's shameful secret? We seem to have moved from super-ego disturbance – self-punishing guilt – to ego disturbance, or at least from guilt to the narcissistic wound of shame which threatens the ego ideal.[36]

Having looked at the words that trigger Congo's most violent and uncontrollable bodily responses as he plays a role in the film-within, what of the responses themselves? In the cannibalism scene, Congo's blenches come in response to something being forced into him, something of his own which is toxic. In psychic terms, this could be read as Congo's desperate attempts to refuse the return of something from the outside; the return of his own projections of toxic guilt. But on the rooftop, Congo seems to be trying to expel something. His body tries again and again to throw something up that is already inside him, but to no avail. If Congo's body is acting out some sort of unconscious struggle, what has he taken in that he is now desperate to expel but is failing to expel? Introjective theories in psychoanalysis often treat the introjected good or bad object as either being annihilated or fully assimilated into the introjecting psyche, restructuring the ego or the super-ego, and becoming an integral part of the psyche. The psyche is altered through the act of introjection becoming a "new" psyche. But Congo's bodily struggles on the rooftop suggest that there is something inside him which is not integrated, something which is separate from him and alien to him,[37] which could be (or at least *feels* as if it could be) expelled.

The work of Nicolas Abraham and Mária Török offers a way to read these struggles. In a series of essays published from the 1950s to the 1980s, Abraham and

Török took up the notion of introjection and, in a radical move, placed it at the heart of psychoanalysis: introjection is made 'the driving force of psychic life in its entirety' (Rand 1994: 8). At the core of Abraham and Török's reworking of introjection was a critical distinction between introjection and incorporation[38]; manifestations of two sorts of psychic *taking-in.* In their 1972 essay, 'Mourning or Melancholia: Introjection versus Incorporation' (1994 [1972]: 125), they propose a crucial distinction between the two. 'Incorporation denotes fantasy, introjection a process' and '[i]n our conception fantasy is essentially narcissistic; it tends to transform the world rather than inflict injury on the subject.' Introjection, by contrast, changes the subject (the psyche), which adjusts to reality through a slow, painful process of transformation, until the introjection is fully integrated. It is in the notion of incorporation, the notion that something is taken in that remains undigested as an alien within the psyche, which offers a way to read Congo's blenches – his dry-retching – in the climatic final scene.

In an essay on mourning as illness, Török (1994 [1968]) uses the distinction to differentiate between a successful and a failed process of mourning. In successful mourning, the lost love object is gradually, slowly and painfully over a period of time taken into the self and eventually the *introjecting* psyche comes to a less painful accommodation with the loss. In failed mourning, on the other hand, the traumatic loss is not worked through. It happens instantaneously and magically. The lost love object is taken into the *incorporating* psyche as if it still existed. Incorporation can have a number of troubling consequences including hallucination (as the reality of the loss is denied) and the erotic charge of possessing the love object which secretly still exists and is available, creating a kind of sentimental sickness (melancholy). The love object is locked away as a troubling, shameful secret. Abraham and Török developed this concept of failed mourning – of incorporation – to describe recurring and unresolved trauma both in the life of the individual and in the transmission of trauma between the generations.

In transgenerational trauma, the *unworked through* trauma of one generation passes unconsciously to the next (and is most comprehensively explored in Török's essay (1994 [1975]) 'Story of Fear: The Symptoms of Phobia – the Return of the Repressed or the Return of the Phantom?')

> [T]he "phantom" is a formation in the dynamic unconscious that is found there not because of the subject's own repression *but on account of a direct empathy with the unconscious or the repressed psychic matter of a parental object.*
>
> (1994 [1975]: 181; Török's italics)

The disturbance remains hidden away like a *ghost* or a *phantom* in the psyche capable of bursting out and overwhelming the subject, like the eruption of an alien being from within. In individual life, the unresolved trauma is locked away inside the individual in a *crypt* where it is hermetically sealed off from the rest of the psyche but with the ever-present danger that it might escape its vault and overwhelm the subject. Both phantom and cryptic behaviour can manifest themselves in bizarre ways (such as verbal and non-verbal para-speech)[39] as if the subject was possessed and controlled and *spoken-through* by the repressed material experienced as an alien being.

The parallel seems irresistible between Török's conception of the crypt, as a hermetically sealed off part of the psyche, and Bessel van der Kolk's construction of traumatic memory as sealed off from ordinary subjective memory (a conception that Cathy Caruth borrows and subsumes into "trauma theory"). Both Török and van der Kolk seem to be pointing to unintegrated elements within the psyche/memory produced by traumatic experience. But where van der Kolk and Caruth conceive of traumatic memory as a 'reality imprint' (van der Kolk *et al.* 1996: 52) or as an 'unprocessed fragment of the thing itself' (Luckhurst 2008: 13), Török takes cryptic behaviour to be a hallucinatory mis-recognition of reality prompted by a melancholic failure to mourn. For Török (and for me), cryptic behaviour is symptomatic, not a trace of the unvarnished, noumenal truth and so, at least in theory, subject to the possibility of change through a process of mourning.

Returning to Congo on the rooftop, the body of Congo the reenactor behaves in bizarre ways suggestive of cryptic behaviour. The very suddenness of the onset of extreme bodily blenches is striking. He moves from a relatively calm narration from memory of his activities of fifty years ago to extreme bodily convulsions as if suddenly possessed. And the dry heaving that ensues graphically suggests that something powerful and toxic has been ingested and needs to be expelled, but nothing will *come up* despite the muscular contortions. If we read this as a bad object that has been taken-in, it has not been annihilated or fully assimilated as we might expect from Karl Abraham's or Freud's accounts of identification through ingestion. The bad object is inside Congo but is still distinct and alien.

But if the toxic object locked in the crypt cannot be expelled, what is the nature of that object? In their 1975 essay 'The Lost Object', Abraham and Török describe it as

> a memory [...] buried *without legal burial place*. The memory is of an idyll, experienced with a valued object and yet for some reason unspeakable. It is a memory entombed in a fast and secure place, awaiting resurrection.
>
> (Abraham and Török 1994 [1975]: 141; authors' italics)

Carrying over Abraham and Török's insight to what we observe of Congo as a character in the film, the memory is unspeakable as it is a memory of his murderous acts, which if fully confronted would unleash overwhelming guilt or shame. In his confrontations with his past in the film-within (and in his reflections on the film-within in the film-without) some of this guilt or shame has begun to be unkennelled.

But the psychic structure is able to endure as it is not only a memory of horror but also the treasured memory 'of an idyll, experienced with a valued object'. The failure to confront the past can be read as a failure to confront the loss of the dead love object. The memory of his unmourned victims is potent as it carries an erotic charge, expressed in the evident joy Congo takes in recalling his sadism: he boasts that he killed 'happily'; he boasts that he and his friends were more sadistic than the Nazi killers they watched in Hollywood films in the 1960s; his final instruction to Koto before he plays his part in the cannibalism scene is to say, 'You should be angry, sad. Sadistic'. Congo's victims seem constantly available, unmourned, undead, and the source of libidinal (sadistic) pleasure. Even in the role-reversal scenes where Congo plays the "communist" victim (a scene that starts to unravel the idyll by bringing Congo into an empathetic encounter with his victims), the perverse structure of the idyll is simultaneously maintained. Congo is alone amongst the killers in choosing to play the victim and we might ask why. Perhaps he is seeking to understand the past. But we might also read this choice as simply choosing to invert the perverse, erotically-charged structure, exchanging the sadistic thrill of the perpetrator for the erotically-charged masochistic thrill of being persecuted. Just as a direct 'empathy with the unconscious or the repressed psychic matter of a parental object' does not undo but rather maintains the phantom of inter-generational trauma, so Congo's direct empathetic encounter with his victims might not start a process of mourning and working through but instead strengthen the structure of the crypt.

In her essay on *The Act of Killing*, Homay King (2013) compares Congo and the various roles he plays to the child in Freud's essay *'A Child Is Being Beaten': A Contribution to the Study of the Origin of Sexual Perversions* (1919a). In the fantasy of the films-within, Congo (like the child) successively occupies 'all three of the classic positions in Freud's beating fantasy: aggressor, onlooker, and finally victim' (King 2013: 33). King argues that 'fantasy [...] is an incredibly malleable instrument, one that allows its subjects to imagine themselves occupying a range of mutually exclusive positions' (2013: 32), and that these fantasised alternative perspectives have a protean potential in documentary to reveal things that would otherwise remain hidden. She concludes that 'fantasy can paradoxically be the route back to reality, performing the difficult work of opening doors to the past that were previously locked shut' (2013: 35). King's argument supports the idea that the deployment of fictions or fantasies in documentary may be a route to meaning for the protagonist and a way to understand and work through a traumatic past; or, in the words of Shakespeare (and Freud), they are a 'bait of falsehood' that might, paradoxically, be able to take the 'carp of truth'. Different fantasised perspectives might provoke identifications (empathy for example) which loosen or challenge rigid psychic structures. But this does not seem to be the case with the Congo we see in *The Act of Killing*. Central to Freud's essay is the sado-masochism of the child (something that King is not particularly interested in in her essay). And central to my reading of the filmic Congo through Abraham and Török's notion of the crypt, is the sado-masochistic (libidinal) nature of Congo's attachment to his victims. It is the sado-masochistic charge he seems to derive from the memory of his victims and his crimes that may prevent him from escaping from the repetitions of his trauma, as the repetitions are horrifying yet simultaneously deeply pleasurable. He is trapped in an 'unspeakable' idyll (in Abraham and Török's terms), possessed by the ghosts of the dead. It is a psychic structure that even a panoply of perspectival fantasies seems powerless to loosen.[40]

In this my second incorporative/introjective reading of Congo, his victims are alive inside him, locked away in an unspeakable crypt. The Hungarian-born French psychoanalyst Judith Dupont (2000) wrote in a gloss of Abraham and Török's work, that when grief cannot be recognised, then the trauma and all the emotions it provokes are locked away in a vault as a shameful secret, shared only with the lost object of love. If the idea of a shameful, live, secret, sado-masochistic love shared with his victims seems far-fetched or even morally repugnant, one can look to Freud's work on cannibalism to find some justification: 'The cannibal [...] has a devouring affection for his enemies and only devours people of whom he is fond' (1921: 105). But Abraham and Török perhaps best capture the strangeness of what we witness on the rooftop; their words reading like a description of the scene that unfolds before the viewer:

> Sometimes [...] when libidinal fulfilments have their way, the ghost of the crypt comes back to haunt the cemetery guard, giving him strange and incomprehensible signals, making him perform bizarre acts, or subjecting him to unexpected sensations.
>
> (1994 [1972]: 130)

The 'bizarre acts' Congo performs for Oppenheimer's camera on the rooftop suggest a moment when the crypt opens ever so slightly to reveal its toxic contents. The 'memory entombed in a fast and secure place, awaiting resurrection' is for a few brief seconds resurrected. The resurrection of Congo's buried love – the breaking open of the crypt within him – is accompanied by the non-verbal para-speech characteristic of cryptic behaviour. In an interview, Oppenheimer describes the moment on the rooftop when Congo begins to retch.

> He had his back toward me, and I, at first, didn't realize that he was choking [...] To clarify this word *choke:* the sounds Anwar makes in this scene imitate the sounds his victims made as he killed them, expressing in phantom ways how it might have felt to have your neck garroted with a wire and pulled tight until it cuts into your windpipe. The choking that Anwar experiences is exactly that, and it is a terrible sound, indeed.
>
> (Oppenheimer in interview with: Cohn 2012; Cohn's italics)

The sounds that emanate from Anwar Congo are the sounds of his victims – his shameful love objects – for so long buried in their crypt. The lid of their tomb has opened far enough for us to hear their groans from beyond the grave or, if one prefers, Congo has become an unwitting ventriloquist "speaking" with the voice of his victims. Congo is indeed 'expressing in phantom ways' his terrible secret; he is proclaiming his malefactions in para-speech: 'For murder, though it have no tongue, will speak with most miraculous organ' (Hamlet in: *Hamlet*: Act II Scene II).

For Congo, there may be no redemption. The crypt within him momentarily opens in his dynamic encounter with his past in the film-within, and we both hear groans from within the crypt and see his body contorted in its struggle to eject the toxic object he has incorporated. In Oppenheimer's words, 'he starts to retch and it's as though, I think, he's trying to vomit up the ghosts that haunt him' (Oppenheimer in interview with Goodman 2013). But Congo cannot eject that object: he cannot vomit; nothing will come up. We could take this as merely a filmic metaphor for his predicament but to me it feels more than that. Bodies do speak in *miraculous* ways and the deeper and more profound the psychological disturbance, the more likely perhaps that the disturbance can only express itself somatically.

In an interview with Pamela Cohn, Oppenheimer expressed a similar view of Congo and his chances of redemption. On the rooftop, on hearing the 'miraculous organ' speak, Oppenheimer knew he was in the presence of something dreadful and deathly.

> That space that Anwar was occupying belonged to the dead. It's filled with ghosts. I could not walk in that space with him [...] That space of the dead is his space, he is of that space, because he's also died somehow. It's a terrible thing to witness that in someone you've come to care about. It's a very difficult scene for me to watch, as well. The final statement is the understanding that he's in a total limbo. And that's where he'll probably stay for the rest of his life.
>
> (Cohn 2012)

What seems to have been unkennelled in Congo through the vehicle of the film-within is perhaps his 'occulted guilt' but, for me, a more complex and a more troubling interpretation is that it is his *occulted shame* that has been unkennelled. What is briefly revealed at the end of *The Act of Killing* is the shameful secret Congo shares with his unmourned victims – his eroticised love objects locked away inside him for fifty years – who cry out from the tomb, whilst Congo in jaunty, yellow suit paces the suburban rooftop in downtown Medan. And what is unmourned probably cannot be escaped; it will continue to haunt him in a perpetual, "timeless", melancholic circle of repetition.

A clinical vignette: Congo's teeth

As a brief afterword, I want to mention Congo's teeth.

A visual metaphor that snakes its way through *The Act of Killing* is Congo's obsession with his teeth and his dentures. The first time I watched *The Act of Killing*, I was struck by the number of shots of Congo "playing" with his teeth: putting in and taking out the line of three dentures that fill a gap between his natural teeth; making sure his teeth look good in any available mirror; making a trip to the dentist[41]; and one almost unwatchable occasion when Congo (alone in his room) takes a pair of woodworking pliers and pulls out a broken section of one of his natural teeth without anaesthetic. Initially, I read these recurring scenes as an astute piece of observational filmmaking. Most of the sequences demonstrate Congo's vanity and narcissism. But the scene with the pliers suggests another facet of Congo; that for all the vanity and conceit, Congo is a man who is disintegrating.

Although these sequences made a powerful impression on me as filmic metaphors, I was not going to write about them here until I re-read Török's essay, 'The Illness of Mourning and the Fantasy of the Exquisite Corpse'. In a clinical vignette, Török describes a patient called Thérèse whom Török presents as a classic case of blocked, incorporative mourning. Unable to mourn her father in the ten years since his death, Thérèse sought an analysis. Török writes:

> In the course of her analysis Thérèse brought a dream triptych that I also found in other patients of mourning: marriage with an inaccessible man, an indictment for having eaten a corpse, a dentist predicting the exposure of her receding gumline, followed by the total loss of her teeth.
>
> (Török 1994 [1968]: 122)

In her analysis with Török, Thérèse also described in highly disguised form, the 'much desired though deeply repressed union in love with her father' which was 'consummated hallucinatorily during the last rites'. Török goes on to make it clear that, far from this case being bizarre or unique, Thérèse's dreams are typical of patients with blocked (incorporative) mourning: dreams about eating and burying a corpse and dreams about teeth, especially their growth or loss, or about receding gumlines (Török 1994 [1968]: 123). I mention Török's clinical observations here because of the uncanny echoes with the Congo we see in *The Act of Killing:* the consumption of a corpse, the disintegrating teeth and the highly disguised but plainly erotic desire for a lost, unmourned love object. If one takes seriously Sobchack's conjecture that documentary gives us access to the real life of the protagonist beyond or behind the screen, then the behaviours Congo displays within the diegesis are suggestive of someone suffering from the clinical symptoms of blocked incorporative mourning as described by Török.

The emergence of meaning: documentary film as analytic process

There are a number of implicit questions in this chapter. Can the creation of (and the reflection on) filmed fictional constructions within the non-fictional frame of a documentary help to bring understanding of a real, non-fictional traumatic past? Or, in the terms in which Freud framed it in *Constructions in Analysis* (1937b), can a 'bait of falsehood' – a play-within-the-play, a forgery – take the 'carp of truth'? If understanding does emerge, for whom does it emerge: for the traumatised protagonist, for the director, for "us" the viewers who constitute the extra-diegetic audience, or perhaps for all three as Errol Morris suggests (2013: 2) in his essay on the *The Act of Killing*? If some sort of meaning does become available to the traumatised protagonist, does it have a curative function – does it lessen the psychic pain attendant on the trauma? And, finally, can parallels be drawn between the filmmaking process and an analytic process where fictions are deployed to represent traumatic histories and begin a process that might over time create or find a meaningful account of a trauma that has all but 'vanished into a crepuscular past' (Morris 2013: 2)?

Anwar Congo: the traumatised protagonist

Measured by the yardstick of Congo's two re-enactments of his killing methods on the rooftop in Medan – one shot at the beginning of the filmmaking process and one at the end – it would be impossible to claim that Congo's involvement in making a film about his past had been "curative". A man troubled by his past at the start of the film ends it on the brink of physical and psychic collapse. Congo appears to have spiralled further into the trauma he sought to escape. But this is not to suggest that the creation of fictional films about his past did not bring a greater understanding. In making, and especially in watching back these films on a screen after the event, Congo is forced to confront his past and to recognise his past actions for what they were. Playing a role in the film-within brought Congo into an empathetic encounter in his imagination with the victims of his violence; a deeply disturbing encounter that at first could only express itself in bodily form as blenches but blenches that were witnessed and then interpreted by Congo as he watched back his own performance on a screen. It is Congo as a member of the intra-diegetic audience (as an inner Winnicottian viewer), watching himself perform in the film-within that finally allows him to speak his guilt and ask Oppenheimer, 'Have I sinned?'. Like Claudius watching Hamlet's production of *The Murder of Gonzago*, Congo blenches; his 'occulted guilt' is unkennelled and later he is able to name (to symbolise) what has been unkennelled.

In interview, Oppenheimer described this process and the central, catalytic role played by the film-within, stressing the essential non-fictionality of the film-within's fictions (non-fictional in the sense that they reveal something that is "true")

> The thought was to look not only at the characters, but the whole regime, through a prism where we see the stories and are also able to create the second- and third-hand stories in which they imagine themselves – and fail to know themselves. We see the way they construct themselves. But I think everything we see is nonfiction. Everything is true. Something true is revealed through this process. However desperate Anwar's fantasy, his visions of the victim, his rewards in heaven, all have a truth – through artifacts, through emotional and poetic force, through his personal process. The village massacre scene was something really problematic to shoot. It's a misbegotten icon of this terrible time of genocide when genocide shouldn't really have an icon. But that's why it's deconstructed – not only by me, but also by the participants.
>
> (Oppenheimer in interview with: Cohn 2012)

What Oppenheimer describes as the participants' deconstruction of their own productions is the reflective process where meaning emerges. A process that begins for Congo in an identificatory encounter with his imagined victims. Bill Nichols recognises how radical *The Act of Killing* is in affording the protagonists an interpretive role.

> Normally, reenactments represent an interpretive gesture by the filmmaker, but that is one of many documentary conventions this remarkable film flouts. In this case, the filmmaker enables his subjects to offer their interpretation of past events.
>
> (Nichols 2013: 25)

But there are limits to what Congo is able to understand of his traumatic past. Whatever horror Congo is experiencing on the rooftop at the end of the film, it is only able to find somatic expression. There is no sense that he understands why he can scarcely complete his re-enactment as his body contorts and retches; he offers no interpretation of these blenches. As the analyst-theorist Joyce McDougall writes: '[t]he body speaks no known language, yet it serves, time and again, as a framework for communicating the psychic scenes of the internal theatre' (1986: 53). Congo seems to be performing a part in McDougall's 'psychosomatic theatre' where 'actors tend to draw attention to themselves by means of gestures or abrupt physical displacements' (1986: 12). Congo is finding a way to communicate the nature of his trauma even if there is no sense that *he* knows the language his body is speaking.

Anwar Congo and Joshua Oppenheimer: the protagonist in interpersonal relation

But if these bodily contortions are a communication, who is the recipient of these communications? The moments of revelation for Congo and his bodily performances occur in the context of his relationship with the director Joshua Oppenheimer. It is through Oppenheimer's prompting – as Congo watches himself on a monitor close to wordless paralysis in the interrogation scene – that Congo finally comes to speak his guilt. And it is for Oppenheimer and his camera that Congo's body puts on its bizarre performance on the rooftop. Oppenheimer acts not just as an ear and an eye – as a passive witness to Congo's trauma – but as an active secondary witness, as another mind, that helps Congo to process what emerges from his engagement in his various films-within.

Oppenheimer fulfils a role not dissimilar to that of the analyst in the analytic encounter. In the question and answer session at the end of a masterclass Oppenheimer gave in London in May 2016, an audience member said, 'Anwar's scenes are like therapy' and asked Oppenheimer to comment. Oppenheimer rejected the idea, saying it could only be therapy if his primary responsibility was to Anwar Congo rather than to the human-rights agenda which he states was his primary goal (Oppenheimer 2016). *The Act of Killing* is indeed a film with a primarily political, human-rights agenda but this does not prevent the relationship at the heart of the film taking the form of, and perhaps performing some of the functions of, the analytic encounter. Congo, at least, seems to have entered into this joint-filmmaking project with the hopes and expectations of an analysand entering therapy, as Oppenheimer confirmed in interview: 'He was working out his own pain, and I was trying to expose a regime of impunity for Indonesians themselves' (Oppenheimer in interview with Fortune 2013). And as the project continued, these hopes and expectations became more pronounced:

> After Anwar decided to explore through the filmmaking his own brokenness, his own trauma, his own pain, he stopped asking when the film would be ready. This happened midway through the production, when he started to suggest we go deeper into his bad dreams.
>
> (Oppenheimer quoted in: Cooper 2013)

So, despite Oppenheimer's reservations, the Oppenheimer-Congo relationship could even be described as an ideal analytic relationship, where critical distance is maintained by the director/analyst whilst retaining the capacity to think empathetically[42] about the protagonist/analysand within a relationship of mutual love.[43]

The close and empathetic relationship between Oppenheimer and Congo is clearly legible to the extra-diegetic audience and it also clearly facilitates the complex communications that take place between the two, including the emergence of a more meaningful (if traumatising) account of the past that comes from Congo's engagement with his own film-within, and he asks 'have I sinned?' That said, much of the complexity of this relationship is not available to us on screen, even in this highly self-reflexive film.

To more fully understand the relationship, one has to have recourse to a more extensive paratext (especially to comments made about the film in interviews subsequent to its release). The analyst/analysand relationship of Oppenheimer/Congo is perhaps exemplified in Congo's increasing dependence on Oppenheimer and in Oppenheimer's predicament in hearing troubling material and being subject to disturbance in the counter-transference (the mutual implication of the Freudian pair in the messy middle). Reflecting on witnessing Congo's 'real descent into hell' (Cohn 2012) in playing the victim in the interrogation scene, Oppenheimer said in interview that he found himself deeply embroiled in Congo's traumatic world:

> I felt so implicated because suddenly we were re-living something, and it felt very, very real. And it felt like the flimsiest cover that it was being played as a gangster scene. I had nightmares and was experiencing intense feelings of guilt. To go really deep into that kind of pain just made me feel dirty, really awful. So much of what eventually constituted the story of the film didn't exist yet. It was a really hard time. I couldn't sleep throughout that period which lasted about six months.
>
> (Oppenheimer in interview with: Cohn 2012)

At this same period, in a separate interview, Oppenheimer (Barnes 2013) described the nightmares he had of a 'family reunion transforming gradually into a scene where somebody I loved was being tortured or killed'. As a member of a family that had lost many close relatives in the Holocaust, Oppenheimer was deeply troubled by making a film with men who had committed genocide but who continued to be celebrated as heroes in Indonesia: 'It dawned on me that I had walked into Germany 40 years after the Holocaust, and found the Nazis still in power' (Oppenheimer quoted in Barnes 2013). At least in the counter-transference, Congo is the ageing Nazi torturer and murderer of Oppenheimer's family and we might speculate that Oppenheimer was drawn to this project in the first place as a way of working through his traumatic family history.

These speculations about the counter-transferential encounter between Oppenheimer and Congo (speculations which gain credence in the light of what Oppenheimer has said in interview), undermine the moral case mounted against *The Act of Killing* by a number of critics. One of the most vociferous of these critics is Nick Fraser, commissioning editor from 1997 to 2016 of the BBC's flagship documentary strand, *Storyville*. Fraser refused to allow the film to be shown on the BBC as he felt the re-enacted scenes were trivialising, deeply ethically flawed and in very bad taste. He suggested that Oppenheimer had only been able to escape moral censure because 'such goings-on in Indonesia are acceptable merely because the place is so far away, and so little known or talked about, that the implications of such an act can pass unnoticed.' To try to persuade his readers that this film should be shunned, he goes on to say, imagine a director 'rounding up a bunch of aging Nazis and getting them to make a film entitled "We Love Killing Jews." That is what the film is about...!' (2013: 21–4). Fraser's provocative rhetorical gesture backfires if we take into account what Oppenheimer has said about his film: it seems Oppenheimer did not intend the implications of his filmmaking act to pass unnoticed – quite the contrary. It is indeed 'what the film is about'. Oppenheimer is, quite deliberately, drawing a parallel between Indonesia and a re-imagined and victorious Nazi Germany both to make a political point about present-day Indonesia and, we might assume, to work through his own troubled family history. Our judgement as to whether this puts the film beyond the ethical pale will depend upon the individual viewer's attitude to the representation of traumatic events and their judgement as to the ethical intent of the director.

But whatever ethical conclusions viewers may come to, it is clear that *The Act of Killing* (like so many filmic trauma texts), has echoes well beyond the apparent personal, geographical and chronological boundaries of its ostensible subject, demonstrating the palimpsestic and/or multidirectional nature of traumatic memory.[44] To borrow the language of Abraham and Török, the making of this film may have been Oppenheimer's way of wrestling with his own inter-generational phantoms.

But the precise details of the transference/counter-transference that Oppenheimer experienced are not available to the viewer in the film as cut and edited. As Agnieszka Piotrowska (2014) has argued, the key relationship that drives and shapes so much of documentary filmmaking – the director-protagonist relationship with its unconscious desires and complex identifications – often leaves few concrete traces in the final film.[45] This relationship, that I argue, has certain parallels to the relationship of analyst and analysand in the consulting room, 'is a ghostly presence, that the spectator may be unaware of, or may intuit, but struggles to reconstruct with any confidence' (Eadie 2017: 381).

If the precise details of this key relationship are hidden, its effects are palpable. It is *with* Oppenheimer that Congo is able to find representational forms for his trauma and when, on occasions, he is only able to respond with bodily blenches (non-representational symptomatology), it is Oppenheimer who steers Congo towards an understanding of his performance. The intense counter-transferential relationship between Oppenheimer and Congo allows Oppenheimer to both grasp the horror of the trauma (the inside of traumatic experience) as he has felt it himself in the counter-transference, whilst also remaining outside the trauma as a mind able to process Congo's nameless anxiety and bodily distress.[46]

The structure of The Act of Killing *and the structure of the analytic encounter*

If the counter-transferential encounter between Oppenheimer and Congo mirrors something of the encounter between analyst and analysand but remains semi-submerged,[47] then much more clearly visible are the structural elements of *The Act of Killing* that mirror structural aspects of the analytic encounter.

Oppenheimer as director/analyst did not try to determine or propose what narratives Congo or the other killers should present, or to modify them. The narratives they came up with mirror the sort of narratives that the analysand might present in analysis: attempts to recount personal history from memory (a conventional history that starts gradually to unravel, to unknot, revealing deeper meanings); descriptions of dreams or nightmares; fantasies in which the analysand desperately tries to evade troubling aspects of their past; the gradual emergence of unconscious fantasies into representational form; the patient beginning to hear what it is that they are saying, etc. The self-reflexive structure of *The Act of Killing* – the protagonist and Oppenheimer watching back on a monitor, scenes that have already been shot – mirrors the analytic encounter where stories told in earlier sessions are picked up, reflected on, and reformulated in the light of later examination.

We could view the film-within in documentary as a kind of *play space*, akin to Donald Winnicott's idea (1990 [1971]a) of the analytic space as a play space (mirroring the transitional or potential space that exists between mother and child). The *film-within-the-film* is a *play space* in documentary, where many plays (many narratives) can be performed: plays of psychic and metaphorical significance that may reveal otherwise hidden "truths"; or, as I would prefer to argue, plays that in the witnessing may allow the construction of otherwise unavailable meanings. These meanings would not have become available without the freedom to fantasise and to lie and to remember and to play with the traumatic past without restriction.

More broadly, and to turn my analogy on its head, the clinical encounter between analyst and analysand and what emerges between them in successive sessions can be read as a particular form of the play-within-the-play. The representations and interpretations that emerge within analysis are all fictional forms that emerge out of the "factual" frame of a life lived (or perhaps more accurately, emerge between the two lives lived of analysand and analyst): dreams; free associations; constructions in analysis; the recounting of personal history through memory in a dynamic present; screen memories; reflections on the transference and counter-transference; and all the various enactments and projections and introjections that take place in the analytic space. The narratives that emerge in analysis are not judged either by their conformity to historical objectivity (an external measure of their truth-value) or by their conformity to a normative moral code but are valued for their capacity to reveal or generate psychological meanings or insights.

The meaning-generative, amoral, *a*-factual space of the analytic encounter is mirrored in the amoral, *a*-factual space opened up in documentary through the film-within. Sometimes the stories told might conform to something like the notion of objective historical "truth", as Hamlet hopes the retelling of his father's murder in fictional form (in *The Murder of Gonzago*) will be.[48] But elsewhere in the play *Hamlet*, it is clear that *baits of falsehood* might equally well *take the carp of truth* and that it is *by these very indirections we find directions out*. The film-within introduces some miching malicho into documentary, not for the sake of mischievousness in and of itself, but to uncover meanings or allow the construction of meanings that are not otherwise available.

Sometimes in analysis and in life, the fictional narratives that are created or found might have a curative function. In Freud's story of his grandson's game with cotton reel and string, the fictive, enacted narrative repeated over time both brings the trauma of maternal separation (loss) into representational form and is simultaneously a representation of the process of working through that trauma. The terror of the loss of the love object is bridged by a fiction; the fiction that the mother is always available now as an introjected good object (the internalisation of the *idea* or *representation* of the mother) which is securely held even when the "real" mother is absent. The outcome for Congo, though, looks much more bleak, as for all his fictive narratives, the object he seems to have introjected (incorporated in Török's terms) is a very *bad* "good object": a fantastical, unmourned, undead version of the actually dead love object. The fictive, enacted narrative that Congo performs on the rooftop both brings the trauma of his murderous past into representational form and is simultaneously a representation of his failure to work through that trauma. For Congo, a meaningful and possibly curative process would involve the recognition that the love object is really dead; killed by him. This would entail a renunciation of the erotic, sadistic charge he draws from his "undead" victims and a much fuller appreciation of his own shame. The incorporated love object carries within it the very trauma he seeks to escape; an object he cannot dislodge; an object that contains his undead victims who cry out for revenge. Congo's fictive narratives seem to carry him only so far in constructing a meaningful, "truthful" account of his trauma before the narratives themselves become traumatising and his capacity to symbolise breaks down.

"Us" – the extra-diegetic audience

In considering the film-within-the-film and its function in catalysing or provoking the emergence of meaning for Congo,[49] I have offered readings, which emerge from within the diegesis. They are readings that explore the potential for a reflexive and self-reflexive filmmaking process to act like the analytic process, as a meaning-making process that might be able to lessen the psychic pain of trauma.

But the ultimate locus for meaning-making is the viewer, "us" as the extra-diegetic audience. And, as it is hard to find a theoretical justification to aggregate viewers together as a collective "we", the ultimate locus for meaning-making is each individual viewer of *The Act of Killing*. In the personal reading offered by this particular viewer, the meanings I have assigned to Congo and the unconscious processes he seems to reveal as he re-enacts scenes from the traumatic past must be owned by me as my personal projections onto the filmic object.

I offered a theoretical justification for this approach arguing from both the film phenomenology of Vivian Sobchack (Chapter 2) and through an elaboration of Phyllis Creme's notion of the *Winnicottian viewer* (Chapter 3). Sobchack argues that the viewer of documentary perceives the filmic object very differently from the viewer of a fiction film and although the documentary viewer is dependent upon the screen for knowledge, he or she also looks through or behind the screen to gain access to aspects of the life of the on-screen protagonist beyond the screen. Phyllis Creme's notion of the Winnicottian viewer performs a similar theoretical function by positing a viewer who does not just passively receive the film but actively enters the potential space of the film on (or through) the cinema screen and so both finds and creates the film and its meanings through their active, playful spectatorship. With the complex structure of *The Act of Killing*, there is a doubling of this filmic potential space. As an *outer* Winnicottian viewer actively finding/creating meanings in my engagement with *The Act of Killing* and imagining (or directly experiencing through forms of identification) the unconscious processes going on inside the "virtual", filmic Congo, I also see another Winnicottian viewer – Anwar Congo within the diegesis – who (like me) reacts to and enters into the film that he is watching. I watch the documentary, and within that documentary I see Congo, the *inner* Winnicottian viewer, watching his own films, imagining what his victims were feeling (or directly experiencing what his victims were experiencing in non-conscious, non-cognitive bodily identification), and actively creating or finding meanings.

In engaging with his own film, Congo, as inner Winnicottian viewer, seems to create or find a meaningful account of his own past to the extent that he begins to speak his own guilt. But this same inner Winnicottian viewer appears unable to find/create a meaningful account of what he experiences in the cannibalism scene or in his near physical collapse on the rooftop at the end of *The Act of Killing*. Of course, in *The Act of Killing* there is no opportunity for Congo to reflect back on the final rooftop scene *with* Oppenheimer (as the filmmaking process ends) and so unlike Winnicott's child patients, there is no opportunity for a dialogue and a process of reflection to take place between "analyst" and "patient". But this notwithstanding, I find it hard not to concur with Oppenheimer's own assessment of Congo's chances of reaching a meaningful account; namely, a very slim chance. The meaning I have assigned to the final scene – Congo's incorporation of an unmourned, undead love object – is a reading that I, as outer Winnicottian viewer, have created or found through my active engagement with the film object as a whole. Or, in Sobchack's terms, I have looked through the screen to speculate about the real psychic life of the on-screen protagonist.

Ultimately, my reading of *The Act of Killing* emerges out of my own transference/counter-transference onto the filmic object. Watching the film was a disturbing, vertiginous, disorientating experience as I found myself drawn into an empathetic encounter with Congo (and the other killers). I am not alone in experiencing the film in this way. For Bill Nichols (2013: 25), 'the killers' vision of reality creates a deep disturbance in the viewer. Oppenheimer intensifies a sense of what it feels like to enter a world without a moral compass'. Whilst Oppenheimer himself offers an even more unsettling reason for our (my) feelings of disturbance, suggesting that those viewers with the courage to do so, will 'see a small part of themselves in Anwar [...] and thereby see themselves as much closer to perpetrators than we would normally wish to see ourselves' (Oppenheimer quoted in Crichlow 2013: 42; footnote 6).[50] These are troubling identifications, as even in feeling empathy I simultaneously felt as if I should be condemning the killers absolutely and out of hand. I was left feeling both tainted by my engagement with the film and guilty for identifying so closely with a mass killer. It is out of this counter-transference onto the filmic object that my reading of Congo emerges as, working backwards from my initial feelings to my later detailed interpretations, my interpretations of what is going on inside Congo replicate my own initial feelings of awfulness and guilt or shame.[51] Whether I have simply projected my feelings on to Congo as filmic object or have felt something of what Congo was feeling whilst making *The Act of Killing* is an open question. For my part, I assume that these countervailing currents cannot be untangled and I cannot know if I have found or created the meanings I have gleaned.

Meaning in all the frames of The Act of Killing

In all the frames of *The Act of Killing*, the meanings that emerge – for Congo, for Oppenheimer, for me as an extra-diegetic viewer – all emerge in the space between two subjects (in an inter- or intra-personal space playing out over time) whether those subjects are real, imagined, the virtual creations of role play and role reversal, or simply filmic avatars. They are all essentially meanings gleaned from reflection on the transference/counter-transference between two subjects. But the meanings that emerge are all set in motion by the mischievous device, the 'false fire', of the film-within; a fictional play-space where trauma is explored in any way and without limit. The device of the fictional film-within-the-film generates powerful affective and somatic responses in all the frames of the complex structure of this documentary: in the players in the film-within; in the intra-diegetic audience (as Congo in the film-without watches himself performing in the film-within on a monitor); in the director as a character in the diegesis and as an extra-diegetic witness after the completion of his film; and in the extra-diegetic audience. The fictional representations of the trauma – the *baits of falsehood* – are not meaningful in themselves but, if they have some purchase, they will precipitate new representations or somatic and affective responses (often bizarre and obscure non-representational symptomatology)[52] which are forms of communication that are open to interpretation (symbolisation). As Freud maintained in *Constructions in Analysis* (1937b), the value of the fiction – its worth – is to be gauged by whether it *touches* the patient, a *touch* that then requires interpretation. Or in the words of Hamlet, we must rivet our eyes on Congo to see 'if he blench' and then use 'our judgments [...] in censure of his seeming' (Act III Scene II).

Notes

1 The film is conventionally catalogued as directed by Oppenheimer alone but was co-directed by Oppenheimer, Christine Cyn and an anonymous Indonesian director (whose name was withheld to protect him/her from reprisals in Indonesia). What follows draws largely on the 115-minute theatrical release of the film although I will refer to some scenes that only appear in the 159-minute director's cut.
2 I mean 'primitive' in a psychic and not an anthropological sense: psychic distress that only seems to register somatically.
3 I am aware of Stef Craps's (2013, 2014) powerful critique of the application of Western trauma categories to non-Western subjects and acknowledge that Congo himself describes his experience in categories drawn from Indonesian culture (possession, haunting, being cursed) but these seem to map very closely onto the categories of trauma theory and other Western constructions of trauma.
4 For Winnicott (1953), separating out the created and found elements of the transitional object is not some impossible *ideal*, in fact quite the opposite: the power of the transitional object resides in not questioning the paradox of it being both created and found.
5 Oppenheimer (2016) argues that non-fiction films require the maker only to give the audience the facts they *need* to understand the core story. It is not necessary to tell all the facts.
6 Oppenheimer (2016) also described *The Act of Killing* as a document of a dynamic process and not simply a single snap-shot of a particular moment in time.
7 Rouch is the most direct influence on Oppenheimer, as Oppenheimer attests in numerous interviews. See, for example, Feldman (2013).
8 Oppenheimer does not appear in shot in *The Act of Killing* but is a powerful presence throughout, intervening as a disembodied voice from behind the camera.
9 A persistent criticism, from a sizeable minority of scholars, is that the film fails to adequately explore the events of 1965–66. The demand seems to be for a more conventional historical documentary despite the film never pretending to be about 1965–66 and explicitly stating that its concern is with the present-day consequences of those events (it is a film about the here-and-now). Albertina Carri's *The Blonds* (2003) has been subject to similar (misplaced) criticism (see Chapter 6). For these critics of *The Act of Killing*, see Fraser (2013 & 2014); Rayns (2013); Tyson (2014); Beckett (2014); Godmilow (2014); Wandita (2014); Critical Asian Studies (2014); Meneghetti (2016).

10 An assumption confirmed by Oppenheimer in several interviews (see, for example, Cohn 2012).
11 In an interview with Amy Goodman (2013), Oppenheimer revealed that the first visit to the roof happened on the very first day Oppenheimer met Congo and the second visit (which was one of the last scenes to be shot) occurred five years later.
12 This is Slavoj Žižek's (2013) reading of *The Act of Killing* (which I explore below in conjunction with Thomas Wartenberg's reading of the re-enactments of the film-within-the-film).
13 Compare another guilty, traumatised protagonist, Lady Macbeth in *Macbeth*: 'Out, damn'd spot! out, I say!'
14 As Oppenheimer allows the Indonesian killers to do (quotation from *The Act of Killing*'s opening on-screen texts).
15 I am referencing Polonius's method for flushing out the truth, which he describes in *Hamlet* Act II Scene I: 'Your bait of falsehood takes this carp of truth; / And thus do we of wisdom and of reach, / With windlasses and with assays of bias, / By indirections find directions out'.
16 Congo is not the first documentary protagonist to be surprised by the destabilising intensity of the experience of re-enacting. In Werner Herzog's film *Little Dieter Needs to Fly* (1997), principal protagonist Dieter Dengler returns to Laos to recreate his capture by the Pathet Lao. As his arms are tied, Dieter is terrified and says 'Uh, oh, this feels a little bit too close to home.'
17 In screen time, Congo returns four minutes after the torture scene. In the real time of the production schedule, we are not sure whether days or months have elapsed.
18 Guattari does also recognise "autochthonic" affect when he cites Daniel Stern's work on 'shareable' (i.e. transitivist) and 'non-shareable' (i.e. autochthonic) affects.
19 I am referring in particular here to post-structuralist 'affect theory' and the so-called affective turn in the humanities in the mid-1990s, conventionally traced back to the publication of an essay by Eve Kosofsky Sedgwick and Adam Frank (1995b) called 'Shame in the Cybernetic Fold: Reading Silvan Tomkins' (see also, 1995a) but prefigured in earlier work by Lawrence Grossberg (1980), Vivian Sobchack, Linda Williams and Steven Shaviro (1993) in the fields of music and film, and also deeply influenced by Deleuze and Guattari's *A Thousand Plateaus* (1988 [1980]) and Brian Massumi's gloss of their work for an anglophone readership.
20 It also stands in contrast to Heidi Maibom's (2017: 24) version of affective empathy which entails an emotion which has '"an object" or "representational content". It is about something.' Affect or affective states are generally considered both to lack this content and (by some including myself) to also lack any readily identifiable object. André Green has stressed the profound difficulty in interpreting affect precisely because of its lack of a readily identifiable object (Green 2005a; especially Chapter 9: 125–64).
21 Shouse draws on the work of Massumi (for example, 1995), Deleuze and Guattari in this essay.
22 For example, in Freud's essay on *Group Psychology and the Analysis of the Ego* (1921). Introjection is *the* central concept in the work of Abraham and Török, which will be explored later in this chapter.
23 The child who is sexually abused by a parent will often desperately try to hold on to the parent as a good object and will introject the bad object – the guilt of the parent – feeling guilty themselves for somehow having asked for or provoked the unprovoked parental assault.
24 The Indonesian scholar and novelist Intan Paramaditha (2013: 44) places the scene in context for the non-Indonesian viewer: 'Aminah, a scantily clad, liver-eating woman whose sexual monstrosity is overemphasized through Herman's unruly body, reminds us of the merciless Gerwani woman who slashes a general's forehead with a razorblade in *Pengkhianatan*.'

25 This opening part of the sequence is in the director's cut *only* but the essentials of the scene are the same in both cuts of *The Act of Killing*.
26 Freud's comments in *Mourning and Melancholia* anticipate his articulation of the tripartite division of the psyche in 1923, where he formally introduces the idea of the super-ego (and indeed the id).
27 One could characterise this moment in this scene as *another* role reversal in which Oppenheimer takes the place of Koto as Congo's interrogator, mirroring in the play-without the earlier interrogation scene from the play-within.
28 Hamlet in *Hamlet*: Act III Scene II: 'If his occulted guilt / Do not itself unkennel in one speech, / It is a damnèd ghost that we have seen, / And my imaginations are as foul / As Vulcan's stithy'.
29 Here (following Freud 1917a) my argument is about the super-ego. I will amend this a little when I look at Abraham and Török's work on the 'crypt', where it is the ego that does the taking-in and the focus is on shame rather than guilt.
30 Koch is using metalepsis in Gérard Genette's sense of 'any intrusion by the extradiegetic narrator or narratee into the diegetic universe (or by diegetic characters into a metadiegetic universe, etc.) or the inverse' (Genette 1980: 234–5).
31 These critics include Fraser (2013); Crichlow (2013); Tyson (2014); Meneghetti (2016).
32 In an earlier scene from the film-within, Congo has dramatised this recurrent nightmare.
33 In the theatrical cut of the film (not the director's cut).
34 Congo's body is 'performing the drama of stupefaction' (Walker 2013: 16).
35 In an early scene in the film, Zulkadry accuses a journalist (Saoduon Siregar) of dissembling and pretending he saw nothing during the murders of 1965–66 even though his office was next to a room in which scores of killings took place. Zulkadry says to Oppenheimer: 'I'm not calling him a liar, Joshua. But this man, a journalist, distancing himself from these things … That's predictable. But logically something we didn't hide, how could he not know? Even the neighbours knew! Hundreds were killed. It was an open secret.'
36 Here, I am distinguishing between super-ego and ego ideal, or between what Otto Fenichel and Sándor Radó describe as two facets of the super-ego, that is between its self-punishing aspect (guilt), and its self-protective aspect (shame), which if threatened inflicts a narcissistic wound (Fenichel 1928: 47–70; Radó 1928: 420–38; Fenichel 1946: 399).
37 As if he is "possessed".
38 Abraham and Török were highly critical of the confusing and imprecise way in which the term introjection had been deployed by Freud, Klein and others (and the random interchanging of the terms introjection and incorporation), leading Török to exclaim: 'the term "introjection" has undergone so many variations in meaning that its mere mention is enough to arouse in me the suspicion of a confused idea, not to say verbiage' (Török 1994 [1968]: 110).
39 This aspect of Abraham and Török's work has been developed by others (for example Cyrulnik 2009).
40 It is a psychoanalytic commonplace that perverse psychic structures (such as sadomasochistic structures) are notoriously persistent and impervious to attempts to shift them.
41 This appears only in the director's cut of the film.
42 Oppenheimer has said he did not *sympathise* with Congo (by which he implied that to feel sympathy would be to condone Congo's past actions) but he did *empathise* with Congo (Oppenheimer 2016).
43 Oppenheimer has spoken about the troubling nature of this relationship in several interviews but is unblinkingly honest about 'love' being at its centre. In a *Guardian* interview (one of several examples) Oppenheimer said: 'I care about him. It's hard to call our relationship a friendship […] I may not exactly like him, but I have love for him as another human being' (Barnes 2013).

44 See Silverman (2013); and, Rothberg (2009).
45 Piotrowska (2014: 9) is talking specifically about the 'type of documentary [...] in which a verbal testimony of the other is at the heart of the work' mostly involving 'a trauma and a profound loss of some kind'.
46 In terms of Bion's theory of infant development, Oppenheimer acts as the mother in her maternal reverie.
47 Of course, it also remains semi-submerged in the analytic encounter.
48 But, of course, these narratives are never "true" in a strict historical sense.
49 Or, more precisely, for Congo as a facet of the dynamic analytic pair of Congo-Oppenheimer.
50 The film draws us into a world of moral degradation and makes us, through identification, through our counter-transference, inhabit the world of the killer. I think it is this aspect of *The Act of Killing* that has led a (sizeable) minority of critics to condemn the film in the most extreme language (e.g. Fraser 2013). Jonathan Dollimore in *Radical Tragedy* (2010) makes a very similar observation about *The Revenger's Tragedy* (Thomas Middleton 2018 [1607]), which has been condemned in the most violent terms by many critics. Dollimore's explanation for all this critical bile is that the play implicates its audience in its deceptions and horrors – it makes the audience morally complicit – and some critics will not countenance being disturbed and challenged in this way.
51 Counter-transferential "feelings" that echo those described by Oppenheimer when making the film (as quoted above): 'intense feelings of guilt [...] that kind of pain just made me feel dirty, really awful' (Cooper 2013).
52 As Janet Walker (2013: 14) puts it in her essay on *The Act of Killing*: 'Body language, gestures, vocal inflection, and the "microphysiognomy" of the face are all crucial.'

Chapter 6

Albertina Carri's *The Blonds* (2003) '(like an outsider)'

First-person documentary or documentary-making as self-analysis

'I can analyze myself only with the help of self-knowledge obtained objectively (like an outsider).'
Sigmund Freud in a letter to Wilhelm Fliess, 24 November 1897
(Freud and Masson 1985)

The analyst's 'task cannot be to remember anything.
What then is his task? His task is to make out what has been forgotten from the traces which it has left behind or, more correctly, to construct it.'
Sigmund Freud *Constructions in Analysis* (1937b)

Albertina Carri's 2003 documentary *Los Rubios* (called *The Blonds* in the English-speaking world) is an autobiographical exploration of the psychic ramifications for the director of the abduction and murder of her parents in the mid-1970s when she was three years old. Like *The Act of Killing*, *The Blonds* approaches historical trauma through fictions and fictionalisations which the traumatised protagonist creates and witnesses within the diegesis. Again, I ask whether the filmmaking process – like the analytic process – can ameliorate the pain of traumatic experience, with evidence for this change gleaned from what can be witnessed within the evolving diegesis.

However, *The Blonds* differs profoundly from *The Act of Killing* in that the traumatic events in question are beyond the reach of the protagonist's memory and so have to be given both form *and* content – some representational expression even if that expression is only to define an absence – before they can become objects of reflection. The problem that confronted Carri in making her film is similar to the problem Freud explored in *Constructions in Analysis* (1937b) where a fiction must be created to take the place of the missing memory, or the problem the Botellas (Botella and Botella 2013: 96–8) pursue though their notion of dreaming the missing content of the analysand's traumatic experience in the counter-transference.

Both these approaches are predicated on the complex interactions between the traumatised protagonist and an outsider, the analyst, who dreams or constructs the fictions *for* the analysand. Carri, by contrast, must construct or dream her own

DOI: 10.4324/9781003657187-8

fictions as her documentary is autobiographical: she is both director and protagonist and (by analogy) both analyst and analysand. In *The Blonds*, Carri adopts practices similar to the self-analytic practices that Anzieu (1986 [1959 & 1975]) and others describe: finding external others and generating internal others. Carri finds external others (in the absence of a physically and psychically separate director) in members of her film crew and in an audience she imagines for her finished film. And she generates internal others – self-observing aspects of the self – in an attempt to view herself 'like an outsider' (to borrow Freud's phrase). Perhaps the closest model for Carri's radical approach in generating internal others is to be found in the literary practice of autofiction, where the author creates fictionalised versions of the self that can be viewed with at least some of the objectivity that Freud sees as a requirement of a self-analysis.[1]

In *The Blonds*, Carri deploys two sorts of fiction: animated segments that reproduce the content of childhood memories or nightmares that occurred some time after the original traumatic events; and a film about the making of a documentary about Carri's past in which Carri is played by an actress, Analía Couceyro.[2] It is through this fictionalisation of herself that Carri attempts to gain the distance necessary to view herself 'like an outsider', borrowing one of the key performative techniques of psychodrama: having one's role taken by another to make oneself visible to oneself. In what follows, I will try to describe the complex role Carri's fictionalised self plays in *The Blonds*: helping to define her traumatic past; allowing her to slough off constructions of herself and her traumatic history that have been foisted upon her by others; and implicitly providing a critique of the conventional practices of realist documentary. *The Blonds* is not merely a self-reflexive search for a meaningful and less painful accommodation with the past through the deployment of fictional films-within-the-documentary but is simultaneously a filmic argument for a new form of documentary that is capable of saying something about traumatic experience that comes without memory.

Throwing away the rule book: *kamikaze* filmmaking[3]

In 1977, Albertina Carri's parents Ana María Caruso and Roberto Carri were abducted and murdered. They were victims of Argentina's so-called "dirty war" of 1976–83, prosecuted by Argentina's right-wing military junta (after the death of Juan Perón in 1974) against left-wing guerrillas, political dissidents and anyone associated with socialist ideas or organisations. Carri's parents were targeted as vocal, revolutionary, Peronist intellectuals: her father was a well-known academic sociologist; her mother a professor of literature. Their deaths left three orphaned daughters: Albertina aged four (three at the time of the abduction) and her elder sisters, Andrea aged thirteen and Paula aged twelve. Following their parents' deaths, the girls moved from the city to a farm in the country to be raised by an aunt and uncle. Between 9,000 and 30,000 people were murdered in Argentina's dirty war, often after torture; many victims (Carri's parents included) were taken in secret abductions and so the victims came to be known as *los desaparecidos* (the disappeared).

Many of the initial reviews of *The Blonds* criticised the film for failing to adequately explain these events. It was deemed to have failed as a historical or investigative documentary of the sort that is familiar to viewers and reviewers. Shortly after its US premiere, Douglas Singleton wrote:

> It is frustrating in its inability to ever really confront the material it purports to explore—the political murder of its filmmaker Albertina Carri's leftist parents by the Argentine secret police in 1977.
>
> (Singleton 2004)

But the film never claims to be an exploration of political murder. The demand that the film should be something that it did not purport to be is a common criticism of recent documentaries that try to explore the experiential "inside" of a traumatic event.[4] It is perhaps because this form of documentary does not fit long-established preconceptions of what a documentary *is* or indeed *should be*. That *The Blonds* is criticised on these grounds is perplexing, as Carri deals with these normative demands directly within the film itself.

About a third of the way into the film, there is a scene in which Carri shoots herself and her film crew discussing a letter they had received from the state body, *The National Film and Audiovisual Arts Institute*; a body Carri hoped would fund the continuation of work on the film. Actress, Analía Couceyro, reads extracts from the letter to the others. The film is deemed to be 'worthy' but in need of 'revision' in 'a more rigorous documentary fashion', and continues:

> The story as it is shown, fictionalizes life experiences when pain can fog the interpretation of harmful facts. The main character's claim for her parents' absence conforms [*sic*] the spine of the story but it requires a more accurate search for "proper documents", like the participation of your parents' comrades, in agreement or not. Roberto Carri and Ana María Caruso were two committed intellectuals in the 1970s. This project deserves to be made.

But Carri is adamant that the film the film institute wants and expects is not her project: 'They need it. I understand that. It's not my place to do it or I don't want to.'[5]

So, what is Carri's project? Very broadly, it is an exploration of the impact on Albertina Carri of the murder of her parents. It is only about the murders themselves to the extent that those events have affected her. *The National Film and Audiovisual Arts Institute* suggests that Carri's *pain* has *fogged* her ability to interpret the historical facts. But Carri's subject is the *pain* and is the *fog*, and not the historical facts *per se*. Fictionalising life experiences is Carri's route to try to understand the pain and fog. Carri said in a 'Director's Statement' that accompanied the film's release, my aim

> was not understood by any fund or producer that read my project. History, for them, lies in my parents' "disappearance" and not in my constitution as a person starting from an absence.
>
> (Women Make Movies Release 2004: 7)[6]

Carri's statement captures the film's vastly ambitious quest: to find out how Carri has come to be who she is in the wake, not of two political murders, but in the shadow of an absence; an absence that *The Blonds* attempts to define. The film is an exploration of the inside of a traumatic event as that event has echoed through the filmmaker's life. As Kerry Bystrom argues (2009: 35), *The Blonds* is an attempt to 'wrest politicized narratives from the public sphere and locate them within the private one'. Politicised narratives are disrupted by this private perspective, challenging long-cherished views, such as the left-liberal vision of Carri's parents' generation as heroes. From Carri's private perspective, she was abandoned by her parents for a political cause, and this generates anger as much as admiration. The film is Carri's attempt to describe to herself and to an audience what it is to be Albertina Carri, the daughter of "disappeared" parents; an ontological quest for what constitutes her as a person.

In pursuit of this nebulous quarry, the overall structure of *The Blonds* is both reflexive and self-reflexive. We see protagonists in the documentary viewing on screen other protagonists who have been recorded at an earlier point in the production and we see Carri herself as a character in the film, not as a documentary interviewee but directing the crew making the documentary. Throughout the film, the crew including Carri are shot on one camera – often in black and white – whilst a second camera – often shooting in colour – records the more standard documentary material (but with the twist that the principal documentary protagonist has been replaced by an actress). This reflexivity led Diego Papic and Jorge Bernárdez to describe the film as 'un meta-documental' (quoted in Page 2009: 168) and Gabriella Nouzeilles (2005: 269) to describe it as 'a self-referential documentary about a "failed" documentary, in which the trace of the real corresponds to the process of making and assembling the film'. For the director, the filmmaking process is a dynamic, meaning-seeking process unfolding over time; a process that viewers of the film can witness in the film as edited.

Within this unconventional structure, fictions or fictionalisations are key. There are two fictional plays-within: one "spoken", the other "dumb", in an intentional or unintentional echo of the two plays staged by the players under Hamlet's direction. The dumb play is broken into several, discontinuous scenes scattered throughout the film and uses Playmobil figures, buildings and accessories[7] to produce stop-motion animated scenes from Carri's childhood: some historically "real"; some of childhood fantasies. The scenes are without dialogue but use sound effects and music. The spoken play-within constitutes much of the screen time of *The Blonds*. Rather than film herself investigating her own past, Carri casts actress Analía Couceyro to play Albertina Carri making a documentary about her traumatic past. As Couceyro announces near the start of the film: 'My name is Analía Couceyro. I'm an actress and in this film. I play the part of Albertina Carri.' Couceyro is seen reviewing taped interviews before editing, setting up film shoots, interviewing old comrades of Roberto Carri and Ana María Caruso, etc. Analía Couceyro is not a conventional autobiographical double – a character who might re-enact scenes from the director's past – rather she plays the director in the present making the very documentary Carri herself is making. With the exception of one scene (where Carri conducts an interview in a suburb of Buenos Aires where her parents last lived) Albertina Carri only appears in the film as the director of *The Blonds* (itself of course a documentary) whilst Couceyro plays the part of "Albertina Carri" making a documentary about Albertina Carri's traumatic past. The scenes with Couceyro making the documentary could even be viewed as a *play-within-the-play-within-the-play.* The film as a whole is structured like a nest of *Matryoshka* dolls.

A. O. Scott, in a *New York Times* review, captures this complexity:

> It is not so much a documentary as a fictional film about the making of a documentary, or perhaps a documentary about the making of a fictional film about the making of a documentary.
>
> (Scott 2004)

Although one struggles to describe the complex structure of the film, it is certainly a film where the director has gone to enormous lengths to conduct a self-exploration and a self-analysis which has the perspective of the 'outsider': to produce a self that can look at the self; to have the self embodied in a double who mirrors and fails to mirror the self. There is the unseen, non-celluloid Albertina Carri whom we know to be the director of *The Blonds* who was responsible for the final cut of the film and its promotion, there is the Albertina Carri we see in the film playing "Albertina Carri" the character in *The Blonds* who directs the framing film and the films-within, and there is Analía Couceyro whom we see in the spoken film-within, playing the character "Albertina Carri" who is directing a documentary about Albertina Carri. Hamlet's own account (Act III Scene II) of the plays he "directed" seems pertinent here: 'Marry, this is miching malicho. It means mischief.'

The mischief runs throughout the film, not just in its formal structure. It is, in Joanna Page's words (2009: 167), 'an experimental and often ludic reflection on the loss of the director's parents'. The film is peppered with tiny visual clues (half-hidden signifiers) and embedded intertextual references – easy to miss on a first viewing – that serve as comments on the film's structure and style, or on Carri's psychological state or ambitions in making the film. One of these is a film poster for John Waters's cult movie, *Cecil B. Demented* (2000), seen fleetingly and unremarked (but frequently) in the background of shots of Analía Couceyro playing Carri in her production office and makeshift editing suite for *The Blonds*. The poster is never featured – there is no cut away – and only sections of the poster can be seen in any one shot. But, in its persistent inclusion, Carri is signalling her intention to throw away the documentary rulebook, just as the anarchic, self-styled movie-makers the 'SprocketHoles' and their unstable leader, Cecil B. Demented (aka Sinclair), do with the Hollywood rulebook in Waters's film. Janis Breckenridge, in an article on the performance of memory and identity in *The Blonds*, makes much of the parallel with *Cecil B Demented*, arguing that Carri takes similar liberties to those taken by Waters with her chosen genre, overthrowing the 'almost suffocating tradition of high seriousness' typical of "trauma" documentaries. But there is a deep seriousness behind the levity:

> As the film advances, it seemingly runs adrift with what might at first appear to be poor filming techniques, random juxtapositions or disjunctures and unwarranted fragmentations; however, the cumulative effect of these cinematic strategies proves these ruptures to be both intentional and revealing.
>
> (Breckenridge 2008: 13)

Carri's ambitions perhaps match those of the fictional director Sinclair (Cecil B. Demented) in Waters's film, who declares: 'I've had a vision. And that vision is called ultimate reality.' For Carri, that 'ultimate reality' is the psychic reality of trauma. Carri and her documentary crew (whom we see and hear many times in the film) are a tight-knit and committed group of friends and collaborators who, like the SprocketHoles, work with and for a strong-willed and determined director and break many of the rules of filmmaking.[8]

The Blonds as vacuum: the limitations of memory and conventional documentary technique

For much of the film, Carri uses her double to define what belongs to Carri or what is meaningful to Carri and what is not. Conventional documentary techniques and practices – of the sort demanded by *The National Film and Audiovisual Arts Institute* – are not excluded from *The Blonds* but are often set up and presented in such a way as to demonstrate their failure. Their failure to move the Albertina Carri we see in the diegesis closer to her nebulous quarry (to comprehending her trauma) through their failure to have any meaningful or affective impact on her double. The double expresses to us (as viewers of *The Blonds*), and more crucially to Carri as a character within the diegesis (as an inner Winnicottian viewer), the failure of these conventional devices.

In two scenes – shot in the back of a taxi and in the production office – Analía Couceyro examines old photographs of the Carri family. Couceyro flicks through the pages of a photo album in the cab or shuffles individual prints on her desk in a desultory fashion, as if looking for something that is not there. Often, in more conventional documentaries about traumatic pasts, family photographs are used to create poignant and affecting moments, as viewers are invited to see – and to feel – the loss that the protagonist has suffered: moments when the photograph of those once alive is able to suspend us, according to Roland Barthes (1984: 79), between life and death; or to allow us to identify with the protagonist (after all we all have family photos) across national, ethnic and other barriers of difference, as Marianne Hirsch claims (1997: 252). In these two scenes in *The Blonds,* there is no attempt to elicit any affective connection or response in the audience, and Couceyro under Carri's direction as Carri's double, remains impassive, so defamiliarising these conventional archive objects, distancing the audience from what they are seeing.

Conventional documentary interviews are treated in an even more alienated, arm's-length fashion. The earnest words and reminiscences of old friends and comrades of Carri's parents are shown without introduction and without naming the interviewee. The interviews do not even appear full-screen but are presented as elements of scenes in which Couceyro is dispassionately reviewing VHS tapes of "her" rushes on a poor-quality monitor in the production office; sometimes she is not even looking at the screen or finds what the interviewees are saying mildly amusing. When Couceyro does interview an old colleague of Carri's parents on one occasion, she shows little interest. Kerry Bystrom (2009: 43) sees this as an attempt to 'downplay [...] testimony's usual claim to unmediated truth'. I think Bystrom is right but these scenes are also a demonstration of the lack of connection Carri feels to other people's memories, alien memories, and she expresses this through her double. However significant these memories are for the interviewee, they are not Carri's memories. And through the double's lack of interest in the heroic stories of her parents' "comrades in arms", Carri is beginning to be able to *act out* (by proxy) her anger with her parents for deserting her in the name of a political cause. It is an anger that Carri does not (or is not able to) express "as herself", torn between loving her parents and feeling deserted by them. In the early scenes of the film, this anger is expressed obliquely through the double's cool, lack of interest in conventionally affecting encounters and objects. Later, Carri finds ways to use Couceyro to express – to enact – her anger more explicitly.

Perhaps the strangest of these affectless interactions with the past through conventional – and what should, by convention, be affecting – documentary material, is enacted near the beginning of the film. Analía Couceyro sits and reads aloud from a book whose title we can just make out on the cover as *Isidro Velázquez*. It is read in a monotone. The text is a piece of utopian, revolutionary prose. In Couceyro's rendition of the text, and in its placement in the structure of the film without context or provenance, it is reduced to gobbledygook. It is a perplexing and alienating experience for the viewer: we have no idea why we are hearing these words; we have no idea who Isidro Velázquez is or was; and we cannot see from the cover of the book who the author of this biography might be.[9] Much later in the film, this same book appears in a shot of Couceyro's production office but again the author of the text is not legible. A little research reveals that the book was written by Carri's father, Roberto. Our genre expectations when presented with a work by a much-loved, murdered father would be, at the very least, for a poignant moment of connection, communicated through the reactions of the reader or perhaps through music or other filmic technique. Carri eschews these conventions, all but burying the significance of the book and its author. A.O. Scott felt it is in moments like this one, where Carri's film fails:

> The film's open-ended, recursive structure is central to Ms. Carri's intellectual agenda, which is to emphasize the deceptive, indeterminate nature of the truth. It is sometimes hard to tell, though, whether she wants to explore the ways that individual and collective psychology contrive to blur and distort painful or shameful aspects of the political past, or whether her concern is with the grander, more abstract and ultimately more banal tendency of any representation to falsify what it tries to depict. Too much of the film is in a mood of chin-scratching detachment, and this creates a vacuum in which its powerful, confrontational moments lose their force, the trauma of the past pushed nearly out of reach.
>
> (Scott 2004)[10]

On first watching *The Blonds*, my reaction was similar to Scott's. I found the film frustrating, even irritating, like an overly ambitious student production. In subsequent viewings, I questioned my transference/counter-transference onto the filmic object, as my initial feelings of frustration and irritation intensified into an almost unbearable sense of desperation; an excruciating sense of trying to reach something that keeps receding as it is approached. Catharsis is withheld. Reflecting on my counter-transference, I now think that Scott's description of the film is acute but I no longer share his negative gloss. That 'the trauma of the past' is 'pushed nearly out of reach' seems to reflect Carri's experience of her trauma. Through her fictionalised double, Carri provides the viewer with a representation of how *she* experiences her traumatic past. And Carri herself – the Carri we see in the film (Albertina Carri playing "Albertina Carri") – does not behave as we expect victims of trauma to behave in documentary films: either emotionally broken down or breaking down under the gaze of the camera and the act of representing the trauma in words. The irony, the humour, the intellectual distance that are evident in *The Blonds* are indeed markers of the distance Carri feels from the traumatic event in her life; for her to pretend otherwise would be dishonest and so at times she finds it difficult to take her own plight seriously. But the vacuum that Scott identifies – a vacuum that undermines 'powerful, confrontational moments' – is not a vacuum of failed filmic representation and failure to establish affective connections but rather Carri's filmic representation of the ontological vacuum that she has described as her 'constitution as a person starting from an absence'. This filmic representation is created in the performance of her double, Couceyro, in the fictional documentary-within-the-documentary and is available both to us as the extra-diegetic audience and to Carri herself within the diegesis. In her attempt to view herself 'like an outsider' – as Freud advocated for the successful practice of self-analysis – Carri seems to view herself like Camus's outsider, Meursault: alienated from her own experience.[11] But unlike the psychopathic Meursault, the alienation Carri feels and her double enacts is deeply painful, frustrating, even excruciating and is available in the intensely similar feelings the film generates in the viewer (or in this viewer).

The sense of alienation and disconnection that pervades much of the documentary is hinted at in the very name of the film, *The Blonds*. The title refers to an outsider's memory of the Carri family; not merely an alien memory with which Albertina Carri cannot engage but a demonstrably false memory. Whilst filming in the neighbourhood where Albertina, her sisters and her parents lived before the parents' abduction, an interview is conducted with the Carris's old neighbour, an elderly woman with jet-black hair. She says she remembers the family well and that they all were blond: 'The girls were blondes. The father was blond, the mother was blonde. All blonds.'[12] Photographs we see of the family, the physical presence in the film of Albertina and the testimony of Albertina's aunt Andrea, all confirm the inaccuracy of the neighbour's memory; the Carris had dark hair. Naming the film *The Blonds* is a powerful indication that the film as a whole has been conceived as an exploration of the fickleness, the falsity and the impossibility of memory.

There is a political dimension to this misremembering. It suggests that the family were viewed as middle-class interlopers in the working-class *barrio* of La Matanza in Buenos Aires where they lived in the mid-1970s. At that time, middle-class Argentinians were frequently blond whilst their poorer compatriots were frequently dark-haired. The neighbour's inaccurate memory is an accurate recollection that the Carris were viewed with suspicion and as outsiders by others in the *barrio*. Much can be made of the politics of this misremembering[13] but here I am more interested in the psychic dimension for Carri and how she treats the misremembering in the film-within. In a later scene in *The Blonds*, Couceyro is taken by Albertina Carri to buy a blonde wig which the director has Couveyro wear in almost all the subsequent scenes in the film. The wig becomes an icon of the impossibility of memory, of the trap of being defined by other's memories. In forcing her double to wear the wig, Couceyro becomes the *not-Carri* double (alongside her role as the Carri double or mirror). The *not-Carri* double is a receptacle for – or an embodiment of – the false or alien memories of others, carrying off elements that are not "Carri" so she can find what really belongs to her.

The double in film, literature or in psychoanalytic theory has played many roles. Which of these does Couceyro most resemble? She is never the traumatising, frightening double we know from literature or from the film *The Student of Prague* (Wegener and Rye, German Empire, 1913) that Otto Rank writes about in *Der Doppelgänger* (1971 [1914]): in fact she is neither of the doubles Rank articulated over his career – neither a narcissistic, morbid manifestation of self-love nor a harbinger of death. She is neither the uncanny, disturbing double of Freud's essay *Das Unheimliche* (*The Uncanny*) (1919b), nor the herald of madness and breakdown that marked the appearance of the clerk's *Doppelgänger* in Dostoevsky's *The Double* (2005), nor the traumatising double that Anwar Congo devises and encounters in the form of his own headless corpse in *The Act of Killing*. And for most of the film, Couceyro is not the double of psychodrama who takes the original participant's place and attempts to make conscious, under-expressed material in an earlier performance by the original participant (although she does perform this role later on in *The Blonds*). Couceyro is so closely directed and coached that she is closer to being the "mirror" of psychodrama, who re-enacts the scene the original participant has just devised.

In wearing the wig, Couceyro most closely resembles Honey Whitlock, whose giant image dominates the poster for John Waters's film *Cecil B Demented* that we catch so many fleeting glimpses of on the production office wall in *The Blonds*. In this image, we see Honey Whitlock (played by Melanie Griffith) bound to a chair and gagged, with the director character, Cecil B Demented (played by Stephen Dorff) holding a gun to her head. In Waters's film, Whitlock is a Hollywood star who has been kidnapped by Demented and the SprocketHoles and is coerced into playing the lead in their *kamikaze* movie. Couceyro plays a very similar role in *The Blonds* in as much as she is very closely and minutely directed and allowed very little agency. To underscore the idea that Analía Couceyro *is* Honey Whitlock, Carri provides the viewer with a brief but wonderfully comic moment in the production office when Couceyro passes the *Cecil B Demented* poster and comes between the camera and the poster. From the camera's point of view, Couceyro's head and body completely mask the poster image of Honey Whitlock's head and body, leaving us with the indelible image of the director, Cecil B. Demented, holding a gun to Couceyro's head.

Crucial to the parallel Carri is drawing between Waters's film and *The Blonds*, is that the Honey Whitlock we see on the poster is red-headed and is depicted just before the moment in Waters's film when she is forcibly "peroxided" by the SprocketHoles; for the rest of the film Whitlock is *very* blonde. Couceyro suffers the same fate in Carri's film; forced to wear a blonde wig as a sign of her subjugation to the will of others. Of course, as with all doubles, they are both mirror and inverse, and highly unstable – which is the "original", which is the double? – and so Honey Whitlock is both Analía Couceyro *and* Albertina Carri. Whitlock is the creature and creation of others, forced to play a role that is not really "her".[14] That is Couceyro's relation to Carri but it also mirrors Carri's predicament; kidnapped by her past and then forced to play a role that others define. The recollections of others seem to conspire to tell her what her past is: *The National Film and Audiovisual Arts Institute* wants to foist on to her other people's memories of her parents and their place in a heroic struggle that the *Institute* defines; old neighbours insist she and her sisters and her parents were blond. This same violence is replicated in some of the academic work on *The Blonds*, where Carri is conscripted to agendas that are not hers – kidnapped by other people's agendas. At this juncture in my argument, Carri has at least managed to foist the *not-Carri* blondness onto her double, Analía Couceyro, who plays the forcibly peroxided Honey Whitlock whilst Carri plays the role of Cecil B Demented. It is part of the process of trying to slough off the *adiaphora*, so Carri can find the core of her very personal trauma. Kerry Bystrom (2009: 42) argues that *The Blonds* focuses on 'the appearance of the subject' and 'the power that narratives framed by others have to shape the self'. But this is not something Carri meekly accepts, rather she tenaciously resists these powerful narratives. Through the fictional device of a double, Carri is able to observe herself as she is in the narratives other people have constructed for her. She is able to watch these "fictions" play out within the diegesis and respond to them.

A harsh reading of Carri's deployment of her double might suggest an element of the narcissism that Otto Rank detected. Carri will not release her double to confront and disturb her – to be fully "other" and to face her 'like an outsider' – and so defuses the potential power of the double; a manifestation of the more general danger of solipsism that always haunts the self-analysis or autobiographical documentary. An alternative reading is that Carri uses the double to try to define what Albertina Carri *is* and what Albertina Carri *isn't*, in an attempt to fill in – or rather to define the edges and borders of – the constitutional absence at her core. In a scene late in *The Blonds*, Carri uses her double to be "Carri" rather than to be the *not-Carri* who wears the blond wig. Couceyro (without the wig for this scene) is very closely coached and directed, Carri telling Couceyro between takes in minute detail how she should play the part and deliver the lines. I found the scene low key and touching, as the things that Carri *knows* to be Carri's are so slight, particular and inconsequential: 'I hate ladybugs, shooting stars, train tracks, going under bridges, flocks of birds, I hate the way your eyelashes fall out…'. This list seems to go to the heart of Carri's existential problem: an aching sense of loss and very little of her own to fill the void. It could be argued that all of Carri's "hates" are items or events which conventionally permit one to make a wish. This modifies my reading: less a case of owning very little and more a case of hating any mechanism that allows a wish, as to wish is to hope and Carri knows these hopes will be dashed. Either reading exposes an aching desire that cannot be met. Even this list of things that Carri either knows to be hers or permit her to make futile, painful wishes is thrown into question by the words the sound recordist utters before the first take (as she "marks" the DAT sound tape with a verbal reference point for the edit):

'Fiction… We are shooting a fiction. Today is […] July seventh 2002'. And as Couceyro's recital of this short list of Carri's "hates" moves on, we are soon drawn back towards the core of the trauma:

> and especially I hate candles […] having to make a wish at your birthday, blowing the candles, because I spent many birthdays wishing the same wish: that my mom would come back, that my dad would come back, that they'd come back soon. And it still happens to me, I blow out birthday candles and I can't help wishing my mom and my dad would come back soon. Actually, it was just one wish but I make it into three wishes, so my wish becomes stronger.

As Couceyro finishes, Carri – who we have seen in shot throughout this scene smiling gently as she looks through the camera's viewfinder and silently mouthing the words Couceyro is speaking – says in a very quiet voice 'Very good…Cut.' This scene seems to touch Carri more than many others in the film. Here in the spoken play-within with Couceyro as her double, Carri's trauma seems to gain some affective content; her desperate desire to be reconnected with her parents.[15]

Carri has used her double to filter out the false and alien memories of others, but what of her *own* memories of her parents and of their disappearance? It seems she remembers very little. The list of hates is an attempt to define something that is definitively hers. When she does reach back to the few memories she has of her parents, she is not sure if they really are her own. In a scene outside a suburban house in Buenos Aires, Couceyro as Carri tells us:

> This was our last house. I lived here with my parents and my sisters [...] I was three so I don't remember much. [...] I don't know if some of my memories are real or they're my sisters'.

The central problem remains. Carri is unsure whether she really remembers anything at all of her parents. As the fiction writer Carlos Gamerro observes in his essay 'Remembering without Memories' (2013: 113), Carri's investigation 'achieves nothing more than making absence present'.[16] And this absence – this void of memory – is a profound existential problem for Carri and a problem for the film (as Carri tells us through Couceyro):

> I have to think of something. Something that will be a movie. All I have are vague memories contaminated by so many versions. Whatever I do to get to the truth, will probably take me further away.

It is in this context that one needs to view the *avant garde* devices and *kamikaze* techniques that Carri deploys in *The Blonds*. They are not superficial, tricksy, stylistic choices but baits of falsehood: traps that Carri sets in a desperate effort to take a carp of truth, to try to find something meaningful in the absence at the centre of her life (and, by extension, at the centre of her film).

Glimmerings of meaning: circling the vacuum

It is one of these *avant garde* devices that begins to reveal the first glimmerings of memories that Carri seems to securely own. Carri employs stop-motion animation of Playmobil figures – in what I am describing as the "dumb" play-within – to try to recreate the world of her childhood both in fact ("real" memories of events) and in fantasy.[17] The memories and fantasies that we see in the animated film-within are not her memories of her parents or of their disappearance but memories of how in childhood Carri tried to deal with their absence.

The importance of this device is established at once, as it is a scene from the dumb play that opens the film. We see a Playmobil house lit from within and beyond the house, and dimly lit, a garden, cows (with mooing on the soundtrack), horses and farm equipment. As the camera pans from the garden towards the house, we hear a voice (a voice that we will learn is Carri's as the film progresses) calling out: 'Make sure I'm not in frame', with this directorial intervention layered over the artificially created sounds of a farm at night (the sounds have been laid on in post-production but give the impression of diegetic sound recorded on *this* farm at night). Over these pictures and soundtrack, we then hear an intimate, close exchange between two female voices in which one instructs the other (a young woman or a girl?) in the art of riding a horse: 'She's a good horse. Do you want to mount her?', etc. This exchange would suggest that the dumb play is not so dumb. But in the very last scene of the film – live-action footage shot on the farm where Albertina Carri grew up – we realise that this verbal exchange takes place between Carri and Couceyro as Carri teaches Couceyro how to ride. It is an exchange from the filmic present of the end of the film and not the reproduction of spoken dialogue from a filmic "past".

What is established in this opening scene are three ideas, which will run throughout the film (and they are established with great economy).[18] This is not a conventional documentary (it employs stop-motion animation). The farm of Carri's aunt and uncle where she spent her childhood is a happy and loving place. The film will be highly self-conscious, as Carri's directorial instruction ('Make sure I'm not in frame') breaks the fourth wall of documentary practice, revealing the constructedness of the film in an act of Brechtian estrangement (*Verfremdungseffekt*).

As the film progresses, we see several more Playmobil scenes set on the farm where Carri grew up: most are happy family scenes, with people partying and having fun. My initial reaction to these scenes was one of confusion, as it confounded my expectation of how Albertina Carri *should* feel after the loss of her parents. How could these scenes of idyllic family life come in the wake of their disappearances? The scenes feel pre- not post-lapsarian. Later in the film, over live-action shots of the farm, Couceyro provides the explanation. The family remained in the city for some time after the disappearance of Ana María Caruso and Roberto Carri and the children continued to receive occasional letters from their parents. When the letters stopped, Albertina and her sisters, Andrea and Paula, moved to their aunt and uncle's farm in the country. Couceyro tells us in voice-over:

> Andrea was fourteen. Paula thirteen. It was a huge cultural and social shock for them. I was five and I fell in love with the horses, the cows, with my uncle Federico and with getting up early [...] My sisters were very depressed when we moved here but I enjoyed being a spoiled child.

Carri's age at the time of the "disappearances" emerges as a key factor in her experience of the loss. Her elder sisters had no difficulty in remembering their parents. They were old enough to have secure and indelible memories, and their reaction to the disappearances was the essentially adult response of depression. Albertina Carri was so young at the time her parents disappeared forever – too young to have securely laid down memories – that by the time she was five and living on the farm, her parents had receded almost entirely from conscious memory.

In the scene that follows directly after the one in which we hear of the sisters' depression and Albertina's happiness on the farm, we see Couceyro in the production office – her desk covered in family photos and Playmobil figures – and are told in voice-over:

The farm was a land of fantasy, where all my memories begin.

I would see my parents arriving by car, by bus, on horseback.

The edge or the border of the constitutional absence at the core of Carri's adult life is beginning to gain some definition. A shape is being defined but a shape without any representational or narrative content. What content the loss appears to have is supplied by others – as Carri hears other people's recollections of her absent parents – and these recollections were then reshaped by the little girl Albertina in her world of fantasy and play. The dumb play is the vehicle Carri devises to unpick this complicated world of fantasy and "memory". The Playmobil figures – whether the young Albertina Carri actually played with these particular toys or not – connect her and her audience back to Carri's childhood world; "childish" vehicles for recollections of childhood. In a literal sense, Carri has adopted a technique that both Klein and Winnicott used in their analysis of children. It is an attempt to unearth something of a trauma that has evaded representation but that might emerge in games with dolls, and teddy bears and pieces of string. More broadly, these scenes are Carri's Winnicottian potential space or play space where fragments of childhood memory and fantasy can be given form and become objects of contemplation for Carri as an 'outsider'. The scenes from the Playmobil play-within are at once both memory and fantasy, history and fiction. Carri's memory reaches its limits in her recollections of her childhood on the farm long after her parents disappeared. To replace the "missing" memories of her early childhood and her "real" parents, fantasy took over. But the fantasy is of course also a version of the historical "real"; her later childhood fantasies about her parents are not memories of the once real and later murdered parents, but they are the "real" of Carri's childhood world where she constructed fantasies about her "forgotten" parents: real memories of childhood fantasies; historically real fictions constructed in childhood to take the place of what was missing. They have the status of what Heidegger called the 'factical' (1962 [1927]) and are a version of reality that Castoriadis was pursuing when he wrote: 'I want to see what being is, what reality is. Now, here is my memory of my dream last night' (1997: 5).

This recollected fantasy world – developed amidst her ostensibly happy childhood life on the farm – was a confusing and perplexing one. Couceyro tells us in voice-over:

> First they told me they were working in another country. At that age I thought "working" meant being a doctor or a lawyer. But they told me my mother had a degree in literature and my father was a sociologist and journalist, which seemed suspicious. When I was twelve they tried to tell me about good guys and bad guys, the Peronists, the workers, the Army, the Montoneros. I didn't understand a word of what they said. What I remember, is I started thinking about guns, shoot outs and heroes.

The scene encapsulates the "problem" of memory – the void – that Carri faces. The child Carri filled the void with representational, narrative memories that were other people's memories she had picked up second-hand and in a garbled form, and then re-worked in fantasy and play. Her parents cease to be academics and writers and are re-worked as the eponymous hero of her father's book *Isidro Velázquez:* Robin-Hood figures and outlaws, shooting it out with the police.[19] But the void of memory is not, I think, the void that is familiar from much writing on trauma – the absence of memory as a consequence of the trauma – rather it is a developmental issue: at only three years old when her parents disappeared, Carri retains no narrative, representational memories of her parents. It is an example of what Freud describes as *infantile amnesia* that begins at the end of the Oedipal stage. By the time Carri arrived on the farm, tangible memories of her parents are likely to have succumbed to this amnesia. As Freud put it: 'The majority of experiences and mental impulses before the start of the latency period now fall victim to infantile amnesia – the forgetting [...] which veils our earliest youth from us and makes us strangers to it' (1917b: 326). Carri, herself, confirms this when she tells us 'all my memories begin' with the family's arrival on the farm when she is five. By then it was almost half her lifetime ago since her parents disappeared.

The developmental issue comes sharply into focus in the only sinister fantasy of the dumb play. In reaching back to her childhood construction of her parents' abduction, Carri creates a Playmobil scene in which a spaceship hovers over an isolated country road and captures one figure and then another (her parents we assume) and takes them into the ship. The ship then flies off into the night sky. A little later, three female Playmobil figures are seen on the same isolated road (Albertina and her sisters we assume) as if searching, but the two abducted figures are nowhere to be seen; they are gone forever. This Playmobil scene seems to be a recreation of Carri's childhood attempts to represent and understand the loss of her parents. For me, it has the feel of a traumatic reworking of the *fort-da* game that Freud's grandson played (throwing away a cotton reel and then retrieving it by pulling on a string) as he negotiated the transition from unsymbolised maternal non-existence to symbolised maternal absence and entered the temporal, spatial and representational world: the world of memory; the world of "self" and "other".

Aged three at the time of her parents' abduction, Albertina Carri was much older than Freud's infant grandson when Freud observed his game, and so would doubtless already have negotiated this transition in her own way. This is not a speculation on my part about Carri's *actual* childhood: I have no knowledge of Carri's childhood beyond what I see and hear on screen in *The Blonds*. Instead, it is a generic comment about a developmental stage that Carri *must* have passed through before the age of three *if* we accept that Freud's account of his grandson's game is a particular instance of a universal phenomenon. In whatever way the infant Carri had negotiated the transition, the negotiation would have been broken or traumatically undone by the disappearance of her parents. Rather than being able to hold on to an old, comforting symbolisation of temporary absence constructed in infancy, the three-year-old Carri was brutally (re-)confronted with endless, permanent absence (loss).[20] When the little Albertina shouted 'da' and pulled on the string, there would be no reel on the other end, the string limp and without agency. We can surmise from *The Blonds* that Carri tried to symbolise this absence later in childhood by playing with ideas of alien abductions but these abductions were in themselves traumatising as they were *one-way* only (in her scenario the "reel" has flown away into outer space and however many times she shouts 'da' or makes birthday wishes whilst blowing out candles, her parents did not come back). The adult Carri tells us she is predicated on, constituted by, an absence. And that absence for Carri, given her age at the time of the abductions, had no secure representational content; it was destined to become a gaping, formless hole. The alien abduction scene feels like an *ex post facto* symbolisation of an inescapable traumatic loss and so is quite unlike Ernst's symbolisation, which helped him to gradually spiral out of and away from the originary trauma. Carri's symbolisation fixed the absence as a permanent reality, as she spiralled back into the originary trauma.

If the Playmobil "dumb" play-within allows Carri to move closer in time to the traumatic loss of her parents by allowing her to represent her childhood responses to the loss, it is through the spoken play-within that the unrepresented trauma is able to find affective expression. Later on in the film, there is a scene shot on the farm near a wood, in which Couceyro screams, unrestrained and in anguish, whilst the camera either focuses on Couceyro or spins round and round in the wood, dizzying the viewer. In voice-over, Couceyro as Carri tells us:

> It's hard for me to understand my mother's decision. I've often asked myself why she never left the country. Sometimes I wonder why she left me here in the world of the living. And when I ask myself, I feel enraged.

Gonzalo Aguilar (2008, 2011), in his book on new Argentinian cinema, locates Carri's anger within a larger and recent tendency in Argentinian film- and documentary-making, to question the formerly unquestioned acceptance of the political rightness of the revolutionary left of the 1970s and 1980s. As Aguilar says of Carri's parents' generation: 'By committing the whole of their lives to political militancy, they dragged along their children, who were neither in a position to choose nor to understand that commitment' (2011: 187).

But having expressed her rage, Couceyro's voice-over becomes more reflective (but still heard over the image of the screaming, anguished figure of Carri's double): 'Are the souls of the dead in those who follow? In those who try to remember them? And how much of that memory is preservation, how much whim?'. So, despite the rage expressed towards her internal mother, the scene ends back at Carri's fundamental problem; the internal mother has no shape or form other than whim, and beyond that is yawning absence. It is perhaps Carri's most affectively powerful use of her double in the whole film as Couceyro seems to embody the anguish, the pain and indeed the rage that Carri feels but, in the screen personae of "Albertina Carri" that Carri plays, is too restrained and contained to convey. Couceyro here, as very much the *Carri* rather than the *not-Carri* double, enacts the anguish, the affect, that Carri cannot express. Here we see the *doubling* technique of psychodrama, where the double makes conscious and manifest, the unspoken, repressed or under-expressed material in the principal protagonist's own performance, giving voice to latent material. Perhaps the film's emotional eloquence is achieved through its combination of moments when anger breaks through only for these moments to be undercut by ironic distance which, far from dissipating the agony, makes it more acute. The Albertina Carri we see in the film may ruthlessly control her double and her crew but she reserves her most ruthless treatment for herself, never allowing herself for long to own her own pain or her own memories, cruelly undoing them through her forensic questioning of everything. Couceyro's unrestrained screaming at the top of her voice is perhaps the only possible representation of this excruciating, agonising predicament.

The nature of the vacuum: bodily connection/disconnection

Attempting to represent an 'event-affect complex without representational content'

For all the experimental, *avant garde* filmic devices that Carri deploys – doubles, Playmobil toys, plays-within, the comradery of a committed film crew pursuing a goal in defiance of potential funding bodies and documentary conventions, the breaking of the "wall" that usually separates the documentary crew from their filmic subjects – the core of Carri's trauma as elaborated in *The Blonds* is to be found in the most basic of human connections: that of one body to another. Or, rather, it is to be found in bodily *dis*connection. The foundational trauma of Carri's life is the unwished for, forcible disconnection from the parental body; a body torn away from her, never to return. It is where the playful, ludic,[21] iconoclastic methods of *The Blonds* and the 'chin-scratching detachment' (Scott 2004) reach their limits and strike something very real: the missing bodies of Carri's parents. It is also the point where Carri's fictionalisations reach their limit and fictionalisation is refused.

In this section, I will seek to establish that it is this missing parental body – and not her missing memories of her parents – that is the absence that haunted Carri's childhood and haunts her adult life. The founding absence – 'my constitution as a person starting from an absence' (Women Make Movies Release 2004: 7) – that Carri pursues and tries to make sense of, is the missing, irrevocably-lost parental body; a body that finds expression in the film as hair, as blood, as DNA. And it is through the fictional provocations of the spoken play-within that this connection-disconnection is unearthed, witnessed by Carri (the director within the diegesis), and given expression as the theatre of the body takes over the stage of the play-within.

If the heart of Carri's trauma is a bodily sense of absence and disconnection, it will inevitably struggle to find representational form. The "sense" I am invoking is what is sometimes referred to colloquially as a "body memory"[22]; an unarticulated and never-articulated sense or feeling that persists and is best understood under Freud's descriptive model of the unconscious: that is *not* a repressed memory (a memory that once had a definite form but underwent repression by the dynamic unconscious) but a feeling which carries with it no narrative structure and so is profoundly difficult to translate into a representable form. It is what Christopher Bollas describes as children experiencing 'in their own bodies […] traumatic events for which they had no language or memory' (Perez 2013: 10).[23]

In a case study dealing with the difficulty of approaching traumatic events in the life of a tiny child, César and Sara Botella write:

> The limits of traditional therapeutic intervention came from two sides: word-presentations could no longer fulfil their role of communication; on the other side, there was the impossibility of connecting the pain to the recollection of the past, because the past was simply blank. Properly speaking, in such cases the notion of a transference of the forgotten past onto the analyst does not meet the actual clinical fact. It is, rather, the actualisation of an "event-affect complex without representational content" that has no history and is incapable of taking the form of represented memories.
>
> (Botella and Botella 2013: 108)

The Botellas's case, of course, differs in two important ways from Carri in search of her trauma. First, the Botellas's patient was still a small child when they undertook the analysis and so the child's lack of word-presentations is not something that hampers the very articulate Carri. That said, the child patient's inability to put its pain into words may well hold true for Carri because adult articulacy is unlikely to gain much traction on an "inarticulate" childhood trauma. The trauma can only be re-felt or re-experienced and then, by accepting that this feeling *is* the memory of the historical event, some understanding might struggle into words. Secondly, Carri's filmic analysis is a self-analysis and so she is attempting to pull off the trick of actualising the 'event-affect complex' without having a truly "other" other (a truly alien other) with whom to interact.

With adult patients in mind, Howard Levine has also dealt with the huge difficulties entailed in traumas of this sort.

> In the presence of the *represented* unconscious [i.e. Freud's dynamic unconscious] […] the analytic process moves via free association and interpretation from conscious and preconscious surface to unconscious depth. In the analysis of unrepresented and weakly represented mental states, *the elements of mind – conscious, preconscious, and unconscious – must first be created by a work that begins in the analyst's psyche and is then offered to and inscribed in the psyche of the patient as part of an interactive, intersubjective relationship and process.*
>
> (2013: 70; Levine's italics)

Levine, like the Botellas, highlights the importance of a creative or empathetic "other" in bringing certain traumas – which must include the traumas of early childhood – into some sort of representational form. In search of her largely wordless, weakly represented or unrepresented trauma, Carri has the difficulty of not having access to 'an interactive, intersubjective relationship and process', and so she must try to create those intersubjective relationships within the structure of a self-analytic filmic process by creating a self that can view the self as an outsider. Of course, the external others of film crew and imagined audience are still available to Carri but, if we follow Anzieu's (1986) account of Freud's self-analysis, an internal other is also required alongside the external others.

The missing parental body: 'trying to rip my parents' absence (as if it were a corpse)'

I will try to substantiate my argument that the core of Carri's trauma is an unrepresented bodily connection/disconnection to her parents from two statements Carri made about her film after its completion (the paratext) and from several clues within the film itself (the text). In an interview, Carri was asked: 'Why did you decide to have yourself played by an actress at certain points in the film?'

> I thought about this a thousand times. At one point, I thought about fictionalizing everything, but I could not have actors taking the parts of my mother and father. So I decided instead to fictionalize my present. To me it seemed important that the viewer be left with the feeling that it is impossible to reconstruct the memory. And that the memory is more a state of mind than anything else.
>
> (Ministerio de Educación, Argentina (Bibliteca y Materiales Didácticos) 2010)[24]

A key part of this reply is the refusal to trespass on the bodies of her parents; Carri could simply 'not have' actors playing her parents. The refusal to fictionalise her parents is *not* a refusal of their fictionalisation in the representational sphere. Again and again in the film, people describe, remember and reminisce about Carri's parents. None of these depictions, these fictionalisations, seem to make much impression on Carri (as played by Couceyro); they remain alien descriptions of unknown people with whom "Carri" seems to feel no connection. Carri treats these depictions with ironic distance or bafflement but does not refuse them a place in her film; there is no effort to 'not have' these depictions. In presenting these fictionalisations, these representations, the double once again has a double function. First, to allow Carri through Couceyro to express her disconnection from other people's "versions" of her parents; and secondly, and conversely, to allow Carri to view her parents dispassionately as the Couceyro double is not emotionally vulnerable to what she is hearing (as Carri herself, doubtless would be). The double is the mirror that allows Carri to see the reflection of the "Medusa" rather than confronting the Medusa directly. But what Carri absolutely refuses is the corporeal impersonation of her parents – a bodily substitution – in the body of an actor. It is this that generates a red line that cannot be crossed.[25]

The director's statement that accompanied the exhibition of *The Blonds* at various international film festivals gives a little more insight into the centrality of the parental body to Carri. At the Pesaro Film Festival in Italy in the summer of 2006, audiences were provided with this statement of Carri's:

> In 1999, I began doing research on the fiction of memory – objective facts placed before fantasies, fragmented stories placed before the impossibility of remembering certain elements and forgetting certain details. I immersed myself in this tunnel, and my erratic, ambitious and desperate search became the first half hour of *Los Rubios*. Later, trying to break up the absence of my parents (like a body), I was able to unite the past and present. Connecting my present as a director with my past, which was marked by this absence, seemed to me like an ambitious job, as well as impertinent and provocative.
>
> (Fondazione Pesaro Nuovo Cinema Onlus, 2006: 42)

Carri's statement was issued in a different translation by the organisation 'Women Make Movies' for a US showing of *The Blonds* in 2004. It is worth reproducing in part for its rendering of the key phrase about the parents' bodies:

> While I was trying to rip my parents' absence (as if it were a corpse), I managed to put the past together with the present.
>
> (Women Make Movies Release, 2004: 7)

Carri's connection to her past is through the bodies of her parents. The difficulty both translators appear to have had in clearly rendering the key sentence – *ripping* or *breaking up* the *body* or *corpse* of the parents – seems to me less evidence of poor translation skills and more revealing of the difficulty in trying to represent in words, an essentially wordless, bodily connection. One may assume that the translators have merely carried over into their translations the opacity of Carri's original words in Spanish and her struggle to represent in words her "unrepresentable" feelings.[26] Or, as the Botellas put it, the difficulty in actualising an 'event-affect complex without representational content'.

The search for the parental body in the film is the search for an 'absence' (as Carri has called it) at the core of her adult life. Carri describes this absence as a *black hole*: 'My feeling is that no-one [in other accounts of the "disappeared"] has reached deep into that black hole that is the absence'[27] (quoted in García 2003) and goes on to say the black hole was the starting point of her quest that became *The Blonds*. Like a black hole in the physical universe, we know it is there because we can detect nothing of it; we have to conjecture its presence from its absolute "absence". Its presence is presumed from the odd effects that occur around it.[28]

Confronting the parental body: the limits of fictionalisation

These effects are apparent in *The Blonds* in a scene shot at the *Center for Forensic Anthropology*. This non-government organisation (*Equipo Argentino de Antropología Forense* or *EAAF*) has been investigating the plight of the "disappeared" since the mid-1980s: collecting written and oral accounts of victims and attempting to locate and identify corpses at various mass burial sites through the matching of DNA taken from the bodies of the disappeared to that of surviving relatives.

Very soon, after we enter the offices of the *EAAF*, the soundtrack becomes a dull roar – a kind of white noise – and all external sounds are not just muffled but obliterated. The strange soundtrack starts as soon as the camera begins to pick out photographs on the office walls of human skulls (presumably excavated from mass graves of the disappeared). The soundtrack continues as we see the *EAAF* representative talking to "Carri" (Analía Couceyro). His lips move in speech and he presses the end of a retractable ballpoint pen but we hear no click when the button on the top of the pen is pressed and we hear no recording of what the representative is saying, just the roaring sound. It is akin to that sound of the rushing of our own blood in our ears. I think we must assume it is a recreation of the roaring sound inside the head of Carri as she films and observes the scene – an internal diegetic sound – not an extra-diegetic sound effect (although technically, of course, it is the latter). The absence of synchronised sound brings an uncanny, disquieting feel to this scene. We, as viewers, are plunged into deafness and trapped inside our own heads. The moving footage we are watching recedes as if it were a disturbing dream. Our eyes tell us we are present but our ears make us feel a long way away. There is the sensation of an *out-of-body* experience or, perhaps, an *absolutely locked into our own body* experience.[29] This scene is the first in the film in which Carri comes close to the bodies, the corpses, of her parents. The corpses on the walls of the Center are a far cry from the verbal descriptions, the photographic images from life or the academic texts that have so far represented her parents. And although the Carri we see in this scene remains calm as ever, the soundtrack tells a different story and has been designed, we must assume, to convey to the viewer the terror or disturbance Carri felt during filming.

There is then an abrupt cut back to synchronised sound as the *EAAF* representative takes a blood sample from Couceyro, who then signs the required paperwork. At this point, Albertina Carri breaks in and says: 'Aren't you going to stick me?' (meaning *Aren't you going to take my blood sample?*). The whole procedure is undertaken again using the blood from the real Albertina Carri's finger and her samples are bagged up to go to the lab. Although, again, Carri remains calm during these exchanges and procedures, what is striking is that Carri has broken a rule of her own notoriously rule-breaking film. Carri's interventions elsewhere in the film are all essentially acts of Brechtian estrangement that unmask the constructed, artificial nature of the documentary-making process and serve to distance the viewer from the narrative. Without exception, Carri's other interventions in *The Blonds* – her continual breaking of documentary's fourth wall – are the interventions of a director as she makes a film: Carri's voice saying 'Make sure I'm not in frame' heard over the first Playmobil scene; Carri instructing Couceyro in how to recite her list of "hates"; etc. Here for the first and only time, Carri breaks into the scene being shot and insists that she has to replace her double. She is saying my double *isn't the real thing*; *only I am the real thing*, or, to put it another way, everything can be fictionalised including myself in the body of Analía Couceyro but not the blood that ran in the veins of Ana María Caruso and Roberto Carri. Carri's unbreakable bond to her parents – a bond of blood, of DNA – crashes through the fourth wall of Carri's film not in an act of distancing disconnection but as a revelation of an unbreakable bodily connection between parents and daughter. I cannot decide from watching the scene whether Carri's intervention was a spontaneous act that occurred, unrehearsed in the filmic present or whether Carri had planned her intervention. I actually do not think this really matters as either way it reveals, through presentation or *re*-presentation, the power of the visceral, bodily connection.

There is then a cut back to Analía Couceyro playing "Albertina Carri". She is looking at a drawing on the wall of the Center; it is a diagram with crudely drawn human figures spread out in various positions across two sheets of paper. It is hard to know what it depicts but it appears to be a map of the positions of bodies within a geographical space, and I assume it is a map of a mass burial site the *EAAF* has excavated. The soundtrack changes once more over these pictures. Again, it is disconcerting although no longer the roaring sound heard earlier but distorted, high-pitched, screeching sounds reminiscent of distant screams.

The sound track was probably created by running sound tape of human speech in fast-forward and/or rewind through a tape recorder with the volume turned on. This hypothesis gains veracity when we become aware of the mechanical "clunks" that punctuate the recordings; "clunks" that sound like the stop button being pressed on the recorder/player and then the fast-forward or rewind button being pressed again to allow the resumption of the high-pitched screeching sound. If these disturbing sounds, these screams, were created by tampering with audio tapes of speech (as I suspect) then they could be construed as another comment on documentary testimony. The voices of interviewees have been reduced to meaningless screeches, but screeches filled with affect and pain when juxtaposed against the images of the dead on the walls of *EAAF* Center. For all the recordings of people's memories of Carri's parents – accurate memories, false memories, other people's memories – Carri is no nearer to a coherent, meaningful picture. When we approach the bodies of the disappeared in the Center – the bones and blood of the dead – all these representations in words disintegrate into an inarticulate wail of pain; the screams of the dead or the screams of the living who have been left behind.

Two other scenes later in the film also make this bodily connection; and in both, as in the scene at the *EAAF* offices, it is in part through the sound edit that Carri signals their importance. In the first of these, Couceyro visits the police station and the cells where Carri's parents were detained and tortured. As Couceyro approaches the cells, a much more muted version of the "roaring" sound effect that we heard over the opening scene at the *EAAF*, is used. Although more muted and layered over synchronised sound, it is nevertheless fully audible and is reprised in this scene where again Couceyro/Carri comes close to the bodies of her parents. Here the bodily proximity is a geographical proximity, as she visits the very site and the very room in which her parents were imprisoned and tortured.

The other "scene" is really a quite complex series of scenes in which the bodies of cows being beaten, prodded and herded into pens come to represent – to stand in for – the tortured bodies of Carri's parents (and remind the viewer that political prisoners of the 1970s were routinely tortured with electric cattle prods). The concluding scene of the series with the cattle is set up earlier when Couceyro (in her role as Albertina Carri) recounts an uncanny story. She says that she and a friend were in a picture-framing shop when by chance she came across some incredible photographs of cows in a slaughterhouse. The photos really moved both Carri and her friend. Couceyro (playing Carri) recalls:

> My friend said: "The person who made these has been tortured."
>
> And I thought: "The photos are great, my friend's nuts."
>
> The photographer's name was Paula. Just Paula.
>
> [...]
>
> My sister called me weeks later, crying, and told me that she had met the only survivor from the detention center where they'd held my parents. The survivor was the same photographer.

After a short break, the story continues:

> She [Paula, the photographer] doesn't want us to film her. She refuses to talk. She said: "I never talked when they tortured me [...] I'm not talking on camera." I wonder how does a camera resemble electric torture? [...] How does a camera resemble a hatchet for killing cows?

Shortly after this scene, Couceyro is back at the farm where Carri grew up, helping the gauchos to herd cattle into a pen. The gauchos use force to beat the bullocks into line so they can be injected (presumably with antibiotics). The bullocks show signs of pain and distress as they are "sticked" (injected). In the middle of the scene, the strange, disturbing sound effects – similar to those heard at the *EAAF* offices – begin again. The pictures we see of the cattle also become stranger at this moment; they are slowed down and jumpy (a number of frames have been removed from the original footage to achieve this effect). As a viewer, we are back in the same, disturbing territory we inhabited at the *EAAF* office. We are in no doubt that the sweating, terrified bodies of the bullocks on the farm are the same terrified bodies of cattle depicted in Paula's photographs (which we never see) and they in turn are the bodies of Carri's parents at the detention centre as they were tortured. As Couceyro/Carri comes close to these bodies on the farm, we as viewers experience Carri's terror or disturbance through the careful manipulation of the sound and the pictures we hear and see on screen.

Each time Carri comes close to the bodies of her parents – at the *EAAF*, in the police cells, with the cattle on the farm – strange and disturbing effects occur. It is on these occasions when the film is furthest from A.O. Scott's (2004) description of it as 'a vacuum in which its powerful, confrontational moments lose their force, the trauma of the past pushed nearly out of reach'. These are the powerful moments, when the viewer is made to feel the disturbance and to know they are in the presence of trauma. But the *thing itself*, the core, is indeed a vacuum or, better, a black hole whose presence we can detect only from the odd effects that occur around it. And these effects are not spontaneous occurrences caught on camera or sound tape in the filmic present (as is the case in *The Act of Killing*). They are filmic effects, engineered in the edit or signalled by the breaking of a convention that had been established elsewhere in the film. They are mediated, constructed, conscious attempts to represent the "unrepresentable" core of Carri's constitutional absence; attempts to convey the intense feeling of absence, of connection to and disconnection from the parental body, that Carri feels. If one is open to these moments, they have a live and affective impact on the viewer.

Taking stock: suspended between fictions at the mid-point of the self-analytic process

The intensity of Albertina Carri's affective response to the proximity of the parental body is the key to understanding the film and also the key to understanding the film as a self-analytic, meaning-seeking process that unfolds over time. But, at this juncture in the film, meaning has yet to emerge for the Carri we see in the diegesis. The deployment of fictional films-within has revealed the black hole of absence in all its starkness: the fictions stripping away both false and alien memories (other people's memories) and childhood attempts to understand the loss of her parents, leaving (for Carri I think, and this viewer certainly) an intense, aching sense of absence. This is the black hole that opened up when the parental bodies were wrenched away from the infant Carri. But it is these parental bodies that offer a way to understand the trauma, as whatever Carri loses and discards in representational content over the course of the film, she recovers (or reveals to the viewer and herself) as affective content through her intense bodily connection to her lost parents.

At this point in my film analysis – a point that coincides with a certain juncture in the film as I have yet to analyse the last few scenes in the last fifteen minutes of *The Blonds* – we have moved closer and closer to the essence of Carri's constitutional absence, but still it evades us and her. It is a point in the film that corresponds to the moment in Freud's *Constructions in Analysis* (1937b) when the analyst has offered a fiction, a bait of falsehood, and the analysand has been *touched* or the moment in *Hamlet* when Claudius is watching the play-within and he *blenches.* The protagonist's powerful affective, somatic response to the fictional play or fictional construction suggests that we are approaching something of importance – a 'carp of truth' as Polonius calls it – but what that might be remains to be interpreted and understood. It corresponds to those moments in *The Act of Killing* when Anwar

Congo confronts one of his own filmic fictions – whether in playing a role or in witnessing himself playing a role – and this elicits a powerful affective or somatic response. At these moments, Anwar Congo has yet to understand what these bodily blenches might mean (and apparently, even after reflection, he is only able to do so to a limited extent with much remaining as symptomatology). It is a point that we might see as suspended between fictions. Fictions have brought the unrepresented core of the trauma into view. For Carri, that core seems to be the unshakeable connection to the missing parental body that cannot be trespassed upon and cannot and must not be fictionalised. If Carri can understand what this means for her – if she can interpret her own affective responses – she may be able to find a less painful accommodation with her past. But this accommodation itself might require the creation of new fictions, soothing fictions, symbolisations, like the one Ernst constructed out of a cotton reel and a piece of string as he gradually came to terms with maternal absence.

The picture and the frame

Finding a secure psychic frame or how to theorise a black hole

But before considering whether Carri is able to construct a meaningful account of her traumatic past, I want to offer an interpretive structure for thinking about the parental body. It draws on the work of André Green and Donald Winnicott and provides a way to conceptualise the black hole, the void, of parental absence.[30] It begins with André Green's ideas on 'the work of the negative' and more specifically on what he calls 'the framing structure'. In this work on the psychic development of the child, Green argues that whilst the mother's representation may be replaced by substitutes, the crucial thing is the introjection of a secure bodily sense of the mother, which acts as an empty frame, holding psychic space, and providing the foundation for all later secure psychic development.

> When we think of the early mother-child relationship in Winnicottian terms, we realise the importance of holding. When a separation occurs, the baby is left alone. The mother's representation may be suspended and replaced by many substitutes. What is of the greatest importance is *the introjected construction of a framing structure [structure encadrante]* analogous to the mother's arms in the holding. This framing structure can tolerate the absence of representation because it holds the psychic space, like Bion's container. As long as the framing structure holds the mind, the negative hallucination can be replaced by hallucinatory wish-fulfilment or fantasy.
>
> (2000: 102–3; Green's italics)

Taking Green's theoretical speculations and placing them alongside the screen character, Albertina Carri, we see a principal protagonist who has an intense sense of connection to her parents. Is this an indication that the framing structure has held?

Could the powerful sense of bodily connection felt by Carri to her parents be taken to be a bodily sense (although it is of course psychic) of a mother's arms holding and containing her?[31]; a sense that can, not without difficulties and pain, 'tolerate the absence of representation' and hold 'the psychic space'? The black hole that Carri has said is at her core (and is revealed more starkly over the course of the film as she strips away and discards the representations of others) is the absence of representation. We might take this for the negative hallucination as described by Green but we have also witnessed Carri's ability to bear the process of stripping the past back to the negative and this could be construed as a sign of psychic strength (an ability to tolerate the negative). An increasingly blank canvas is revealed but one that may sit within a secure psychic frame. In Winnicottian terms, does Carri have enough *good-enough* mothering inside her to tolerate the negative? But the film tells us nothing about the parenting Carri received as an infant (and the adult Carri is without memory of this time). What we do discover in the film is that Carri's aunt and uncle were able to provide a happy home for Carri on the farm after her parents' deaths (and we see this environment reproduced in the early Playmobil scenes in *The Blonds*). Is this the firm ground and the base on which she *might* be able to build? Is this a solid frame into which Carri *might*, eventually, be able to place a picture (a 'substitute' representation)?

Green, though, reminds us of what can go wrong (and this quotation follows on directly from the one above):

> But when the baby is confronted by the death experience, the frame becomes unable to create substitute representations – it holds only the void. This means the non-existence of the object or of any substitute object. The negative hallucination of the object cannot be overcome; the negative does not lead to an alternative positive substitution. Even the badness of the object and fantasised destructiveness will not do. It is the mind, that is, mental activity giving birth to representations, which is under threat of being destroyed, in the frame. At other times it is the framing structure itself that is damaged; here we have disintegration.
>
> (Green 2000: 103)

In Carri's ruthless stripping away and questioning of representations that once stood in for her parents – discarding all the *not-Carri* representations – there feels a very real danger that she will be left with nothing but the void, with a traumatising, unshiftable negative hallucination. Carri does rail at 'the badness of the object' in the scene where Couceyro enacts Carri's rage at the mother who deserted her (Couceyro spinning and screaming) but as the rage subsides, Carri's mother (parents) returns to intangibility, to absence, with Carri describing her parents as a 'whim': a void of unfulfilled desire; a wish as impotent as her birthday wishes. Perhaps the danger for Carri (which Green outlines in a further gloss of Winnicott's speculations) is that 'non-existence, will become, the only thing that is real' and that it will take 'possession of the mind, erasing representations of the object that preceded its absence. This is an irreversible step, at least until treatment' (Green 2000: 104). Is this Carri's fate and predicament? Is there only a black hole – a negative hallucination – that has become 'the only thing that is real'?

My reading of *The Blonds* suggests otherwise. To ground this argument, I will need to take a detour back through the work of Freud and Winnicott. As so often with Freud, he had already stumbled across the notion of the negative hallucination long before Green seized upon it, but consigned it, unelaborated, to a footnote in an essay that was driving in a different direction. In *A Metapsychological Supplement to the Theory of Dreams*, he writes, 'I may add by way of supplement that any attempt to explain hallucination would have to start out from *negative* rather than positive hallucination' (1917 [1915]: 232; footnote 3; italics in *Standard Edition*). More directly relevant to my purposes here is Freud's observation of his two-year-old grandson's *fort-da* game, where the traumatising *absence* of the mother – experienced as *non-existence* – precipitates representation and symbolisation: absence (non-existence) precedes representation; representation is a response to traumatic absence; and a representation has the potential to catalyse the emergence of a meaningful account (a symbolisation of the trauma). Winnicott takes a step back from Freud's chronological point of observation and asks how the child is able to develop a mind that can use a cotton reel and two words (*fort/da*) in this way? He takes a perhaps surprising direction, insisting that the infant needs a comforting illusion (a fiction) and that illusion is a normal, non-pathological phenomenon (Chaplin 2016: 2). He even suggests that it is the mother's task to support the infant in the illusion that what the infant creates really exists. This sounds like *folie à deux* and indeed '[t]here is madness here which is permissible' (Olive Stevenson quoted in Winnicott 2017: Volume 4: 298). The symbolising ego grows through or out of illusion, temporarily sanctioned and protected. Illusion provides:

> an intermediate area of *experiencing*, to which inner reality and external life both contribute. It is an area that is not challenged, because no claim is made on its behalf except that it shall exist as a resting-place for the individual engaged in the perpetual human task of keeping inner and outer reality separate and yet interrelated.
>
> (1990 [1971]b: 3; Winnicott's italics)

Winnicott then takes this theorisation one step further. If illusion is necessary for symbolisation, so is gradual disillusion arrived at through failure. As the mother progressively fails to adapt to the infant, the infant butts into external reality, the otherness of the mother, the world outside its omnipotence. This is another "impossible" parenting task, to fail the infant at the right speed. Too fast a disillusionment and the infant is traumatised; too slow and the *folie à deux* persists (Chaplin 2016: 3).

The Blonds could be read as Carri's third attempt to negotiate maternal (parental) absence. The first attempt, as I have said, is a conjecture on my part that the infant Carri – like *every other* infant – must have negotiated this traumatising absence in her own way with her own illusions. The second attempted negotiation was precipitated by the sudden disappearance of Carri's parents when she was three; an event that must have undone any soothing illusions the little Carri had developed to cope with absence (and the thoughts that had gradually superseded those initial, soothing illusions) re-exposing the negative hallucination beneath it. This second, terrifying encounter with "non-existence" was a confrontation with what Green calls 'the death experience', which begs the question of whether the little Albertina Carri would be left with the *void*, where the 'negative hallucination of the object cannot be overcome' and where 'the negative does not lead to an alternative positive substitution'. This second negotiation is represented in the film in various scenes from the dumb play (the Playmobil play-within), as Carri stages the struggle of her younger self to find a soothing illusion or a positive substitution to fill the void. We see a pair of Playmobil figures arriving at the farm whilst Couceyro tells us in voice-over: 'The farm was a land of fantasy, where all my memories begin. I would see my parents arriving by car, by bus, on horseback.' This fantasy is echoed in Carri's recurrent birthday wish for her parents' return as she blows out her birthday candles (which Carri presents in the spoken play-within through her double Couceyro). But this attempt at a positive substitution fails as it crashes into the brute facts of *outer reality* – her parents never return – and it gives way to the Playmobil scene of alien abduction. The fantasy has now adapted itself to outer reality but in so doing, it has fixed the traumatic absence as permanent and irreversible. For the child Carri growing up on the farm, the illusion of alien abduction could never have been soothing but seems instead to be a representation of her *too fast a disillusionment* as her mother (parents) literally "disappeared", leaving her trapped in a perpetual, melancholic repetition of the moment of the traumatising disappearance. The little Albertina Carri did manage to fill the void but the substitution she achieved was a traumatising substitution. And as an adult, Carri puts other traumatising pictures into this empty frame: Paula's photographs of cattle in an abattoir representing the bodies of the tortured "disappeared"; and the tortured bodies of the bullocks on her uncle's farm. The adult Albertina Carri who decided to make the film that came to be *The Blonds* presents herself as caught in a trap of perpetually repeating (and re-traumatising) substitute representations of the parental disappearance.

This brings us to what theoretically we might imagine to be Carri's third attempt to negotiate maternal (parental) loss, which we witness in great detail; that negotiation is the film *The Blonds* itself. The film as a whole is a search for a representation, a positive substitution which can replace the failed and traumatising substitutions of childhood. But, for most of the film, Carri rejects all substitutions: the failed historic and psychic residues of her childhood substitutions are ruthlessly stripped away along with the substitute representations and alien memories of others, as she pares her past back to the bare bones of what she really knows or what she really feels. It is as if Carri is aware that she has to start again from the negative hallucination, a psychic *ground zero*, as arguably she had done twice before. For me as a viewer, Carri's ruthlessness, lack of sentimentality and use of ironic distance in achieving this ground zero seemed fraught with dangers. I feared that she would be left only with the void, reconfronting the death experience and unable to replace the negative hallucination with a positive substitution. It is an interpretation that developed out of my initial counter-transference onto the filmic object; an agonising sense of frustration where nothing felt tangible or certain, where there seemed to be nothing but a void. It is a fear of this "nothingness" that Carri herself expresses in the film when she says 'I have to think of something. Something that will be a movie'. She is desperate to find a substitute representation to put in the frame that is her documentary project.

But by the end of the film, this feeling has dissipated and it finishes on a guardedly optimistic note.[32] I reached this conclusion both by contemplating the filmic object itself (*The Blonds* viewed from the outside as a single coherent text) and from the specific content of the film, and especially from the scenes in the film's concluding fifteen minutes. The filmic object as a whole is a picture of a mind representing itself in the act of representing; a mind representing and failing to represent a psychic predicament. But the *failing to represent* is itself represented in the film; it is not the void of non-representation. From this perspective, the secure frame is not a psychic capacity we search for in the filmic character "Albertina Carri" but the frame of the documentary, which is a container for all these representations including the failed representations. The frame seems to have held.

And turning away from the film object as a whole to the specific narrative content of scenes within the film (the pictures Carri places in the frame), by the end of the film we do not witness the protagonist's disintegration but a protagonist working through and coming to terms with the past.

Putting a picture in the frame (or bridging the void)

In the last few scenes, we see what appear to be positive substitutions – non-traumatising pictures are placed within the frame of the documentary – which suggest there is a possibility of escaping the traumatising void: that it might be possible to find or create a soothing (meaningful) account to lay over the traumatic past and fill the void. The film's closing sequence of scenes begin with Carri and her crew back at her aunt and uncle's farm, standing outside in the depths of the night, with a single, dim light throwing long shadows of their bodies onto the ground. It is, in a literal sense, the darkest point of the film. But the sound track moves in a slightly different direction; it is of cicadas and other night-time country sounds, and recalls, through sound, the film's relatively positive opening scene of the Playmobil farm at night. At this point, a series of cryptic texts float across the screen:

> If all the world could be like that
> like memories
> I would love all mankind
> and happily die for it

It seems that Carri craves memories (positive memories) and so seems to be searching for something positive to fill the void; something like the happy childhood memories she formed on the farm where 'I fell in love with the horses, the cows, with my uncle Federico and with getting up early.' In the next scene, night time has given way to the first glimmerings of dawn; the red glow of the morning sun still below the horizon. There is a cut to the crew waking up in an out-building on the farm with the early dawn still visible through the windows. They prepare coffee. All of them now possess blond wigs, which they brush, before heading out into the new day with their film equipment. The crew chats happily to each other, laughing (although we cannot make out the words). A male voice then begins to sing a ballad, which continues throughout the remaining scenes shot at dawn on the farm, throughout the closing credits and on through a final ("post-end") scene that comes in the middle of the closing credits. The song's lyrics act as a commentary on what we are seeing at the end of the film and, to some extent, on the film as a whole. Although this is not announced to the viewer, the song is called *Influencia* by the hugely popular Argentinian singer and rock star, Charly García (a fact that would not be lost on an Argentinian audience).[33]

As the song continues, the pre-credits closing scene begins with Analía Couceyro, in blonde wig, walking away from the camera into the distance down a long, muddy, farm track. We then cut back to Albertina Carri saying to the crew: 'It's better. The film ends with Analía alone. It's more beautiful.' But what we actually see immediately after this is the whole crew of five, including Albertina and Analía, all wearing blond wigs in the dawn sun, walking away from the camera into the distance. The scene has the strangely optimistic feel of a band of friends (an alternative family) walking together towards a new future. The feeling of a positive future and new beginnings is generated in part by the use of that common literary and filmic trope of a new dawn signifying a new beginning, in part by a sense that in dressing up and wearing wigs the crew have become like children happy in their creative play, and in part by the lyrics and the tempo of the song. Is this Carri's *positive substitution*, her *comforting illusion* that can fill the void and rescue her from the danger Green sees when 'non-existence, will become, the only thing that is real'?

In thinking about this question, the temporal dimension is crucial. The dawn scene is not a flight from the past and a rush towards a rose-tinted vision of the future – such a solution would be fragile and liable to collapse back into trauma when the past caught up with Carri – it is rather a scene that links Carri and her crew to the past as well as the future. The five-person crew mirrors or "doubles" Albertina Carri's nuclear family with its five members: the parents, Ana María Caruso and Roberto Carri, and the three daughters, Andrea, Paula and Albertina. The connection is made explicit in that the crew all wear blond wigs, echoing the old neighbour's comment: 'The girls were blondes. The father was blond, the mother was blonde. All blonds.' Carri seems to be making a link between (trying to integrate) her traumatic past and an optimistic vision of the future; a future with friends and with possibilities. It is perhaps the moment when Carri recovers what Eric Brenman (1980: 53–60; and 2006) calls 'the lost good object'.

In Chapter 3, I argued that Ernst's *fort-da* game was not merely a soothing illusion that could fill the void of maternal absence and rescue little Ernst from the nameless, shapeless agony of his mother's "non-existence". To be able to create a soothing illusion, Ernst had to enter the spatial and temporal world: to understand that if his mother was not *here* she still existed somewhere else; and to understand that if his mother was not present *now*, she had been present in the past and would be again in the future. In Rosine Perelberg's gloss of the developmental moment Freud observed in his grandson, she argues it is in this moment that 'the whole of psychic reality, in its positive and negative aspects, is structured in terms of time and space' (2008: 2). If, as I have argued, the film *The Blonds* is Carri's third attempt to deal with maternal absence, then the temporal integration of past, present and future must form part of this third attempt if it is to be successful.

Carri herself was fully aware of the importance of the temporal dimension in the directorial statement that accompanied the release of the film.

> Later, trying to break up the absence of my parents (like a body), I was able to unite the past and present. Connecting my present as a director with my past, which was marked by this absence, seemed to me like an ambitious job, as well as impertinent and provocative.
>
> (*Fondazione Pesaro Nuovo Cinema Onlus*, 2006)

and in the alternative translation:

> While I was trying to rip my parents' absence (as if it were a corpse), I managed to put the past together with the present.
>
> (Women Make Movies Release, 2004: 7)

Carri does say *past and present* in this statement rather than *past and future*, but I think Carri's statement entails a notion of the future. It is the crew's happy "togetherness" in the present that allows the optimistic vision of the future; a vision that is not yet achieved. The optimism for the future arises out of the putting together – the re-integration – of past and present. The resulting vision of the future is both Winnicott's soothing illusion and Green's positive hallucination; illusion and hallucination, that is, not in the sense of *false and deluded* but in the sense of *unrealised and possible*.

Carri's directorial statement also reminds us that she was only able to achieve this temporal integration by going through the bodies (the corpses) of her parents. In the closing sequence with the crew, Albertina Carri walks alongside her mother and her father (the past), their roles taken by her friends who simultaneously represent a positive vision of the future. The scene is a very concrete and externalised representation of Green's '*introjected construction of a framing structure* analogous to the mother's arms in the holding' (2000: 102–3; Green's italics); her parents are there with her, holding her, as she walks on the farm. The scene suggests that the framing structure has been able to hold Carri's mind and so allow the negative hallucination to be 'replaced by hallucinatory wish-fulfilment or fantasy' (2000: 102–3). Or, in Winnicott's terms, the final scene sees Carri's mother, alongside her, fulfilling the mother's task of supporting the infant (but now adult Carri) in the illusion that what the infant creates, really exists.[34] The introjected, bodily sense of a loving and protective mother has allowed Carri to gain some control over her traumatic past and to create the fantasy, or illusion, or hallucinatory wish for a less troubled future. As Perelberg goes on to say in her gloss of the story: 'The constitution of the individual takes place in the context of the time-space created in the relationship with the mother (and her body)' (2008: 21). By integrating the trauma of the past into a dynamic, temporal frame including the present and the future, Carri seems finally to have begun to come to terms with what she calls 'my constitution as a person starting from an absence' (Women Make Movies Release, 2004: 7). That absence, as it turns out, contained, or rather was contained by, an unbreakable, positive, psychic sense of her mother, expressed in terms of the maternal body.

That everything changes in the last few minutes of the film is evident in Carri's changed attitude to blondness. For most of the film, Carri was fiercely protective of what was hers, forcing the false memory of blondness onto her *not-Carri* double, Analía Couceyro (herself, in turn, a double for the kidnapped and forcibly peroxided Honey Whitlock in the film *Cecil B Demented*). Carri has also spent most of the film refusing to have her parents' bodies fictionalised in any way. This was an absolute red line for Carri. But in the closing, dawn sequence, Carri's parents' bodies are fictionalised, their places taken by members of the crew, who not only impersonate (embody) them but wear blond wigs. It seems that having stripped everything in her past back to what is truly hers, leaving herself with no representations (a void) but with a burning sense of bodily connection to her lost parents, Carri was then able to fantasise again. Having found the outlines of the black hole at the core of her being – having returned to the negative hallucination – she was then able to find 'an alternative positive substitution' (Green 2000: 103). In finding that substitution, it is as if Carri has been released from the prison of her ever-repeating traumatic past, and in finding that freedom she is also free from the strictures she placed upon herself and the anathemas she issued to protect the corporeal integrity of her parents. I am not suggesting that her intense sense of bodily connection to her parents no longer matters – it does profoundly – but it no longer needs to be policed so fiercely as she knows it is secure within her. Her parents can now be impersonated (their bodies replaced with those of "actors") and fictionalised in the wearing of blond wigs.

My reading of the last few scenes of the film is supported by a narrative commentary provided by the words of the song *Influencia*. But just before considering the song's lyrics, it is worth noticing that the mere fact that Carri allows the words of a popular song to provide a commentary on her life and her predicament is deeply surprising (like her surprising decisions to allow the impersonation of her parents and the wearing of blond wigs). The fierce desire to pare everything down to precisely what she knows to be hers and the refusal to borrow the memories of others seems to have gone. I cannot imagine Carri being willing to borrow the generic words of a popular song earlier in the film. It is only possible in the context of her transformation at the end of the film. The song's lyrics – written in the first person – can be read as Carri's commentary on *The Blonds* and her attempt to find a meaningful account of her traumatic past.[35]

As the lyric tells us, throughout the film, Carri has refused to 'run or hide' from her 'destiny' and has faced her troubled past with a ruthless disregard for herself and with a powerful sense that she must 'trust' herself and her 'intuitions'. In finding that deep bodily/psychic connection to her parents (which might equate to Green's framing structure), Carri has found that thing that the song lyric describes as something that's 'hard to see', 'deep inside' her, 'controlling' her. According to the song, the resolution at the end of the film is not a simple-minded vision that everything's fine now but rather a personal accommodation to a traumatic past, where there is 'pleasure' but pleasure as an aspect of 'this sorrow'. And the song conveys a sense of what drives the whole film; Carri's insistence that 'I have to know [...] I have to trust myself, I have to know'. Carri desperately did want to understand and painstakingly worked towards that goal. In so many documentaries that treat trauma, whether films with a separate director and protagonist or first-person films like *The Blonds*, the desire to know and to understand is very often the driving force of the narrative. As Gabriela Nouzeilles (2005: 267) writes of documentary in general and Carri's documentary in particular: 'the director and her crew take advantage of the resources offered by the documentary as an investigative genre driven by the desire to know, and based on the ideal of transparency in opposition to fiction film.'

The Blonds has one final, post-closing scene which comes in the middle of the end titles. This live-action scene sees Albertina Carri on the farm where she grew up, teaching her double, Analía Couceyro, to ride a horse and so reprises the film's opening Playmobil farm scene in which we hear two female voices, one teaching the other how to ride (voices which continue to be heard in a subsequent scene where the picture has switched from the Playmobil farm to the real farm). In the context of these opening scenes, the voices are apparently those of the child Albertina Carri being taught to ride by an older woman (perhaps her aunt but certainly someone who is "mothering" her). The voices are now revealed to be those of Carri and Couceyro recorded during the post-closing scene.

The opening and closing scenes bring a structural symmetry to the film and hint at the tendency of trauma to repeat either in a cycle of exact repetition – a cycle of re-traumatisation (which is essentially melancholic) – or in a cycle of repetition susceptible to tiny changes, suggesting the possibility of the gradual amelioration of the pain of the original trauma and a spiralling out of trauma (a process akin to mourning). For Gabriela Nouzeilles, for all the film's demonstration of the problems of memory, this 'does not make of *Los Rubios* a melancholic project' rather the film 'constitutes in itself a way of dealing with loss'; the film is a 'therapeutic' process (Nouzeilles 2005: 271). Bystrom in part endorses Nouzeilles's view, seeing the "fictional" devices in *The Blonds* as creative and therapeutic strategies that allow Carri to move beyond 'the traumatic bind – a way to mourn rather than to suffer from melancholy' (Bystrom 2009: 44). What has changed between the opening and closing scenes suggests that Carri is able to mourn.[36] The live-action, post-closing scene not only echoes the film's opening, "happy" scene from childhood, but it also echoes (and indeed continues) the optimism of the immediately preceding scene, where Carri and her friends (her new family) walk into the distance in the dawn sun. The two closing scenes together offer the hint of a better future for Carri, now she has put her present together with her past.

The geographical echo between all four of these scenes (the two closing scenes and the film's two opening scenes) also seems significant. If, at the end of the film, we witness Carri's perhaps successful attempt to negotiate maternal (parental) non-existence, then the negotiation – in an echo of the infant's negotiation of the originary trauma – will entail a structuring of the subject in both time *and* space. The structuring in time seems to have been attempted in the integration of past with present and future. But the spatial structuring is also recognised in the setting of all four of these scenes on the farm of Carri's childhood, where she formed her first memories and where she has said she was happy.

The spatial dimension, like the temporal dimension, is structured in relation to the mother's body, as Perelberg (2008: 21) has argued. In the opening scenes, Carri is "mothered" by the woman who teaches her to ride and in the closing scenes there is a return of the mother's body to the same place. In the closing, dawn scene the mother is present on the farm, her part taken by a member of the crew in blonde wig. In the post-closing horse-riding scene, the mother also returns, but this time as a *quality* or a *psychic capacity* embodied in the daughter, Albertina Carri. Carri's capacity to act as a patient and loving teacher to Couceyro suggests that Carri holds enough *good mothering* inside her to be able to use it to care for others (whether or not the source of this psychic capacity is Carri's actual biological mother). One can conceptualise this capacity in Carri either as an expression of the internal mother (in the language of object relations) or as a manifestation of the introjected framing structure of the mother's enclosing and protecting arms (in the language of André Green). Again, there is a sense of doubling here, with Carri taking the role of her mother looking after her daughter, Albertina, represented in this post-closing horse-riding scene (as she is throughout the film) by the actress-double, Analía Couceyro. In this reading, there is a sense of resolution in this scene. Albertina Carri – at least psychically or in fantasy – is reunited with her mother, becoming her mother, embodying her mother. Carri's optimism at the end of the film seems a riposte to, and a resolution of, her own pessimistic despair earlier in the film when she said (through Couceyro): 'To develop yourself without the one who gave you life becomes an obsession, at odds with daily life, disheartening. Since most of the answers have been lost in time.'

That Carri has been able to find a positive substitution to replace the negative hallucination she so ruthlessly exposed earlier in the film suggests that she has not fallen into the desperate trap Green outlined (2000: 104): that 'non-existence, will become, the only thing that is real' and that it will take 'possession of the mind, erasing representations of the object that preceded its absence'. How did Carri avoid this fate? The answer may lie in what Green directly goes on to say after this statement: 'This is an irreversible step, at least until treatment.' *The Blonds*, I would argue, *is* the treatment. The film is an extended exercise in that enormously difficult task of self-analysis, beset by the dangers of failure, collapse into solipsism, self-indulgence, and 'part explanation, behind which resistance may be keeping back something that is more important' (the 'faulty action' that Freud describes (1935: 234)). Despite the dangers, Carri always appeared to be on a quest for 'self-knowledge obtained objectively (like an outsider)' just as Freud prescribed for a successful self-analysis (Freud's letter to Fleiss in Freud and Masson 1985), with her ruthlessness towards herself perhaps just an expression of that necessary, cool objectivity.

The film itself – the film as a whole – could be theorised in a variety of ways. If *The Blonds* is Carri's attempt to (re-)negotiate the disappearance of her parents, it is the equivalent of Ernst's cotton reel and piece of string but a cotton reel and a piece of string devised by a sophisticated, thoughtful, thirty-year-old filmmaker, not an infant just entering the world of representation. The film could be seen as a Winnicottian play space, a potential space between the opening and closing credits in which Carri finds/creates objects and arranges them in an attempt to represent and then symbolise the trauma. The film could also be seen, following Green, as a framing structure. It is a frame into which Carri places and then removes a variety of representations – some old representations of her own, some she borrows from other people – as she excavates her traumatic past before finding her own soothing, "meaningful" picture or fantasy to place in the frame, to *fill in* the blank canvas (the void) that she has systematically revealed in the earlier stages of the film.

In Green's theory of meaning as outlined in Chapter 3, fictions (like Polonius's 'bait of falsehood') are deployed to prompt or catalyse meanings into existence but these meanings, Green reminds us, should not be mistaken for the timeless truth (the thing-in-itself). Instead, the meanings that emerge are perhaps themselves also "fictions", having the ambiguous status of the transitional object: they are both found and created, both the truth and a fantasy, perpetually suspended between Sleeping Beauty and Aphrodite, between a truth awoken and a fantasy created in the process of analysis. The meanings that emerge from *The Blonds* should be approached in the same way as Green approaches the meanings that emerge in analysis. It is not what the meanings *are* (their ontological status as truth or fiction) but what they *do* that matters. If they allow a traumatised protagonist to come to a less painful accommodation with their traumatic past – as seems to be the case for Carri – then their job is done.

Afterlife of *The Blonds*: the re-kidnapping of Albertina Carri

The fate of *The Blonds* in its afterlife as an object of academic and cultural study frequently has been to repeat what Carri struggled so hard to avoid within the film. Carri refused other people's memories and the versions of her history, in order to find or create her own unique and personal version of her traumatic history as experienced from the inside and her own accommodation with that history. In the making of the film, Carri refused to be taken hostage and forcibly peroxided like Honey Whitlock, only for her to be taken hostage once more following the release of the film by friends and foes alike: Carri's film co-opted to support other people's agendas; or used as an illustration of what one is apparently forbidden to do in relation to a traumatic set of events.

Martín Kohan is perhaps Carri's most extreme critic and was one of the first to write about the film. He not only issued the *Bilderverbot* familiar from trauma theory (Kohan was outraged that Carri should *trivialise* the "disappearances" of the 1970s and 1980s by employing animated Playmobil toys as representational tools) but accuses Carri of narcissistic excess, of disrespect towards her parents (a 'régimen de la discortesía') and of having a superficial view of Argentina's past and present, calling the film 'a game of poses and an essay in frivolity' ('un juego de poses y un ensayo de levedad') (Kohan 2004: 28; 30).[37] Kohan, like the *The National Film and Audiovisual Arts Institute* (whose letter Carri and her crew discuss in the film), demands that Carri should employ conventional documentary techniques and must tell the story of the parental generation's heroic struggle. Kohan fails to understand that *The Blonds* is a personal and psychological exploration of Carri's 'constitution as a person starting from an absence' and not a political film about the disappearances and that the games and the poses (the fictions) are Carri's exploratory tools. Beatriz Sarlo (2007: 153) is more measured but criticises the film for its apolitical 'strong subjectivity', failing to understand (or to allow) that what Carri is exploring is her sense of self. And both Sarlo and Kohan attempt to marginalise Carri's film by claiming it is not representative of the views and political stance of most children of the disappeared.

Other more friendly critics try to take Carri "hostage" by co-opting *The Blonds* under the rubric of 'postmemory',[38] Marianne Hirsch's conceptual tool used to describe 'the relationship of the second generation to powerful, often traumatic, experiences that *preceded their births* but that were nevertheless transmitted to them so deeply as to seem to constitute memories in their own right' (Hirsch 2008: 103; my italics). A special issue of the *Journal of Romance Studies* in 2013 was devoted to questions raised by the films, novels, plays, photographs, etc., of the so-called post-revolutionary and post-dictatorship generation of Latin American artists and writers (roughly those of Albertina Carri's generation). The whole issue was called 'Revisiting Postmemory: The Intergenerational Transmission of Trauma in Post-Dictatorship Latin American Culture' (Blejmar and Fortuny, eds., 2013) and several of the contributors place Carri and other "artists" with very similar traumatic histories, into the category of postmemory. This seems to enact a double kidnapping of Carri. First, she is denied recognition of her direct experience of her own past: she is not the child of traumatised survivors but the direct subject of a traumatic loss. Secondly, and more broadly, there seems to be a kidnapping of the Latin American experience of trauma by trauma and memory paradigms developed in the aftermath of the Holocaust. Only one contributor resisted the 'postmemory' label. Marianna Eva Perez points to the intrinsic difference between children 'raised by traumatized parents who survived Nazi concentration camps' and those whose parents 'disappeared'. As she puts it, the Latin-American filmmakers and writers are 'orphans without a corpse' not children of the traumatised; they are victims and witnesses in their own right, not *secondhand* victims and witnesses (Perez 2013: 8–9).

Finally, another set of cultural critics co-opt Carri and her film to a political agenda that seeks to wrest ownership of the traumatic past from the families of the disappeared and to democratise it as the inheritance of everyone in Latin America. At the time of the disappearances in Argentina, the call for justice was led by the 'Abuelas/Madres de Plaza de Mayo' ('The Grandmothers [or Mothers] of the Plaza de Mayo') formed in 1977 and, with the passage of time, that leading role gradually passed to an organisation set up in 1995 by the children of the disappeared, 'HIJOS' ('Children') or 'Hijos por la Identidad y la Justicia contra el Olvido y el Silencio' ('Children for Identity and Justice Against Forgetting and Silence'). The political agenda of both organisations, according to Gabriela Nouzeilles (2005: 265), was 'a claim for justice based on biological identity and family ties'. A number of critics object to this 'discourse of identity and genealogical interpellation' (Nouzeilles 2005: 273) – to this 'DNA performance' (Taylor 2003: 173–5) – as it excludes those without blood-ties to victims and obscures the traumatic legacy as it plays out for all Argentinians. Other critics, like Cecilia Sosa, object to the conservative, catholic, nuclear-family-orientated agenda of (especially) the grandmothers' organisation, and offer an alternative queer reading of Argentinian history and Carri's film:

> For more than thirty years, this bloodline assembly of victims has commanded the experience of mourning, transforming the local landscape of memory struggles into a family issue.
>
> (Sosa 2014: 1–2)

Sosa wants to look instead at 'the experience of mourning beyond the boundaries of those who have been "directly affected" by violence' and '[i]n doing so, [...] seek to illuminate an alternative perspective to understand the transmission of trauma beyond bloodline inscriptions' and so 'contest the biological normativity that has become hegemonic' (Sosa 2014: 1–2). To make her case, Sosa (2013: 77) co-opts Hirsch's latest iteration of postmemory – so-called 'affiliative postmemory' (Hirsch 2012: 36) – which encompasses embodied forms of transmission that transcend familial ties. But affiliative postmemory seems a poor fit with Carri's experience, which *is* 'familial' and *is not* 'post'.

Although one suspects that Carri might not object to the politics of these positions, they do not seem to fit very comfortably with the film Carri actually produced and the film's presentation of her experience of her *constitutional absence*. Of *The Blonds*, Gabriela Nouzeilles writes,

> Against the compulsory demand of genealogical inscription, Carri suggests the desirability of other kinds of communities, beyond the politics of blood and party; that is, flexible, open communities, capable of imagining still undefined, alternative political projects, helping the members of a wounded society to accomplish what Alberto Moreiras has called *el duelo del duelo*, the mourning of mourning.
>
> (Nouzeilles 2005: 266)

The optimistic closing scene of *The Blonds*, as Carri walks towards a new dawn with her crew of friends, supports Nouzeilles's vision of an alternative future, with Carri part of a new, non-biological family (a flexible, open community). But this cannot mask Carri's connection to her past through blood and DNA, through an unbreakable bodily bond to her parents revealed to the viewer in the scene at the *EAAF* offices. This is not the 'politics of blood' – it is not a political position that Carri has adopted – but it is a brute, primitive, psychic connection that finds expression in blood. And certainly, for me, Joanna Page (2009: 175) goes too far when she writes that 'Carri prefers to emphasize the absence of those links. Rather than claiming authority on the basis of blood-ties, *Los Rubios* does what it can to insist on the rupture of the family line.' Whilst I can agree that Carri does not claim *authority* on the basis of blood-ties, she is only able to reclaim something for herself on precisely that basis, even if the tie that expresses itself as blood is ultimately an unconscious, psychic tie. It is all she has left of her parents; it is that profound link that resists rupture.

In their desire to displace the central and conservative metaphor of the 'wounded family' in the process of national mourning (in which 'memory has risked being reduced to a matter of blood'), Carri's film has been seized upon by friendly critics as a disruptive, queer, questioning, open text that offers the possibility of a better future for Argentina's past (Sosa 2013: 76). Sosa argues passionately that placing the *wounded family* at the heart of the national response to the events of the 1970s and 1980s (and making a blood-tie to one of the disappeared into a qualification that permits one to speak about the past), has damaged the national debate, undermining the possibility of an open, communal mourning process. As she writes: 'this is the biological normativity that restrains the resonances of trauma from traveling throughout a wider society', stifling 'a more extensive idea of "us" for postdictatorial Argentina' (Sosa 2011: 66). She writes of the final scene in *The Blonds*

> the crew wearing blond wigs has the lightness of a visionary dream. The embryonic queer family walking towards the horizon has the ability to highlight something that is still in a process of emergence in Argentine society: a new lineage where past and present are joined together through an experience of shared mourning [...] the film enacts a dream that invents its own future.
>
> (Sosa 2011: 78)

I find nothing to argue with in this reading of the film's closing scene itself; it is an optimistic fiction or fantasy or hallucination or wish-fulfillment which Carri places over the blank canvas of absence. But in co-opting this closing vision to a national, political agenda, Sosa scotomises the powerful psychic tie expressed through blood and hair that connects Carri to the 'corpses' of her parents. This is the unrepresented, introjected, psychic framing structure that holds everything else in place; a frame that is required as a container for the optimistic or soothing fantasies, fictions or hallucinations of the closing scene. Sosa sees and celebrates the picture in the frame but cannot see the frame. In doing so, Carri's very personal film about her struggle to find her "disappeared" parents is taken hostage by a political agenda which was not Carri's in making *this* film or at least by an agenda that is not supported by *this* film.[39]

My views are closer to those of Kerry Bystrom for whom *The Blonds* (and a number of other recent Argentinian films)

> present the individual subject, and not the community, society or the nation as the basic unit that needs to be reconstructed. They thus point to the limitations of filmmaking from any side of the political spectrum that threatens to overwhelm individual stories – sublimating individual pain into social catharsis – and suggest instead a documentary politics anchored in the painstaking unraveling of one's own complex subject position.
>
> (Bystrom 2009: 48)

The Blonds is a highly personal, interior exploration of a private trauma in which the director is constantly trying to disentangle her psychic history from other people's histories and from broader political forces that attempt to hijack her story. Carri's vision of the future is important and protean but the core of the film – its profound psychic meaning – lies in a bodily connection between Carri and her dead parents. The route Carri chose to painstakingly unravel her 'own complex subject position' was through fictions – films-within-the-documentary – which she conceived and directed and witnessed within the diegesis as an intra-diegetic audience member. It was a process made possible by the self-reflexive form of *The Blonds:* a process that bears many of the hallmarks of an exercise in self-analysis.

Notes

1 As Jordana Blejmar and Natalia Fortuny (2013: 3) point out, Carri's approach was new to documentary: this 'blending of autobiography with fiction [...] was not common in films, literature and testimonies of the 1980s and 1990s' in Latin America about the 'dictatorial past'.

2 I refer to Analía Couceyro as an *actress* rather than *actor*, following the form, *actriz*, used by Carri in the film.

3 'Kamikaze' is how the characters in John Waters's *Cecil B. Demented* (2000) describe their filmmaking.

4 Nick Fraser and several other scholars make a similar (invalid) criticism of Joshua Oppenheimer's *The Act of Killing*: 'Instead of an investigation, based on such humdrum aspects of the killings as to why and how they occurred [...] we have ended somewhere else' (Fraser 2013: 22).

5 Carri says this on screen in response to hearing the letter.

6 Carri is not alone amongst her generation of orphans of the "disappearances" either in her sense of a formative *constitutional absence* at her core or in her resort to documentary film to explore that absence. Lisa Renee DiGiovanni (2013: 65) writes that in the decade since *The Blonds* was made (c. 2003–13), the documentary genre has provided a platform for the children of the disappeared to contemplate the legacies of loss; what Gabriela Nouzeilles (2005: 265) calls 'the complex sense of identity that they carried with them as a result of the foundational absence that defines their lives'.
7 Playmobil is a line of plastic toys produced, since the 1970s, by the Brandstätter Group in Germany. They were popular in Argentina by the time Carri's parents disappeared in 1977.
8 My description of Carri as 'a strong-willed and determined director' is not intended as a description of the "real" Albertina Carri but of the character "Albertina Carri" as played by Albertina Carri, whom we see in *The Blonds*.
9 It is conceivable that a well-read Argentinian viewer might know something of the book and therefore might have a different take from a non-Argentinian viewer (from this viewer). But it is my reading of the scene, that it was set up to deliberately produce the response I have described in all its viewers.
10 Scott's view fits Stella Bruzzi's description (2006: 185) of the use of performance within a non-fiction (documentary) context, as drawing 'attention to the impossibilities of authentic documentary representation' and acting as 'an alienating, distancing device'.
11 Albert Camus *The Outsider* (1983 [1942]).
12 The neighbour repeats several times the idea that the family were blond and always with complete certainty.
13 The neighbour's "recollection" could be viewed as a parapraxis performed by the political unconscious or as an ideologically prompted mis-remembering.
14 The intertextual echo (or, in Bakhtin's terms, the *dialogic* reach of *The Blonds*) does not end with the figure of Honey Whitlock, kidnapped and bent to the will of others. Waters memorably found room in *Cecil B Demented* for a cameo role for Patty Hearst – arguably the most famous kidnap victim of the twentieth century – who still generates controversy as to whether she was forced by, or conspired with, her kidnappers to commit criminal acts. So, in this dialogic reading of *The Blonds*, Carri/Couceyro is also Patty Hearst who is in turn either an innocent victim or a manipulative deceiver.
15 Here I agree with Shohini Chaudhuri (2014: 110): 'The scene is repeated in a series of takes, which serves not, as Joanna Page claims, to "detract from [the] emotive value of what is recounted onscreen" but to insist on it' (here Chaudhuri quotes and disagrees with Page 2009: 172).
16 Gamerro's observation is not intended as a criticism of the film.
17 Jane Pilling (2012: 2) has written about the creative possibilities of wordless animation: it transcends the 'boundaries of language' and in so doing 'give[s] voice to that which is hard to articulate' namely 'unconscious feelings'. In similar vein, Paul Wells (1998: 184) notes that 'animation can become a vehicle by which inarticulate emotions and experiences may be expressed'.
18 The scene runs for only 46 seconds.
19 Although we are not told this in *The Blonds*, Roberto Carri's life ended with uncanny parallels to that of Isidro Velázquez (whose biography Roberto wrote and which Couceyro reads in an early scene in *The Blonds*). Both tried to help the poor and dispossessed of Argentina and both ended up being murdered by the state.
20 The Playmobil scenes suggest that this traumatic *undoing* may have taken place gradually. Carri's early fantasy of her parents returning to the farm 'by car, by bus, on horseback' might at first have "worked" for Carri but over time it gave way to the traumatising fantasy/nightmare of alien abduction.
21 What Jordana Blejmar (2013, 2016) calls 'playful memory'.

22 By using the term "body memory", I am *not* invoking Paul Connerton's (1989) concept of 'embodied memory' (memory carried in bodily gestures and habits). The unconscious connection between Carri and her parents has not even been able to struggle into the forms of bodily representation (bodily mirroring) that concern Connerton, as Carri was too young at the time of their disappearance.

23 This is Marianna Eva Perez's gloss of Bollas' ideas in *The Shadow of the Object* (1987).

24 Interviewer: '¿Por qué decidiste que por momentos se interpretara una actriz?'
Carri: 'Pasé por mil instancias. En algún momento pensé en ficcionalizar todo, pero no podía llamar a actores para que hagan de mi madre y de mi padre. Entonces decidí ficcionalizar mi presente. Me pareció importante que el espectador se quede con esa sensación de que es imposible reconstruir la memoria. Y que el recuerdo es más un estado de ánimo que otra cosa.'

25 It reminds me of the absolute refusal of the traumatised characters in Luigi Pirandello's *Six Characters in Search of an Author* (1995 [1921]) to have themselves substituted bodily by the actors.

26 I have not managed to find a copy of Carri's original statement in Spanish on which these two translations must be based (despite contacting Carri herself through *Cinemargentino*). The "missing" original Spanish text seems to have replicated in my research, the predicament Carri found herself in. I find myself with plenty of other people's translations floating around the edges of the missing core text, just as Carri had plenty of other people's memories (translations) floating around the edges of the missing core that was her parents. Perhaps this doesn't matter, as it is clear, even from translations, that Carri was only able to put her past together with her present when she came to focus on her parents' absent bodies/corpses.

27 'Mi sensación es que nadie ha metido la mano en ese agujero negro que es la ausencia.'

28 Carri is not alone in reaching for an astronomical metaphor when trying to describe her experience of a "disappearance". The filmmaker and some of the interviewees in Patricio Guzmán's 2010 documentary exploration of the Chilean disappearances, *Nostalgia for the Light*, also look to the stars to find ways to represent and describe the experience.

29 Similar sound techniques were used to disturbing effect in the diving-bell scenes in the film *The Diving Bell and the Butterfly* (2007), as director Julian Schnabel attempted to make the viewer feel the terror of the film's hero Jean-Dominique Bauby, who is left with "locked-in syndrome" after a stroke.

30 My comments on Green and Winnicott in this section are indebted to an unpublished conference paper by Rachel Chaplin (2016).

31 I am following Green's and Winnicott's usage of mother/maternal here, but this does not exclude paternal holding or even extra-parental holding and really designates the crucial early bonding of the baby with whoever is the care-giver.

32 Several critics point to this feeling of optimism at the end of the film, for example, Nouzeilles (2005), Bystrom (2009), Page (2009), Sosa (2013).

33 *Influencia* (released 2002) was originally a Todd Rundgren song, *Influenza* (1982). In the 1970s, García was a member of the band *La Máquina de Hacer Pájaros* whose 1977 album *Películas* (*'Movies'*) contained several political songs directed against the military junta responsible for the disappearances.

34 Winnicott's developmental speculations also describe the nature of film, where there is the illusion that what the *director* creates really exists.

35 For the complete lyrics to the song, type *charly garcia influencia lyrics* into a search engine.

36 Bystrom's characterisation of the process of making *The Blonds* as a therapeutic process of mourning is similar to Laplanche's characterisation of the psychoanalytic process as a process of mourning (see Ray 2012: 56); and Alisa Lebow's (2008) characterisation of her own filmmaking practice as a process of coming to terms with loss.

37 Kohan's criticism of *The Blonds* is reminiscent of the fierce policing of Holocaust representation that was so prevalent in the 1980s and 1990s. Kohan seems to want to set similarly narrow limits to, and impose a list of approved methods for, the representation of the Latin American state-sponsored murders and disappearances of the 1970s and 1980s.

38 For example, Bystrom (2009: 45), Nouzeilles (2005: 265).

39 I am aware that Carri has spoken in support of Sosa's political agenda at conferences organised by Sosa. But my point is that notwithstanding Carri's public political agenda, the film *The Blonds* itself seems to reveal something that challenges or at least complicates this agenda.

Conclusion

This book began as my attempt to understand why a number of recent documentaries that deal with traumatic personal histories have featured fictions or forms of representation, more usually associated with fiction, and broken with the conventions of "realist" documentary practice. These documentaries do not appear to have abandoned the desire to discover something about the "real" world; rather, it seems that something in the nature of trauma demands the deployment of fictions as a route to "truths" or meanings about the real, non-fictional world.

The 'bait of falsehood' emerged as an organising principle. It draws on a clinical technique first suggested in Freud's radical paper *Constructions in Analysis* (1937b) – itself drawing on speculations in *Hamlet* about the power of enacted, embodied fictions – where a fiction is the bait that takes an otherwise unavailable truth about the "real" world. It is a technique that recognises the profound difficulty in representing trauma whilst rejecting the contention of post-structuralist trauma theory, that trauma is irrevocably unrepresentable and beyond the reach of understanding. These fictions can take many forms, from out-and-out fictions to quasi-historical reconstructions of past events. Their function is to bring representational content to otherwise unrepresented aspects of traumatic experience, which can then act as *baits* or *catalysts* to coax out meaning for the traumatised documentary protagonist. Bringing meaning or understanding to the trauma might just help to ameliorate the pain of traumatic experience.

It is a contention that sees the documentary-making process as having the potential to be a dynamic, therapeutic process, which bears comparison with aspects of the analytic and self-analytic process: an inter- and intra-personal exploration, where a trauma rooted in the past is revivified in current relationships. It is an argument that insists that certain documentaries do not just *show* something but *do* something. The edited films that result are records of a creative act playing out over time, in which things that happen in the filmic present, transform (and can be seen by the viewer to transform) fixed and intractable patterns of psychic behaviour. This dynamic process begins with the provocation of the fiction (the bait of falsehood of the film-within-the-film), kick-starting a self-reflexive process of reflection for the filmic protagonist that might lead to symbolisation: to what Freud called a 'carp of truth' and I would describe as a meaningful account.

DOI: 10.4324/9781003657187-9

Drawing on psychoanalytic models, I have theorised the bait of falsehood in a number of ways. The space occupied by the fictional film within the documentary is akin to the potential space that Donald Winnicott opened up for his child patients to play with toys and to create fictional scenarios that might capture aspects of hitherto hidden, lost or unarticulated facets of a trauma. I have also thought of the documentary film as a frame, like André Green's 'framing structure', into which the protagonist places, removes and replaces a variety of "pictures" (fictions) in the struggle to create or find representational content for the trauma. Representations are conjured up and played with and placed in the frame: a process Rithy Panh described as a search for 'the missing picture'; and Albertina Carri experienced as a desperate quest to fill a black hole, a constituting absence, like a blank canvas within the frame of both herself and her documentary. Documentary protagonists use the documentary-making process to stage scenes from their inner psychic theatre as Anna O did on the "stage" of her analysis with Josef Breuer. Sometimes these "plays" are not conscious, intentional constructions – even if they begin as that – but the bizarre performances that Joyce McDougall observed in her patients, where the body stages its own scenes, or where the unconscious acts out troubling, "forgotten" relationships, and the conscious "I" becomes witness to a trauma playing itself out on the stage of their own body. To coax these performances from the traumatised actor in the film-within, documentary makers have reached for a range of imaginative, provocative devices, often (re-)discovering the creative potential of the performative techniques pioneered in psychodrama: role-playing, role reversal, doubling, mirroring, soliloquy. All are attempts to lure the buried trauma onto the open stage.

Though the 'bait of falsehood' is the organising principle of the book, it is ultimately concerned with the 'carp of truth' – with the psychic meanings the falsehood provokes. The 'bait' is not in itself meaningful. It is only in the documentary protagonist reflecting on their emotional, affective and somatic responses to the fiction (described by Hamlet as *blenches* and by Freud as *touches*) – including reflection on the powerful inter- and intra-personal identifications generated both within the fictional film-within and in witnessing it – that meaning might emerge. The carps of truth that emerge from this process of reflection as it plays out over filmic time are perhaps best understood as tentative, contingent meanings that neither conform to an external notion of objectivity nor are they an absolute truth: the psychic "Real" or "O" (the thing-in-itself). It is never possible to know if the meanings that emerge have been created or found (whether they are fiction or truth): instead, their importance lies in their power to transform psychic experience. This is a pragmatic and therapeutic conception of meaningfulness. Guy Maddin certainly thought of his own filmmaking practice as offering this therapeutic potential when he announced at the beginning of *My Winnipeg* (2007), 'What if … I film my way out of here?' (that is, film his way out of his trauma-induced depression) and Ari Folman confirmed this potential when, at the end of the filmmaking process looking back at the making of *Waltz with Bashir* (2008), he described it as 'four years of therapy'.[1]

My main focus in this book has been on the processes through which meanings emerge for the documentary (or diegetic) protagonist. In many documentaries, these processes remain hidden from the viewer but they are at least partially available in the open, reflexive and self-reflexive documentaries I have chosen to consider in this study: documentaries that foreground the processes and the inter-personal mechanisms that generate diegetic meanings through a Brechtian unmasking of the mechanics of the filmmaking process and in allowing the process of mediation involved in the reception of the documentary to play out within the documentary itself.

Beyond the protagonist, I also wanted to understand and theorise a second *locus* of meaning-making. The one with which documentary theory is more usually concerned: that of the person who watches the completed documentary – the extra-diegetic viewer engaging with the film and the on-screen protagonists. I have conceptualised meaning-making in both *loci* as occurring through a counter-transferential process. This counter-transferential model builds on and extends the transferential models of the documentary encounter that have been developed by a number of documentary scholars in recent years. A counter-transferential model best captures the complex back-and-forth movements of affect and somatic effects and forms of identification that take place between viewer and viewed, whether that viewer is the intra-diegetic viewer (the traumatised protagonist) inside the documentary responding to the 'bait' of the film-within or "us", as extra-diegetic viewers, responding to the documentary object. In both *loci*, subject and object, viewer and viewed, are enmeshed with one another through powerful forms of identification.

This counter-transferential methodology, drawn from psychoanalysis, is also implicit in film phenomenology. That is, in phenomenology's refusal of a simple division between subject and object – viewer and viewed – through its positing of a subject who is always an experiencing-subject who views an object which is always an experienced-object. Neither subject nor object exists separately but each is always implied by the other and implicated in the other. More specifically, I have advocated a counter-transferential approach to try to capture the radical nature of the identifications generated in documentary spectatorship where, rather than thinking of a two-way movement between separate objects, we could think of the objects as becoming the same, becoming identical, as they come into contact.

This intermingling of viewer and viewed is also at the heart of Winnicottian approaches to film, where the extra-diegetic viewer both *finds* the documentary out there on the screen and *creates* the documentary in an imaginative encounter with the filmic object as it acts back on the viewer and enmeshes with the viewer's unique subject position (including the viewer's unconscious). This finding and creating of the film by the extra-diegetic viewer also describes the diegetic protagonist/viewer's engagement with the filmic fictions – the *baits* – of the film-within.

The use of fictions in documentary raises the question of which interpretative tools should be deployed. Do we treat documentary as fictional and pursue approaches that were developed with a fictional text in mind or do we treat them as "real" and approach them more in the manner of the historian or sociologist or psychologist or anthropologist rather than the literary critic? I have tried to draw on both of these theoretical tendencies. In speculating about the psychic lives of real on-screen protagonists, I am also fully cognisant of the brute fact that my only access to these protagonists is through a mediated, edited, manipulated filmic text. My approach has been influenced by film phenomenologist Vivian Sobchack, who insists that when we watch documentary, we look both at the screen and through the screen; we are dependent upon the screen for knowledge but are 'also aware of an excess of existence not contained by it' (1999: 246). In looking through the screen, we speculate about the lives – including the psychic lives – of protagonists but when we look at the screen for knowledge, we must interpret a text and understand how that text works. It is an approach to filmic texts and filmic protagonists that places the documentary viewer in a position akin to that of the reader of a psychoanalytic case study: dependent on the on-page text for knowledge of Dora or Anna O or the Wolf Man – dependent on the on-screen text for knowledge of Anwar Congo or Albertina Carri or Rithy Panh – but also attempting to look through the text to a real life beyond.

In taking seriously the idea that these documentaries can open a route to understanding real traumas for both the viewer and the viewed, those conventionally fictional elements within the diegesis – the fictional-films-within-the-film – can be seen to be fictional in only a limit sense. The fictions are the necessary detour, the circuitous route, that enables trauma to take representational form; representations that act, in turn, as a bait to take a truth, to take a meaningful account of trauma that might just prove to be cathartic in a very real, non-fictional life.

> Your bait of falsehood takes this carp of truth;
> And thus do we of wisdom and of reach,
> With windlasses and with assays of bias,
> By indirections find directions out.
>
> (Polonius to Reynaldo:
> *Hamlet*: Act II Scene I)

Note

1 Maddin's comment was made in voice-over in the film; Folman's in an interview (Schäuble 2011: 210).

List of works cited

Abraham, Karl. 1927 [1924]. "A Short Study of the Development of the Libido, Viewed in the Light of Mental Disorders. History of the Development of the Libido." *Selected Papers of Karl Abraham*, 418–79. London: Hogarth Press and Institute of Psycho-Analysis.

Abraham, Nicolas, and Mária Török. 1986. *The Wolf Man's Magic Word: A Cryptonymy*. Translated by Nicholas T. Rand. Minneapolis: University of Minnesota Press.

Abraham, Nicolas, and Mária Török. 1994 [1972]. "Mourning or Melancholia: Introjection versus Incorporation." In *The Shell and the Kernel: Renewals of Psychoanalysis*, edited and translated by Nicholas T. Rand, 125–38. Chicago, IL and London: University of Chicago Press.

Abraham, Nicolas, and Mária Török. 1994 [1975]. "'The Lost Object - Me': Notes on Endocryptic Identification." In *The Shell and the Kernel: Renewals of Psychoanalysis*, edited and translated by Nicholas T. Rand, 139–56. Chicago, IL; London: University of Chicago Press.

Abraham, Nicolas, and Mária Török. 1994. *The Shell and the Kernel: Renewals of Psychoanalysis*. Edited and translated by Nicholas T. Rand. Chicago, IL and London: University of Chicago Press.

Agamben, Giorgio. 2000. *Remnants of Auschwitz: The Witness and the Archive*. New York: Zone Books.

Aguilar, Gonzalo. 2008. *Other Worlds: New Argentine Film*. Translated by Sarah Ann Wells. New York: Palgrave Macmillan.

Aguilar, Gonzalo. 2011. *Otros mundos un ensayo sobre el nuevo cine argentino*. Buenos Aires: Santiago Arcos editor.

Aisenstein, Marilia. 2017. *An Analytic Journey: From the Art of Archery to the Art of Psychoanalysis*. London: Routledge.

Amar, Nadine. 1988. *Formation au psychodrame analytique*. Paris: Dunod.

Amar, Nadine. 2005. "Analytic Psychodrama." In *International Dictionary of Psychoanalysis*, edited by Alain de Mijolla, 77–9. Detroit, MI: Macmillan Reference USA.

Anzieu, Didier. 1986 [1959 & 1975]. *Freud's Self-Analysis*. Translated by Peter Graham. London: Hogarth.

Anzieu, Didier. 2004 [1957]. *Le psychodrame analytique: Chez l'enfant et l'adolescent*. 3rd edition. Paris: PUF.

Arendt, Hannah. 2006 [1963]. *Eichmann in Jerusalem: A Report on the Banality of Evil*. London: Penguin.

Asibong, Andrew. 2022. *Post-traumatic Attachments to the Eerily Moving Image: Something to Watch over Me*. (Psychoanalysis and Popular Culture Series). London and New York: Routledge, Taylor & Francis Group.

Bainbridge, Caroline. 2019. "Box-set Mind-set: Psycho-cultural Approaches to Binge Watching, Gender, and Digital Experience." *Free Associations*, 75 June: 65–83. Freely available at: https://freeassociations.org.uk/FA_New/OJS/index.php/fa/issue/view/25. [Accessed 22 January 2026].

Bainbridge, Caroline, Ivan Ward, and Candida Yates, eds. 2014. *Television and Psychoanalysis: Psycho-Cultural Perspectives*. (Psychoanalysis and Popular Culture Series). London and New York: Routledge, Taylor & Francis Group.

Bainbridge, Caroline, and Candida Yates. 2011. "Therapy Culture/Culture as Therapy: Psycho-cultural Studies of Media and the Inner World." *Free Associations*, 62 September: i–v. Freely available at: https://freeassociations.org.uk/FA_New/OJS/index.php/fa/issue/view/5. [Accessed 22 January 2026].

Bainbridge, Caroline, and Candida Yates. 2014. "Introduction." In *Media and the Inner World: Psycho-cultural Approaches to Emotion, Media and Popular Culture*, edited by Caroline Bainbridge and Candida Yates, 1–16. Basingstoke: Palgrave Macmillan.

Bannister, Anne. 2007. "Psychodrama and Child Development." In *Psychodrama: Advances in Theory and Practice*, edited by Clark Baim, Jorge Burmeister, and Manuela Maciel, 239–46. London and New York: Routledge.

Barnes, Henry. 2013. "Joshua Oppenheimer: 'You Celebrate Mass Killing so You Don't Have to Look Yourself in the Mirror'." Interview. *The Guardian*, 20 June. Available at: https://www.theguardian.com/film/2013/jun/20/joshua-oppenheimer-act-of-killing. [Accessed 11 May 2016].

Barron, James W., ed. 1993. *Self-Analysis: Critical Inquiries, Personal Visions*. Hillsdale, NJ and London: Analytic Press.

Barthes, Roland. 1984. *Camera Lucida: Reflections on Photography*. Translated by Richard Howard. London: Flamingo.

Beckett, Colin. 2014. "Finding a Liberal Form: Oppenheimer, Morris, Godmilow." *INCITE!* (Fall). Available at: https://incite-online.net/beckett5.html. [Accessed 18 November 2019].

Belau, Linda. 2001. "Trauma and the Material Signifier." *Postmodern Culture* 11 (2). https://doi.org/10.1353/pmc.2001.0001. Freely available at: https://pmc.iath.virginia.edu/text-only/issue.101/11.2belau.txt. [Accessed 24 March 2018].

Bennington, Geoffrey. 1987. *Lyotard: Writing the Event*. Manchester: Manchester University Press.

Bergstrom, Janet. 1999. *Endless Night: Cinema and Psychoanalysis, Parallel Histories*. Berkeley and London: University of California Press.

Berman, Emanuel, Timna Rosenheimer, and Michal Aviad. 2003. "Documentary Directors and Their Protagonists: A Transferential / Countertransferential Relationship?" In *The Couch and the Silver Screen: Psychoanalytic Reflections on European Cinema*, edited by Andrea Sabbadini, 212–32. Hove and New York: Brunner-Routledge.

Bion, W. R. 1957. "Differentiation of the Psychotic from the Non-Psychotic Personalities." *International Journal of Psycho-Analysis* 38: 266–75.

Bion, W. R. 1959. "Attacks on Linking." *International Journal of Psycho-Analysis* 40: 308–15.

Bion, W. R. 1962. "The Psycho-Analytic Study of Thinking." *International Journal of Psycho-Analysis* 43: 306–10.

Bion, W. R. 1970. *Attention and Interpretation: A Scientific Approach to Insight in Psycho-Analysis and Groups*. London: Tavistock Publications.

Bion, W. R. 1992. *Cogitations*. Edited by Francesca Bion. London: Karnac.

Bion, W. R. 1994 [1962]. *Learning from Experience*. Lanham, MD, Boulder, CO, New York, Toronto and Oxford: Rowman & Littlefield.

Birksted-Breen, Dana. 2016. *The Work of Psychoanalysis: Sexuality, Time and the Psychoanalytic Mind.* London and New York: Routledge.

Birksted-Breen, Dana, and Sara Flanders. 2010. "General Introduction." In *Reading French Psychoanalysis*, edited by Dana Birksted-Breen, Sara Flanders, and Alain Gibeault, 1–51. London and New York: Routledge.

Birksted-Breen, Dana, Sara Flanders, and Alain Gibeault, eds. 2010. *Reading French Psychoanalysis*. London and New York: Routledge.

Blejmar, Jordana. 2013. "Toying with History: Playful Memory in Albertina Carri's 'Los Rubios'." *Journal of Romance Studies* 13 (3): 44–61.

Blejmar, Jordana 2016. *Playful Memories: The Autofictional Turn in Post-Dictatorship Argentina*. New York: Springer.

Blejmar, Jordana, and Natalia Fortuny, eds. 2013. "Introduction - Revisiting Postmemory: The Intergenerational Transmission of Trauma in Post-Dictatorship Latin American Culture." *Journal of Romance Studies* 13 (3): 1–5.

Bohleber, Werner, Peter Fonagy, Juan Pablo Jiménez, Dominique Scarfone, Sverre Varvin, and Samuel Zysman. 2013. "Towards a Better Use of Psychoanalytic Concepts: A Model Illustrated Using the Concept of Enactment." *International Journal of Psychoanalysis* 94 (3): 501–30.

Bollas, Christopher. 1987. *The Shadow of the Object: Psychoanalysis of the Unthought Known*. London: Free Association Books.

Botella, César. 2014. "On Remembering: The Notion of Memory without Recollection." *International Journal of Psychoanalysis* 95 (5): 911–36.

Botella, César, and Sara Botella. 2005. *The Work of Psychic Figurability: Mental States without Representation.* Translated by Andrew Weller, with the collaboration of Monique Zerbib. Hove, East Sussex; New York, NY: Brunner-Routledge.

Botella, César, and Sara Botella. 2013. "Psychic Figurability and Unrepresented States." In *Unrepresented States and the Construction of Meaning: Clinical and Theoretical Contributions*, edited by Howard B. Levine, Gail S. Reed, and Dominique Scarfone, 95–121. London: Karnac Books.

Boyle, Deirdre. 2014a. "Confronting Images of Ideology: An Interview with Rithy Panh." *Cineaste* 39 (3) (Summer): 33–35.

Boyle, Deirdre. 2014b. "Finding the Missing Picture: The Films of Rithy Panh." *Cineaste* 39 (3) (Summer): 28–32.

Boyle, Deirdre. See also: Panh, Rithy, and Dierdre Boyle. 2015.

Bradshaw, Nick. 2013. "Build My Gallows High." *Sight & Sound*, July: 36–9.

Breckenridge, Janis. 2008. "Performing Memory and Identity: Albertina Carri's 'Los Rubios'." *Letras Femeninas* 34 (2): 11–27.

Brenman, Eric. 1980. "The Value of Reconstruction in Adult Psychoanalysis." *International Journal of Psycho-Analysis* 61: 53–60.

Brenman, Eric. 2006. *Recovery of the Lost Good Object*. Edited by Gigliola Fornari Spoto. London: Taylor & Francis.

Breuer, Josef. 1955 [1893]. "Fräulein Anna O: Case Histories: Case I." In *The Standard Edition of the Complete Psychological Works of Sigmund Freud,* edited and translated James Strachey et al., 24 volumes, volume 2, 19–47. London: The Hogarth Press and The Institute of Psycho-Analysis.

Breuer, Josef, and Sigmund Freud. 1955 [1893]. "On the Psychical Mechanism of Hysterical Phenomena." In *The Standard Edition of the Complete Psychological Works of Sigmund Freud,* edited and translated James Strachey et al., 24 volumes, volume 2, 1–17. London: The Hogarth Press and The Institute of Psycho-Analysis.
Brink, Joram ten, and Joshua Oppenheimer. 2012. *Killer Images: Documentary Film, Memory and the Performance of Violence*. London and New York: Wallflower Press.
Britton, John. 1961. "A. C. Bradley and Those Children of Lady Macbeth." *Shakespeare Quarterly* 12 (3): 349–51.
Brook, Andrew. 2003. "Kant and Freud." In *Psychoanalytic Knowledge*, edited by Man Cheung Chung and Colin Feltham, 20–39. London: Palgrave Macmillan UK.
Bruzzi, Stella. 2006. *New Documentary*. 2nd edition. London and New York: Routledge.
Bruzzi, Stella. 2015a. "Re-Enacting Trauma in Film and Television: Restaging History, Revisiting Pain." In *Therapy and Emotions in Film and Television: The Pulse of Our Times*, edited by Claudia Wassmann, 89–98. Basingstoke: Palgrave Macmillan.
Bruzzi, Stella. 2015b. "Recording Reality, Desiring the Real - The Right to Play Oneself: Looking Back on Documentary Film." Book review of Elizabeth Cowie's 2011 *Recording Reality, Desiring the Real*. *Screen* 56 (3): 384–87.
Butler, Judith. 2005. *Giving an Account of Oneself.* New York: Fordham University Press.
Bystrom, Kerry. 2009. "The Politics of Subjectivity: Notes on 21st Century Argentinian Documentary Film." In *Rethinking Third Cinema: The Role of Anti-Colonial Media and Aesthetics in Postmodernity*, edited by Frieda Ekotto and Adeline Koh, 31–51. Berlin: LIT.
Camus, Albert. 1983 [1942]. *The Outsider*. Translated by Joseph Laredo. Harmondsworth: Penguin.
Candeloro, Jean-Pierre. 2000. *Docu-Fiction: Convergence and Contamination between Documentary Representation and Fictional Simulation*. PhD thesis. Università della Svizzera Italiana Lugano. Available at: https://web.archive.org/web/20110911104733/https://www.bul.unisi.ch/cerca/bul/memorie/com/pdf/9900Candeloro.pdf. [Accessed 3 February 2017].
Caruth, Cathy. 1991. "Introduction to Psychoanalysis, Trauma and Culture." *American Imago* 48 (1): 1–12.
Caruth, Cathy, ed. 1995. *Trauma: Explorations in Memory*. Baltimore, MD: Johns Hopkins University Press.
Caruth, Cathy. 1996. *Unclaimed Experience: Trauma, Narrative, and History*. Baltimore, MD: Johns Hopkins University Press.
Casebier, Allan. 1991. *Film and Phenomenology: Toward a Realist Theory of Cinematic Representation*. Reprinted 2009. Cambridge: Cambridge University Press.
Castoriadis, Cornelius. 1997. *World in Fragments: Writings on Politics, Society, Psychoanalysis, and the Imagination*. Edited and translated by David Ames Curtis. Stanford, CA: Stanford University Press.
Cazenave, Jennifer. 2018. "Earth as Archive: Reframing Memory and Mourning in 'The Missing Picture'." *Cinema Journal* 57 (2) (Winter): 44–65.
Chanan, Michael. 2007. *The Politics of Documentary*. London: BFI.
Chaplin, Rachel. 2016. *The Creation of the Symbolising Mind: An Approach from the Independent Tradition*. Unpublished paper (given at the Interdisciplinary Seminar Series: UCL Psychoanalysis Unit, University College London, Institute of Advanced Studies): 1–6.
Chaplin, Rachel. 2027 (forthcoming). "It's Not a Sin to Fly: Beyond the Pleasure Principle and the Radical Imagination." In *Beyond the Pleasure Principle Revisited: Clinical Explorations in the 21st Century*, edited by Rachel Chaplin, Part Three (Epilogue). London and New York: Routledge, Taylor & Francis Group.

Chaudhuri, Shohini. 2014. *Cinema of the Dark Side: Atrocity and the Ethics of Film Spectatorship*. Edinburgh: Edinburgh University Press.

Cohn, Pamela. 2012. "Joshua Oppenheimer by Pamela Cohn" Interview (with Joshua Oppenheimer). *BOMB*, 18 December 2012. Available at: https://bombmagazine.org/articles/joshua-oppenheimer-1/. [Accessed 11 May 2016].

Connerton, Paul. 1989. *How Societies Remember*. Cambridge and New York: Cambridge University Press.

Cooper, Caroline M. 2013. "On Anwar, from Oppenheimer." Blog. *Caroline M Cooper*, 13 June. Available at: https://carolinemcooper.com/on-anwar-from-oppenheimer/. [Accessed 24 January 2019].

Cousins, Mark, and Kevin Macdonald. 2006. *Imagining Reality: The Faber Book of Documentary*. Revised edition. London: Faber.

Cowie, Elizabeth. 1999. "The Spectacle of Actuality." In *Collecting Visible Evidence*, edited by Jane Gaines and Michael Renov, 19–45. Visible Evidence, v. 6. Minneapolis: University of Minnesota Press.

Cowie, Elizabeth. 2011. *Recording Reality, Desiring the Real*. Visible Evidence, v. 24. Minneapolis: University of Minnesota Press.

Craps, Stef. 2013. *Postcolonial Witnessing: Trauma out of Bounds*. Basingstoke: Palgrave Macmillan.

Craps, Stef. 2014. "Beyond Eurocentrism: Trauma Theory in the Global Age." In *The Future of Trauma Theory: Contemporary Literary Criticism*, edited by Gert Buelens, Sam Durrant, and Robert Eaglestone, 45–61. New York: Routledge.

Creme, Phyllis. 2013. "The Playing Spectator." In *Little Madnesses: Winnicott, Transitional Phenomena and Cultural Experience*, edited by Annette Kuhn, 39–51. London and New York: I.B. Tauris.

Crichlow, Warren. 2013. "'It's All about Finding the Right Excuse' in Joshua Oppenheimer's 'The Act of Killing'." *Film Quarterly* 67 (2): 37–43.

Critical Asian Studies, Editorial. 2014. "The Act of Killing." *Critical Asian Studies* 46 (1): 145–6.

Cross, Karen. 2022. *Toy Story and the Inner World of the Child: Animation, Play and Creative Life*. (Psychoanalysis and Popular Culture Series). London and New York: Routledge, Taylor & Francis Group.

Currie, Gregory. 1990. *The Nature of Fiction*. Cambridge: Cambridge University Press.

Cusset, Catherine. 2012. *The Limits of Autofiction*. Conference paper (delivered at New York University conference on autofiction, April 2012). Available at: https://www.catherinecusset.co.uk/wp-content/uploads/2013/02/THE-LIMITS-OF-AUTOFICTION.pdf. [Accessed 20 July 2017].

Cyrulnik, Boris. 2009. *Resilience: How Your Inner Strength Can Set You Free from the Past*. London: Penguin.

Deleuze, Gilles, and Félix Guattari. 1988 [1980]. *A Thousand Plateaus: Capitalism and Schizophrenia*. Translated by Brian Massumi. London: Athlone Press.

Delourmel, Christian. 2013. "An Introduction to the Work of André Green." *International Journal of Psychoanalysis* 94 (1): 133–56.

Di Iorio, Sam. 2007. "Total Cinema: 'Chronique d'un été' and the End of Bazinian Film Theory." *Screen* 48 (1): 25–43.

DiGiovanni, Lisa Renee. 2013. "Visual Archives of Loss and Longing in Chile: 'Mi Vida Con Carlos' by Germán Berger Hertz." *Journal of Romance Studies* 13 (3): 62–74.

Dollimore, Jonathan. 2010. *Radical Tragedy: Religion, Ideology and Power in the Drama of Shakespeare and His Contemporaries*. Reissued 3rd edition. Houndmills, Basingstoke, Hampshire and New York: Palgrave.

Dostoevsky, Fyodor. 2005. *The Double and The Gambler*. Translated by Richard Pevear and Larissa Volokhonsky. [*The Double* first published in 1846]. New York and London: Everyman.

Doubrovsky, Serge. 1989. *Le livre brisé*. Paris: Éditions Grasset.

Dupont, Judith. 2000. "La notion de trauma selon Ferenczi et ses effets sur la recherche psychanalytique ultérieure." *Filigrane* (Printemps): 19–31.

Eadie, Bruce. 2017. "Psychoanalysis and Ethics in Documentary Film." Book review (Agnieszka Piotrowska's *Psychoanalysis and Ethics in Documentary Film*). *New Review of Film and Television Studies* 15 (3): 381–84.

Eadie, Bruce. 2020. "Baits of Falsehood: The Role of Fiction in Documentary or from Untheorised Practice to Unpractised Theory." In *Creative Practice Research in the Age of Neoliberal Hopelessness*, edited by Agnieszka Piotrowska, 164–82. Edinburgh: Edinburgh University Press.

Eagleton, Terry. 2009. *Trouble with Strangers: A Study of Ethics*. Chichester and Malden, MA: Wiley-Blackwell.

Ebiri, Bilge. 2008. "Guy Maddin on Directing a 'Docu-Fantasia' about His Hometown." *Vulture*, 13 June. Available at: https://www.vulture.com/2008/06/guy_maddin.html. [Accessed 20 November 2017].

Eifermann, Rivka R. 1993. "The Discovery of Real and Fantasized Audiences for Self-Analysis." In *Self-Analysis: Critical Inquiries, Personal Visions*, edited by James W. Barron, 171–93. Hillsdale, NJ and London: Analytic Press.

Evans, Dylan. 1996. *An Introductory Dictionary of Lacanian Psychoanalysis*. London and New York: Routledge.

Feldman, Sally. 2013. "'The Act of Killing': Art, Documentary or Research with Impact?" *Times Higher Education (The)*, August 15. Available at: https://www.timeshighereducation.com/comment/columnists/the-act-of-killing-art-documentary-or-research-with-impact/2006482.article. [Accessed 13 May 2016].

Felman, Shoshana. 1991. "In an Era of Testimony: Claude Lanzmann's 'Shoah'." *Yale French Studies*, 79 (January): 39–81.

Felman, Shoshana, and Dori Laub. 1991. *Testimony: Crises of Witnessing in Literature, Psychoanalysis, and History*. New York: Routledge.

Fenichel, Otto. 1928. "The Clinical Aspect of the Need for Punishment." *International Journal of Psycho-Analysis* 9: 47–70.

Fenichel, Otto. 1946. *The Psychoanalytic Theory of Neurosis*. London: Routledge & Kegan Paul.

Ferencz-Flatz, Christian, and Julian Hanich, eds. 2016. "Editor's Introduction: What Is Film Phenomenology?" *Studia Phaenomenologica* 16: 11–61.

Ferenczi, Sándor. 1949 [1932]. "Confusion of the Tongues between the Adults and the Child (The Language of Tenderness and of Passion)." *International Journal of Psycho-Analysis* 30: 225–30.

Fletcher, John, and Martin Stanton. 1992. *Jean Laplanche: Seduction, Translation and the Drives*. London: Institute of Contemporary Arts.

Fondazione Pesaro Nuovo Cinema Onlus. 2006. "Catalogo Della 42a Mostra Internazionale Del Nuovo Cinema." Film catalogue and press release. *PesaroFilmFestival.it*. Available at: https://www.pesarofilmfest.it/IMG/pdf/catalogo_2006.pdf. [Accessed 29 March 2017].

Fortune, Drew. 2013. "Joshua Oppenheimer and Werner Herzog on 'The Act of Killing'." *AV CLUB*, 30 July. Available at: https://www.avclub.com/article/joshua-oppenheimer-and-werner-herzog-on-ithe-act-o-100900. [Accessed 13 May 2016].

Frank, Adam. See: Sedgwick, Eve Kosofsky, and Adam Frank. 1995a, 1995b.
Fraser, Nick. 2013. "We Love Impunity." *Film Quarterly* 67 (2): 21–24.
Fraser, Nick. 2014. "The Act of Killing: Don't Give an Oscar to This Snuff Movie." *The Guardian*, February 23. Available at: https://www.theguardian.com/commentisfree/2014/feb/23/act-of-killing-dont-give-oscar-snuff-movie-indonesia. [Accessed 2 November 2014].
Freud, Sigmund. 1953–74 [1886–1939]. *The Standard Edition of the Complete Psychological Works of Sigmund Freud.* Edited and translated James Strachey et al., 24 volumes. London: The Hogarth Press and The Institute of Psycho-Analysis.
Specific books, papers, essays and lectures available in the Standard Edition (SE) and cited in the book are as follows (dates given are of first publication in German):
Breuer, Josef. 1893 [1955]. *Fräulein Anna O: Case Histories: Case I.* SE Vol. 2: 19–47.
Freud, Sigmund, and Josef Breuer. 1893 [1955]. *On the Psychical Mechanism of Hysterical Phenomena.* SE Vol. 2: 1–17.
Freud, Sigmund. 1896. *The Aetiology of Hysteria.* SE Vol. 3: 187–221.
Freud, Sigmund. 1900–01. *The Interpretation of Dreams.* SE Vols. 4 & 5: ix–628.
Freud, Sigmund. 1905 [1901]. *Fragment of an Analysis of a Case of Hysteria* [also known as the "Dora" case]. SE Vol. 7: 1–122.
Freud, Sigmund. 1905a. *Three Essays on the Theory of Sexuality.* SE Vol. 7: 123–246.
Freud, Sigmund. 1905b. *Jokes and Their Relation to the Unconscious.* SE Vol. 8: 1–247.
Freud, Sigmund. 1909. *Notes Upon a Case of Obsessional Neurosis* [also known as the "Rat Man" case]. SE Vol. 10: 151–318.
Freud, Sigmund. 1913 *Totem and Taboo.* SE Vol. 13: vii–162.
Freud, Sigmund. 1914a. *Remembering, Repeating and Working Through (Further Recommendations on the Technique of Psycho-Analysis).* SE Vol. 12: 145–56.
Freud, Sigmund. 1914b. *On Narcissism: An Introduction.* SE Vol. 14: 67–102.
Freud, Sigmund. 1915a. *Instincts and Their Vicissitudes.* SE Vol. 14: 109–40.
Freud, Sigmund. 1915b. *The Unconscious.* SE Vol. 14: 159–215.
Freud, Sigmund. 1917 [1915]. *A Metapsychological Supplement to the Theory of Dreams.* SE Vol. 14: 217–35.
Freud, Sigmund. 1917a. *Mourning and Melancholia.* SE Vol. 14: 237–58.
Freud, Sigmund. 1917b. *Introductory Lectures on Psycho-Analysis: Lecture No.* XXI - *The Development of the Libido and the Sexual Organizations.* SE Vol. 16: 320–338.
Freud, Sigmund. 1918. *From the History of an Infantile Neurosis* [also known as the "Wolf Man" case]. SE Vol. 17: 1–124.
Freud, Sigmund. 1919a. *'A Child Is Being Beaten': A Contribution to the Study of the Origin of Sexual Perversions.* SE Vol. 17: 175–204.
Freud, Sigmund. 1919b. *The Uncanny.* SE Vol. 17: 217–56.
Freud, Sigmund. 1920. *Beyond the Pleasure Principle* (especially Section II containing vignette on Freud's grandson's "fort-da" game at pp. 14–7). SE Vol. 18: 1–64.
Freud, Sigmund. 1921. *Group Psychology and the Analysis of the Ego* (especially Section VII "On Identification" at pp. 105–10). SE Vol. 18: 65–144.
Freud, Sigmund. 1923. *The Ego and the Id.* SE Vol. 19: 1–66.
Freud, Sigmund. 1935. *The Subtleties of a Faulty Action.* SE Vol. 22: 231–236.
Freud, Sigmund. 1937a. *Analysis Terminable and Interminable.* SE Vol. 23: 209–254.
Freud, Sigmund. 1937b. *Constructions in Analysis.* SE Vol. 23: 255–70.
Freud, Sigmund. 1939. *Moses and Monotheism: Three Essays.* SE Vol. 23: 1–138.
Freud, Sigmund, and Jeffrey Moussaieff Masson. 1985. *The Complete Letters of Sigmund Freud to Wilhelm Fliess, 1877-1904.* Edited and translated by Jeffrey Moussaieff Masson. Cambridge, MA and London: Belknap Press of Harvard University Press.

Friend, Stacie. 2012. "Fiction as a Genre." *Proceedings of the Aristotelian Society* 112: 179–209.
Gaines, Jane, and Michael Renov, eds. 1999. *Collecting Visible Evidence*. Visible Evidence, v. 6. Minneapolis: University of Minnesota Press.
Gamerro, Carlos. 2013. "Remembering without Memories." *Journal of Romance Studies* 13 (3): 110–15.
Ganteau, Jean-Michel. 2015. *The Ethics and Aesthetics of Vulnerability in Contemporary British Fiction*. New York: Routledge.
García, Lorena. 2003. "Albertina Carri: 'La ausencia es un agujero negro'." Film review (Carri's *Los Rubios*). *La Nación*, April 23.
Gay, Peter. 1988. *Freud: A Life for Our Time*. London: Dent.
Genette, Gérard. 1980. *Narrative Discourse*. Translated by Jane E. Lewin. Oxford: Basil Blackwell.
Gibeault, Alain. 2005. "Process of Symbolization." In *International Dictionary of Psychoanalysis*, edited by Alain de Mijolla, 1712–4. Detroit, MI: Macmillan Reference USA.
Gibeault, Alain. See also: Birksted-Breen, Dana, Sara Flanders, and Alain Gibeault, eds. 2010.
Giffney, Noreen. 2021. *The Culture-Breast in Psychoanalysis: Cultural Experiences and the Clinic*. (Psychoanalysis and Popular Culture Series). London and New York: Routledge, Taylor & Francis Group.
Godmilow, Jill. 2014. "Killing the Documentary: An Oscar-Nominated Filmmaker Takes Issue with 'The Act of Killing'." Blog. *IndieWire*, 5 March. Available at: https://www.indiewire.com/2014/03/killing-the-documentary-an-oscar-nominated-filmmaker-takes-issue-with-the-act-of-killing-29332/. [Accessed 18 November 2019].
Goodman, Amy. 2013. "'The Act of Killing': New Film Shows US-Backed Indonesian Death Squad Leaders Re-Enacting Massacres." Film Review. *Democracy Now!*, 19 July. Available at: https://www.democracynow.org/2013/7/19/the_act_of_killing_new_film. [Accessed 17 September 2019].
Green, André. 1977. "Conceptions of Affect." *International Journal of Psycho-Analysis* 58: 129–56.
Green, André. 1978a. *Between Reality and Fantasy: Winnicott's Concepts of Transitional Objects and Phenomena*. Edited by Simon A. Grolnick and Leonard Barkin. Northvale, NJ and London: Aronson.
Green, André. 1978b. "Potential Space in Psychoanalysis: The Object in the Setting." In *Between Reality and Fantasy: Winnicott's Concepts of Transitional Objects and Phenomena*, edited by Simon A. Grolnick and Leonard Barkin, 169–89. Northvale, NJ and London: Aronson.
Green, André. 1979. *The Tragic Effect: The Oedipus Complex in Tragedy*. Translated by Alan Sheridan. Cambridge: Cambridge University Press.
Green, André. 1980 [1971]. "The Unbinding Process." Translated by Lionel Duisit. *New Literary History* 12 (1): 11–39. [First published in French as "La déliaison" in *Littérature*, No. 3, October 1971].
Green, André. 1986a. *On Private Madness*. Translated by Katherine Aubertin and others. London: The Hogarth Press.
Green, André. 1986b. "Potential Space in Psychoanalysis." In *On Private Madness*, translated by Katherine Aubertin and others, 277–96. London: The Hogarth Press.

Green, André. 1986c. "The Analyst, Symbolization and Absence in the Analytic Setting." In *On Private Madness*, translated by Katherine Aubertin and others, 30–59. London: The Hogarth Press.

Green, André. 1999. *The Fabric of Affect in the Psychoanalytic Discourse*. Translated by Alan Sheridan. London and New York: Routledge.

Green, André. 2000. "The Intuition of the Negative in 'Playing and Reality'." In *André Green at The Squiggle Foundation*, edited by Jan Abram, 85–106. [First published in 1997 in *The International Journal of Psycho-Analysis*, 78: 1071–84, and based on a paper given before the International Psychoanalytical Association Congress in Milan on 6th April 1997]. London and New York: Karnac Books for the Squiggle Foundation.

Green, André. 2005a. *Key Ideas for a Contemporary Psychoanalysis: Misrecognition and Recognition of the Unconscious*. London and New York: Routledge.

Green, André. 2005b. *Play and Reflection in Donald Winnicott's Writings: The Donald Winnicott Memorial Lecture*. London: Karnac Books.

Green, André. See also: Kohon, Gregorio, and Rosine Jozef Perelberg. 2017.

Gregg, Melissa, and Gregory J. Seigworth. 2010a. "An Inventory of Shimmers." In *The Affect Theory Reader*, edited by Melissa Gregg and Gregory J. Seigworth, 1–25. Durham, NC: Duke University Press.

Gregg, Melissa, and Gregory J. Seigworth, eds. 2010b. *The Affect Theory Reader*. Durham: Duke University Press.

Grierson, John. 1966. *Grierson on Documentary*. Edited by Forsyth Hardy. Revised edition. London: Faber & Faber.

Grossberg, Lawrence. 1984. "Another Boring Day in Paradise: Rock and Roll and the Empowerment of Everyday Life." *Popular Music* 4 (January): 225–58.

Guattari, Félix. 1996. *The Guattari Reader*. Edited by Gary Genosko. Oxford and Cambridge, MA: John Wiley and Sons.

Guattari, Félix. See also: Deleuze, Gilles, and Félix Guattari. 1988 [1980].

Halbwachs, Maurice. 1992. *On Collective Memory*. Edited and translated by Lewis A. Coser. The Heritage of Sociology. Chicago, IL: University of Chicago Press.

Hanna, Robert. 2016. "Kant's Theory of Judgement." In *The Stanford Encyclopedia of Philosophy*, edited by Edward N. Zalta, Winter 2016. Stanford, CA: Stanford University. Available at: https://plato.stanford.edu/entries/kant-judgment/. [Accessed 1 January 2018].

Heidegger, Martin. 1962 [1927]. *Being and Time*. Translated by Edward S. Robinson and John Macquarrie. San Francisco, CA: Harper and Row.

Herzog, Werner. 2005. "Filmmaker Herzog's 'Grizzly' Tale of Life and Death." Radio interview (Werner Herzog interviewed by Dave Davies). *'Fresh Air': NPR (radio)*, 28 July. Available at: https://www.npr.org/templates/story/story.php?storyId=4774946. [Accessed 28 March 2020].

Hirsch, Joshua Francis. 2004. *Afterimage: Film, Trauma, and the Holocaust*. Philadelphia, PA: Temple University Press.

Hirsch, Marianne. 1997. *Family Frames: Photography, Narrative, and Postmemory*. Cambridge, MA: Harvard University Press.

Hirsch, Marianne. 2008. "The Generation of Postmemory." *Poetics Today* 29 (1): 103–28.

Hirsch, Marianne. 2012. *The Generation of Postmemory: Writing and Visual Culture after the Holocaust*. New York: Columbia University Press.

Hoffmann, E. T. A. 2004 [1816]. "The Sandman." In *Tales of Hoffmann*, edited and translated by R. J. Hollingdale, 85–126. London: Penguin Books.
Hoffmann, E. T. A. 2012 [1819]. *The Uncanny Guest*. Translated by (not credited). Redditch, Worcestershire: Read Books (Fantasy and Horror Classics).
Husserl, Edmund. 2013 [1913]. *Ideas: General Introduction to Pure Phenomenology*. Oxford and New York: Routledge.
IDFA. 2013. *Masterclass [with] Rithy Panh*. Online. Available at: https://www.youtube.com/watch?v=uGiyN8lOqEc. [Accessed 4 October 2017].
Jameson, Fredric. 1983. "Postmodernism and Consumer Society." In *Postmodern Culture*, edited by Hal Foster, 111–25. London: Pluto Press.
Jameson, Fredric. 1984. "Postmodernism, or The Cultural Logic of Late Capitalism." *New Left Review* 146 (August): 53–92.
Jameson, Fredric. 2015. "In Hyperspace." *London Review of Books*, 10 September.
Johnson, Barbara. 1980. *Critical Difference: Essays in the Contemporary Rhetoric of Reading*. Baltimore, MD: John Hopkins University Press.
Kansteiner, Wulf. 2004. "Genealogy of a Category Mistake: A Critical Intellectual History of the Cultural Trauma Metaphor." *Rethinking History* 8 (2): 193–221.
Kant, Immanuel. 1951 [1790]. *The Critique of Judgment, Theory of the Aesthetic Judgment and Theory of the Teleological Judgment, Critique of the Power of Judgment from the Author of Critique of Pure Reason, Critique of Practical Reason, Fundamental Principles of the Metaphysics of Morals & Dreams of a Spirit-Seer*. Translated by J. H. (John Henry) Bernard [1892]. New York: Hafner.
Kant, Immanuel. 1999 [2nd edition 1787]. *The Critique of Pure Reason*. Translated and edited by Paul Guyer and Allen W. Wood. Cambridge: Cambridge University Press.
Katz, Gil. 2014. *The Play Within the Play: The Enacted Dimension of Psychoanalytic Process*. Hove, East Sussex and New York: Routledge, Taylor & Francis.
King, Homay. 2013. "Born Free? Repetition and Fantasy in 'The Act of Killing'." *Film Quarterly* 67 (2): 30–36.
Klein, Melanie. 1984 [1932]. *The Psycho-Analysis of Children*. New York: Free Press.
Koch, Julian. 2019. *Perpetrating Narrative: Metalepsis and the Fiction-Nonfiction Divide in Oppenheimer's 'The Act of Killing'*. Abstract of conference paper (delivered at Queen Mary University of London conference: *Documentaries and the Fiction-Nonfiction Divide*), 15–16 November.
Kohan, Martín. 2004. "La Apariencia Celebrada." *Punto de Vista* 78 (April): 24–30.
Kohon, Gregorio, and Rosine Jozef Perelberg. 2017. *The Greening of Psychoanalysis: André Green's New Paradigm in Contemporary Theory and Practice*. London: Karnac Books.
Konigsberg, Ira. 1996. "Transitional Phenomena, Transitional Space: Creativity and Spectatorship in Film." *Psychoanalytic Review* 83 (6): 865–89.
Kornhaber, Donna. 2020. *Nightmares in the Dream Sanctuary: War and the Animated Film*. Chicago, IL: University of Chicago Press.
Kuhn, Annette. 2013a. "Little Madnesses: An Introduction." In *Little Madnesses: Winnicott, Transitional Phenomena and Cultural Experience*, edited by Annette Kuhn, 1–10. London and New York: I.B. Tauris.
Kuhn, Annette, ed. 2013b. *Little Madnesses: Winnicott, Transitional Phenomena and Cultural Experience*. London and New York: I.B. Tauris.
Kyd, Thomas. 2013 [c.1587]. *The Spanish Tragedy*. Edited by Clara Calvo and Jesus Tronch. London: The Arden Shakespeare.
Lacan, Jacques. 1966. *Écrits*. Paris: Éditions du Seuil.

Lacan, Jacques. 1977. *Écrits: A Selection*. Translated by Alan Sheridan. New York: Norton.
Lacan, Jacques. 1988. *The Seminar of Jacques Lacan (Book 1): Freud's Papers on Technique* 1953-1954. Edited by Jacques-Alain Miller. Translated by John Forrester. Cambridge: Cambridge University Press.
Lacan, Jacques. 1991 [1960–1]. *Le Séminaire. Livre VIII. Le transfert*. Edited by Jacques-Alain Miller. Paris: Éditions du Seuil.
Lanzmann, Claude. 1995. *'Shoah': The Complete Text of the Acclaimed Holocaust Film*. Revised edition. New York: Da Capo Press.
Lanzmann, Claude. 2007. "Hier Ist Kein Warum." In Claude *Lanzmann's 'Shoah': Key Essays*, edited by Stuart Liebman, translated by Claude Lanzmann. Oxford and New York: Oxford University Press.
Laplanche, Jean. 1999a. *Essays on Otherness*. Edited by John Fletcher. New York and London: Routledge.
Laplanche, Jean. 1999b. "Time and the Other." In *Essays on Otherness*, edited by John Fletcher, 234–59. New York and London: Routledge.
Laplanche, Jean. 2006. *Problématiques IV. L'après-coup*. Paris: PUF.
Laplanche, Jean, and Jean-Bertrand Pontalis. 1988 [1967]. *The Language of Psycho-Analysis*. Translated by Donald Nicholson-Smith. Reprinted. London: Karnac Books and The Institute of Psycho-Analysis.
Launchbury, Claire. 2013. "Animating Memory: Ari Folman's 'Waltz with Bashir'." In *Concentrationary Memories: Totalitarian Terror and Cultural Resistance*, edited by Griselda Pollock and Max Silverman, 193–202. London: I.B. Tauris.
Lebow, Alisa. 2006. "Faking What?: Making a Mockery of Documentary." In *F Is for Phony: Fake Documentary and Truth's Undoing*, edited by Alexandra Juhasz and Jesse Lerner, 223–37. Visible Evidence, v. 17. Minneapolis: University of Minnesota Press.
Lebow, Alisa. 2008. *First Person Jewish*. Minneapolis: University of Minnesota Press.
Lebow, Alisa. 2012. *Cinema of Me: The Self and Subjectivity in First Person Documentary*. London: Wallflower Press.
Lennon-Patience, Siobhan, and Marit Røkeberg. 2014. "Television as "Docutherapy": An Interview with Richard McKerrow and Jonathan Phang." In *Television and Psychoanalysis: Psycho-Cultural Perspectives*, edited by Caroline Bainbridge, Ivan Ward, and Candida Yates, 139–68. (Psychoanalysis and Popular Culture Series). London and New York: Routledge, Taylor & Francis Group.
Levin, G. Roy. 1971. *Documentary Explorations: 15 Interviews with Film-Makers*. Garden City: Anchor Press.
Levinas, Emmanuel. 1998. *Otherwise Than Being, or, Beyond Essence*. Translated by Alphonso Lingis. Pittsburgh, PA: Duquesne University Press.
Levine, Howard B. 2013. "The Colourless Canvas: Representation, Therapeutic Action, and the Creation of Mind." In *Unrepresented States and the Construction of Meaning: Clinical and Theoretical Contributions*, edited by Howard B. Levine, Gail S. Reed, and Dominique Scarfone, 42–71. London: Karnac Books.
Levine, Howard B., Gail S. Reed, and Dominique Scarfone. 2013a. "Introduction: From a Universe of Presences to a Universe of Absences." In *Unrepresented States and the Construction of Meaning: Clinical and Theoretical Contributions*, edited by Howard B. Levine, Gail S. Reed, and Dominique Scarfone, 3–17. London: Karnac Books.
Levine, Howard B., Gail S. Reed, and Dominique Scarfone, eds. 2013b. *Unrepresented States and the Construction of Meaning: Clinical and Theoretical Contributions*. London: Karnac Books.

Leys, Ruth, and Marlene Goldman. 2010. "Navigating the Genealogies of Trauma, Guilt, and Affect: An Interview with Ruth Leys." *University of Toronto Quarterly* 79 (2): 656–79.

Liebman, Stuart. 2007. *Claude Lanzmann's 'Shoah': Key Essays*. Edited and translated by Stuart Liebman. Oxford and New York: Oxford University Press.

Loizos, Peter. 1993. *Innovation in Ethnographic Film: From Innocence to Self-Consciousness, 1955-85*. Chicago, IL: University of Chicago Press.

Luckhurst, Roger. 2008. *The Trauma Question*. London and New York: Routledge.

Lusztig, Irene. 2013. "The Fever Dream of Documentary." *Film Quarterly* 67 (2): 50–56.

Lyotard, Jean François. 1988 [1983]. *The Differend: Phrases in Dispute*. Translated by Georges Van Den Abbeele. Manchester: Manchester University Press.

Lyotard, Jean François. 1994 [1991]. *Lessons on the Analytic of the Sublime*. Translated by Elizabeth Rottenberg. Stanford, CA: Stanford University Press.

Mahon, Eugene J. 2016. "Book Review: The Play within the Play: The Enacted Dimension of Psychoanalytic Process." Book review. *Journal of the American Psychoanalytic Association* 64 (6): 1255–66.

Maibom, Heidi L., ed. 2017. *The Routledge Handbook of Philosophy of Empathy*. London and New York: Routledge.

Margulies, Ivone. 2007. "The Real In-Balance in Jean Rouch's 'La Pyramide Humaine'." In *Building Bridges: The Cinema of Jean Rouch*, edited by Joram ten Brink, 125–33. London and New York: Wallflower Press.

Massumi, Brian. 1995. "The Autonomy of Affect." *Cultural Critique* 31 (October): 83–109.

McDougall, Joyce. 1986. *Theatres of the Mind: Illusion and Truth on the Psychoanalytical Stage*. London: Free Association Books.

McDougall, Joyce. 1989. *Theatres of the Body: A Psychoanalytic Approach to Psychosomatic Illness*. London: Free Association Books.

Meneghetti, Mike. 2016. "Self-Exculpatory Imaginings: Reenactment and Observation in 'The Act of Killing'." *Canadian Journal of Film Studies* 25 (2): 39–61.

Meunier, Jean-Pierre. 1969. *Les structures de l'expérience filmique: L'identification filmique*. Louvain: Librairie universitaire.

Middleton, Thomas. 2018 [1607]. *The Revenger's Tragedy*. Edited by Gretchen Minton. London and New York: The Arden Shakespeare.

Mijolla, Alain de, ed. 2005. *International Dictionary of Psychoanalysis*. Detroit, MI: Macmillan Reference USA.

Miller, Jacques-Alain. 1984. "Jacques Lacan: 1901-1981." *Psychoanalysis and Contemporary Thought* 7 (4): 615–28.

Minh-Ha, Trinh T. 1990. "Documentary Is/Not a Name." *October* 52 (Spring): 77–98.

Ministerio de Educación, Argentina (Bibliteca y Materiales Didácticos). 2010. *Memoria y Derechos Humanos en el Mercosur*. Online. Available at: https://www.memoriaenelmercosur.educ.ar/wp-content/uploads/2009/03/2010_los_rubios_-_propuesta_definitiva.pdf. [Accessed 16 April 2017].

Mitchell, Stephen A. 1993. "Foreword." In *Self-Analysis: Critical Inquiries, Personal Visions*, edited by James W. Barron, xiii–xviii. Hillsdale, NJ and London: Analytic Press.

Morag, Raya. 2012. "Perpetrator Trauma and Current Israeli Documentary Cinema." *Camera Obscura: Feminism, Culture, and Media Studies* 27 Number 2 (80): 93–133.

Morin, Edgar. 2003 [1960]. "Chronicle of a Film." In *Ciné-Ethnography*, edited and translated by Steven Feld [1st published in French in January 1960 in 'France Observateur'], 229–65. Minneapolis and London: University of Minnesota Press.

Morris, Errol. 2013. "The Murders of Gonzago." *Slate*, 10 July. Available at: https://www.slate.com/articles/arts/history/2013/07/the_act_of_killing_essay_how_indonesia_s_mass_killings_could_have_slowed.html. [Accessed 29 May 2016].

Nancy, Jean-Luc. 2000. *Being Singular Plural*. Translated by Robert D. Richardson and Anne E. O'Byrne. Stanford, CA: Stanford University Press.

Neyraut, Michel. 2010. "Countertransference and Psychoanalytic Thought." In *Reading French Psychoanalysis*, edited by Alain Gibeault, Dana Birksted-Breen, and Sara Flanders, 218–32. London and New York: Routledge.

Nichols, Bill. 1994. *Blurred Boundaries: Questions of Meaning in Contemporary Culture*. Bloomington: Indiana University Press.

Nichols, Bill. 2013. "Irony, Cruelty, Evil (and a Wink) in 'The Act of Killing'." *Film Quarterly* 67 (2): 25–29.

Nichols, Bill. 2016. *Speaking Truths with Film: Evidence, Ethics, Politics in Documentary*. Oakland: University of California Press.

Nichols, Bill. 2017. *Introduction to Documentary*. 3rd revised edition. Bloomington: Indiana University Press.

Nouzeilles, Gabriela. 2005. "Postmemory Cinema and the Future of the Past in Albertina Carri's 'Los Rubios'." *Journal of Latin American Cultural Studies* 14 (3): 263–78.

Ogden, Thomas H. 2004. "The Analytic Third: Implications for Psychoanalytic Theory and Technique." *Psychoanalytic Quarterly* 73 (1): 167–95.

Oppenheimer, Joshua. 2012. "Perpetrators' Testimony and the Restoration of Humanity: 'S21', Rithy Panh." In *Killer Images: Documentary Film, Memory and the Performance of Violence*, edited by Joram ten Brink and Joshua Oppenheimer, 243–55. London and New York: Wallflower Press.

Oppenheimer, Joshua. 2016. *Masterclass: Joshua Oppenheimer in Conversation with Francine Stock at the Regent Street Cinema, London.* Unpublished notes (taken by Bruce Eadie at University of Westminster and Cream Screens Masterclass), 10 May. Available at: https://www.dropbox.com/s/zq9lqzvtpzfmgdf/Oppenheimer%20Masterclass_notes.100516.doc?dl=0. [Accessed 26 May 2016].

Oppenheimer, Joshua, and J. Hoberman. 2015. "The Film Comment Podcast: 'Shoah' (J. Hoberman Interviews Joshua Oppenheimer)." Blog. *Film Comment*, 7 October. Available at: https://www.filmcomment.com/blog/podcast-first-episode-shoah/. [Accessed 28 November 2018].

Page, Joanna. 2009. *Crisis and Capitalism in Contemporary Argentine Cinema*. Durham, NC: Duke University Press.

Panh, Rithy. See: IDFA. 2013. *Masterclass [with] Rithy Panh*.

Panh, Rithy, and Christophe Bataille. 2013. *'The Missing Picture': Voice over Narration*. Online. Available at: https://cambodialpj.org/wp-content/uploads/2014/05/DCCAM_CLPJ_Panh1.pdf. [Accessed 3 October 2017].

Panh, Rithy, and Deirdre Boyle. See also: Deirdre Boyle's article and interview with Panh: Boyle, Deirdre. 2014a, 2014b.

Panh, Rithy, and Deirdre Boyle. 2015. "Interview with Rithy Panh on 'The Missing Picture'." Filmed interview (Rithy Panh interviewed by Deirdre Boyle) plus associated paratext. Higher Learning event co-presented with 'Visible Evidence'. *TIFF*. 21 December. Available at: https://www.tiff.net/the-review/rithy-panh-the-missing-picture/index.html. [Accessed 4 October 2017].

Paramaditha, Intan. 2013. "Tracing Frictions in 'The Act of Killing'." *Film Quarterly* 67 (2): 44–49.

Patsalides, Beatrice, and André Patsalides. 2001. "'Butterflies Caught in the Network of Signifiers': The Goals of Psychoanalysis According to Jacques Lacan." *Psychoanalytic Quarterly* 70 (1): 201–30.
Perelberg, Rosine Jozef. 2008. *Time, Space, and Phantasy*. London: Routledge.
Perelberg, Rosine Jozef. See also: Kohon, Gregorio, and Rosine Jozef Perelberg. 2017.
Perez, Mariana Eva. 2013. "Their Lives after: Theatre as Testimony and the So-called 'Second generation' in Post-Dictatorship Argentina." *Journal of Romance Studies* 13 (3): 6–16.
Phillips, Adam. 1988. *Winnicott*. Cambridge, MA: Harvard University Press.
Pigman, George W. 1995. "Freud and the History of Empathy." *International Journal of Psycho-Analysis* 76: 237–56.
Pilling, Jayne. 2012. *Animating the Unconscious*. London and New York: Columbia University Press.
Piotrowska, Agnieszka. 2014. *Psychoanalysis and Ethics in Documentary Film*. London: Taylor and Francis.
Pirandello, Luigi. 1995 [1921]. "Six Characters in Search of an Author." In *Six Characters in Search of an Author and Other Plays*, by Luigi Pirandello, translated by Mark Musa, 1–66. London and New York: Penguin Books.
Plantinga, Carl. 1987. "Defining Documentary: Fiction, Non-Fiction, and Projected Worlds." *Persistence of Vision* 5 (Spring): 44–54.
Plantinga, Carl. 2005. "What a Documentary Is, After All." *The Journal of Aesthetics and Art Criticism* 63 (2): 105–17.
Radó, Sándo. 1928. "The Problem of Melancholia." *International Journal of Psycho-Analysis* 9: 420–38.
Rancière, Jacques. 2006. "Is History a Form of Fiction?" In *The Politics of Aesthetics*, edited by Gabriel Rockhill, 31–37. London: Continuum.
Rancière, Jacques. 2011. *The Emancipated Spectator*. Translated by Gregory Elliott. London: Verso.
Rand, Nicholas T. 1994. "Introduction: Renewals of Psychoanalysis." In *The Shell and the Kernel: Renewals of Psychoanalysis*, by Nicholas Abraham and Mária Török, edited and translated by Nicholas T. Rand, 1–22. Chicago, IL and London: University of Chicago Press.
Rank, Otto. 1971 [1914]. *The Double: A Psychoanalytic Study*. Translated by Harry Tucker (junior). [First published in 1914 as "Der Doppelgänger" in the journal *Imago*]. Chapel Hill: The University of North Carolina Press.
Ray, Nicholas. 2012. "Forming New Knots: Jean Laplanche 1924-2012." *Radical Philosophy* 174 (July/August): 53–56. Available at: https://www.radicalphilosophy.com/obituary/jean-laplanche-1924-2012. [Accessed 7 October 2019].
Rayns, Tony. 2013. "The Act of Killing." Film review. *Sight & Sound* 23 (7), July: 113.
Renov, Michael. 1993. *Theorizing Documentary*. New York: Routledge.
Renov, Michael. 1999. "New Subjectivities: Documentary and Self-Representation in the Post-Verité Age." In *Feminism and Documentary*, edited by Diane Waldman and Janet Walker, 84–94. Minneapolis: University of Minnesota Press.
Renov, Michael. 2004 [1989]. "The Subject of History: The New Autobiography in Film and Video." In *The Subject of Documentary*, [1st published in *Afterimage* Summer 1989], 104–19. Minneapolis: University of Minnesota Press.
Renov, Michael. 2004 [1996]. "Charged Vision: The Place of Desire in Documentary Film Theory." In *The Subject of Documentary*, 93–103. [Chapter first published in 1996]. Minneapolis, MN: University of Minnesota Press.

Renov, Michael. 2004. *The Subject of Documentary*. Visible Evidence, v. 16. Minneapolis: University of Minnesota Press.
Renov, Michael. 2008. "First-Person Films: Some Theses on Self-Inscription." In *Rethinking Documentary: New Perspectives, New Practices*, edited by Thomas Austin and Wilma de Jong, 39–50. Maidenhead, Berkshire: McGraw-Hill Education (Open University Press).
Renov, Michael. 2015. "Documentary and Psychoanalysis: Putting the Love Back in Epistephilia." In *Embodied Encounters: New Approaches to Psychoanalysis and Cinema*, edited by Agnieszka Piotrowska, 147–55. East Sussex and New York: Taylor and Francis.
Renov, Michael. See also: Gaines, Jane, and Michael Renov, eds. 1999.
Rothberg, Michael. 2000. *Traumatic Realism: The Demands of Holocaust Representation*. Minneapolis: University of Minnesota Press.
Rothberg, Michael. 2009. *Multidirectional Memory: Remembering the Holocaust in the Age of Decolonization*. Stanford, CA: Stanford University Press.
Rouch, Jean. 2003. *Ciné-Ethnography*. Edited and translated by Steven Feld. Visible Evidence, v. 13. Minneapolis and London: University of Minnesota Press.
Salmi, Hannu, Asko Nivala, and Jukka Sarjala. 2016. *Travelling Notions of Culture in Early Nineteenth-Century Europe*. New York: Routledge.
Sarlo, Beatriz. 2007. *Tiempo pasado cultura de la memoria y giro subjetivo. Una discusión*. Buenos Aires: Siglo XXI Editores Argentina.
Scarfone, Dominique. 2010. "In the Hollow of Transference: The Analyst between Activity and Passivity." *Sitegeist* 4 (Spring): 7–20. Available at: https://www.the-site.org.uk/4272/sitegeist-issues/sitegeist-issue-4/. [Accessed 24 May 2026].
Scarfone, Dominique. See also: Bohleber, Werner, Peter Fonagy, Dominique Scarfone, et al. 2013.
Scarfone, Dominique. See also: Levine, Howard B., Gail S. Reed, and Dominique Scarfone, eds. 2013a.
Schact, Michael. 2007. "Sponteneity-Creativity: The Psychodramatic Concept of Change." In *Psychodrama: Advances in Theory and Practice*, edited by Clark Baim, Jorge Burmeister, and Manuela Maciel, 21–40. London and New York: Routledge.
Schäuble, Michaela. 2011. "All Filmmaking Is a Form of Therapy: Visualizing Memories of War Violence in the Animation Film 'Waltz with Bashir' (2008)." In *Violence Expressed: An Anthropological Approach*, edited by Maria Six-Hohenbalken and Nerina Weiss, 203–22. Farnham, Surrey and Burlington, VT: Ashgate.
Scott, A. O. 2004. "Personally Political: Fallout from the 'Dirty War'." Film review (Albertina Carri's 'The Blonds'). *The New York Times*, 7 April. Available at: https://www.nytimes.com/2004/04/07/movies/film-review-personally-political-fallout-from-the-dirty-war.html. [Accessed 24 March 2017].
Sedgwick, Eve Kosofsky, and Adam Frank, eds. 1995a. *Shame and Its Sisters: A Silvan Tomkins Reader*. Durham, NC: Duke University Press.
Sedgwick, Eve Kosofsky, and Adam Frank. 1995b. "Shame in the Cybernetic Fold: Reading Silvan Tomkins." *Critical Inquiry* 21 (2): 496–522.
Shakespeare, William. 1982 [c.1600]. *Hamlet*. Edited by Harold Jenkins. London: Routledge.
Shakespeare, William. 2015 [1606]. *Macbeth*. Edited by Sandra Clark and Pamela Mason. 3rd edition. London: The Arden Shakespeare.
Shaviro, Steven. 1993. *The Cinematic Body*. Minneapolis: University of Minnesota Press.
Shouse, Eric. 2005. "Feeling, Emotion, Affect." *M/C Journal* 8 (6). Available at: https://doi.org/10.5204/mcj.2443. [Accessed 24 May 2026].

Silverman, Max. 2013. *Palimpsestic Memory: The Holocaust and Colonialism in French and Francophone Fiction and Film*. New York: Berghahn Books.
Silverman, Max. 2018. "Masterclass: Palimpsestic Memory, Ethics and Performance." Event notification and publicity for Max Silverman masterclass (ANU School of Literature, Languages and Linguistics at the Australian National University). 21 August 2018. Available at: https://slll.cass.anu.edu.au/events/masterclass-palimpsestic-memory-ethics-and-performance. [Accessed 6 April 2020].
Singleton, Douglas. 2004. "The Blonds: Slippery Slope of Truth." Film review. *The Brooklyn Rail*, 1 May. Available at: https://brooklynrail.org/2004/05/film/the-blonds-slippery-slope-of-truth. [Accessed 23 March 2017].
Skogstad, Wilhelm. 2015. "Speaking through Action, Acting through Speech: Acting and Enacting in the Analytic Process." *British Journal of Psychotherapy* 31 (2): 191–206.
Sobchack, Vivian. 1992. *The Address of the Eye: A Phenomenology of Film Experience*. Princeton, NJ: Princeton University Press.
Sobchack, Vivian, ed. 1996. *The Persistence of History: Cinema, Television, and the Modern Event*. New York: Routledge.
Sobchack, Vivian. 1999. "Toward a Phenomenology of Nonfictional Film Experience." In *Collecting Visible Evidence*, edited by Jane Gaines and Michael Renov, 241–54. Visible Evidence, v. 6. Minneapolis: University of Minnesota Press.
Sobchack, Vivian. 2004. *Carnal Thoughts: Embodiment and Moving Image Culture*. Berkeley: University of California Press.
Sobchack, Vivian. 2009. "Phenomenology." In *The Routledge Companion to Philosophy and Film*, edited by Paisley Livingston and Carl R. Plantinga, 435–45. London and New York: Routledge.
Sosa, Cecilia. 2011. "Queering Acts of Mourning in the Aftermath of Argentina's Dictatorship: Mothers of the Plaza Mayo and 'Los Rubios'." In *The Memory of State Terrorism in the Southern Cone: Argentina, Chile, and Uruguay*, edited by Francesca Lessa and Vincent Druliolle, 63–85. New York: Palgrave Macmillan.
Sosa, Cecilia. 2013. "Humour and the Descendants of the Disappeared: Countersigning Bloodline Affiliations in Post-Dictatorial Argentina." *Journal of Romance Studies* 13 (3): 75–87.
Sosa, Cecilia. 2014. *Queering Acts of Mourning in the Aftermath of Argentina's Dictatorship: The Performances of Blood*. Woodbridge, Suffolk and Rochester, NY: Tamesis.
Spaulding, Shannon. 2017. "Cognitive Empathy." In *The Routledge Handbook of Philosophy of Empathy*, edited by Heidi L. Maibom, 13–21, chapter 1. London and New York: Routledge.
Spiegelman, Art. 1992. *Maus II: A Survivor's Tale – And Here My Troubles Began*. London: André Deutsch.
Spiessens, Anneleen. 2014. "The Aim of All Genuine Art Is Always Engaged." *Testimony between History and Memory* 118 (September): 66–73.
Stueber, Karsten. 2017. "Empathy and Understanding Reasons." In *The Routledge Handbook of Philosophy of Empathy*, edited by Heidi L. Maibom, 137–47, chapter 12. London and New York: Routledge.
Sweedler, Milo. 2014. *The Dialectic of Truth and Fiction in Joshua Oppenheimer's 'The Act of Killing'*. Laurier Digital ebook (WLU University Press).
Taylor, Diana. 2003. *The Archive and the Repertoire: Cultural Memory and Performance in the Americas*. Durham, NC and London: Duke University Press.

Thomas, Julian. 2009. "Sigmund Freud's Archaeological Metaphor and Archaeology's Self-Understanding." In *Contemporary Archaeologies: Excavating Now*, edited by C. Holtorf and A. Piccini, 33–45. London: Peter Lang.

Török, Mária. 1994 [1968]. "The Illness of Mourning and the Fantasy of the Exquisite Corpse." In *The Shell and the Kernel: Renewals of Psychoanalysis*, by Nicholas Abraham and Mária Török, edited and translated by Nicholas T. Rand, 107–24. Chicago, IL and London: University of Chicago Press.

Török, Mária. 1994 [1975]. "Story of Fear: The Symptoms of Phobia – The Return of the Repressed or the Return of the Phantom?" In *The Shell and the Kernel: Renewals of Psychoanalysis*, by Nicholas Abraham and Mária Török, edited and translated by Nicholas T. Rand, 177–86. Chicago, IL and London: University of Chicago Press.

Török, Mária. See also: Abraham, Nicolas, and Mária Török. 1986, 1994 [1972], 1994 [1975], 1994.

Tracey, Andrew, et al. 2013, 2019. "The Essay Film." *Sight & Sound* (a 'Deep Focus' feature). 1st published in August 2013 issue and updated 7 May 2019. Available at: https://www.bfi.org.uk/news-opinion/sight-sound-magazine/features/deep-focus/essay-film. [Accessed 30 April 2018; 28 July 2020].

Trezise, Thomas. 2013. *Witnessing Witnessing: On the Reception of Holocaust Survivor Testimony*. New York: Fordham University Press.

Tyson, Adam. 2014. "Multiple Acts of Killing." *Critical Asian Studies* 46 (1): 157–61.

Van der Kolk, Bessel A., Alexander C. McFarlane, and Lars Weisæth. 1996. *Traumatic Stress: The Effects of Overwhelming Experience on Mind, Body, and Society*. New York: Guilford Press.

Van der Kolk, Bessel A., and Onno Van der Hart. 1989. "Pierre Janet and the Breakdown of Adaptation in Psychological Trauma." *American Journal of Psychiatry* 146 (12): 1530–40.

Varvin, Sverre. 2003. "Extreme Traumatisation: Strategies for Mental Survival." *International Forum of Psychoanalysis* 12 (1): 5–16.

Vermeulen, Pieter. 2007. "The Suspension of Reading: Wordsworth's 'Boy of Winander' and Trauma Theory." *Orbis Litterarum* 62 (6): 459–82.

Viderman, Serge. 1970. *La construction de l 'espace analytique*. Paris: Donoël.

Waldman, Diane, and Janet Walker, eds. 1999a. *Feminism and Documentary*. Visible Evidence, v. 5. Minneapolis: University of Minnesota Press.

Waldman, Diane, and Janet Walker. 1999b. "Introduction." In *Feminism and Documentary*, edited by Diane Waldman and Janet Walker, 1–35. Visible Evidence, v. 5. Minneapolis: University of Minnesota Press.

Walker, Janet. 2013. "Referred Pain." *Film Quarterly* 67 (2): 14–20.

Walker, Janet. See also: Waldman, Diane, and Janet Walker. 1999a, 1999b.

Wandita, Galuh. 2014. "Preman Nation: Watching 'The Act of Killing' in Indonesia." *Critical Asian Studies* 46 (1): 167–70.

Wartenberg, Thomas E. 2017. "Providing Evidence for a Philosophical Claim: 'The Act of Killing' and the Banality of Evil." *NECSUS* (Autumn). Available at: https://necsus-ejms.org/providing-evidence-philosophical-claim-act-killing-banality-evil/. [Accessed 24 January 2019].

Wells, Paul. 1998. *Understanding Animation*. London and New York: Routledge.

Wiesel, Elie. 1968. *Legends of Our Time*. New York: Holt, Rinehart and Winston.

Williams, Linda. 1991. "Film Bodies: Gender, Genre, and Excess." *Film Quarterly* 44 (4): 2–13.

Williams, Linda. 1993. "Mirrors without Memories: Truth, History, and the New Documentary." *Film Quarterly* 46 (3): 9–21.
Winnicott, D. W. (Donald Woods). 1953. "Transitional Objects and Transitional Phenomena - A Study in the First Not-Me Possession." *International Journal of Psycho-Analysis* 34: 89–97.
Winnicott, D. W. (Donald Woods). 1989 [1977]. *The Piggle: An Account of the Psychoanalytic Treatment of a Little Girl*. Edited by Ishak Ramzy. London: Penguin.
Winnicott, D. W. (Donald Woods). 1990 [1971]a. *Playing and Reality*. London: Routledge.
Winnicott, D. W. (Donald Woods). 1990 [1971]b. "Transitional Objects and Transitional Phenomena." In *Playing and Reality*, 1–25. London: Routledge.
Winnicott, D. W. (Donald Woods). 1990 [1971]c. "Playing: A Theoretical Statement." In *Playing and Reality*, 38–52. London: Routledge.
Winnicott, D. W. (Donald Woods). 2017. *The Collected Works of D.W. Winnicott*. Edited by Lesley Caldwell and Helen Taylor Robinson, 12 volumes. Oxford and New York: Oxford University Press.
Women Make Movies Release, A. 2004. "Press Release for 'The Blonds' (Including Reviews and Newspaper Articles)". Film catalogue and press release. *wmm.com*. Available at: https://www.wmm.com/storage/films/the-blonds/press/blothe_presskit.pdf. [Accessed 24 May 2026].
Wood, David, ed. 1991. *On Paul Ricœur: Narrative and Interpretation*. London: Routledge.
Zahavi, Dan. 2017. "Phenomenology, Empathy and Mindreading." In *The Routledge Handbook of Philosophy of Empathy*, edited by Heidi L. Maibom, 33–43, chapter 3. London and New York: Routledge.
Žižek, Slavoj. 2013. "'The Act of Killing' and the Modern Trend of 'Privatising Public Space'." *New Statesman*, 12 July. Available at: https://www.newstatesman.com/culture/2013/07/slavoj-zizek-act-killing-and-modern-trend-privatising-public-space. [Accessed 3 November 2014].

List of films cited

Carri, Albertina. 2003. *The Blonds [Los Rubios]*. Argentina. [DVD: 2003. New York: Women Make Movies].

Dauman, Florence. 2011. *A Summer +50 [Un été +50]*. France: Argos Films. [DVD: 2013. London: British Film Institute (packaged with Rouch and Morin's *Chronique d'un été,* 1961)].

Flaherty, Robert J. 1926. *Moana*. US: Paramount Pictures.

Folman, Ari. 2008. *Waltz with Bashir* [*Vals Im Bashir* / ואלס עם באשיר]. Israel, Germany, France: Bridgit Folman Film Gang; Razor Film Produktion; Les Films d'Ici. [DVD: 2009. London: Artificial Eye].

Guzmán, Patricio. 2010. *Nostalgia for the Light [Nostalgia de la luz]*. Chile. [DVD: 2011. New York: Icarus Films].

Herzog, Werner. 1997. *Little Dieter Needs to Fly*. Germany: Werner Herzog Filmproduktion. [DVD: 1998. US: Anchor Bay].

Lanzmann, Claude. 1985. *Shoah*. France: Les Films Aleph; Why Not Productions. [DVD: 2007. UK: Eureka! (The Masters of Cinema series)].

Lebow, Alisa, and Cynthia Madansky. 1998. *Treyf*. US. [DVD: 1998. New York: Women Make Movies].

Lumet, Sidney. 1964. *The Pawnbroker*. US: Allied Artists Pictures Corporation. [DVD: 2003. Los Angeles, CA: Paramount Pictures via Republic Entertainment].

Maddin, Guy. 2007. *My Winnipeg*. Canada: Buffalo Gal Pictures; Documentary Channel; Everyday Pictures. [DVD: 2008. London: Soda Pictures].

McCay, Winsor. 1918. *The Sinking of the Lusitania*. US: Jewel Productions; Universal Film Manufacturing Company. Available at: https://www.youtube.com/watch?v=dyd2KhGFLZg. [Accessed 24 November 2017].

Morris, Errol. 1988. *The Thin Blue Line*. US: The Corporation for Public Broadcasting; National Endowment for the Arts; Program Development Company Productions Incorporated; The Chubb Group of Insurance Companies; various public television stations. [DVD: 2015. New York: The Criterion Collection].

Noer, Arifin C. 1984. *The Treachery of the 30th September Movement of the Communist Party of Indonesia [Pengkhianatan G30S/PKI]*. Indonesia: PPFN.

Oppenheimer, Joshua. 2012. *The Act of Killing*. UK, Denmark, Norway: Final Cut for Real. [DVD: 2013. UK: Dogwoof].

Panh, Rithy. 2003. *S21: The Khmer Rouge Killing Machine [S-21, la machine de mort Khmère rouge]*. Cambodia, France: Arte France. [DVD: 2005. New York: First Run Features].

Panh, Rithy. 2013. *The Missing Picture [L'image manquante]*. Cambodia, France: CDP; Arte; Bophana Production. [DVD: 2013. London: New Wave Films].

Perret, Léonce. 1912. *The Mystery of the Rocks of Kador [Le Mystère des Roches de Kador]*. France: Gaumont. Available at: https://www.youtube.com/watch?v=SYLjxp5CAPk. [Accessed 5 December 2016].

Resnais, Alain. 1959. *Hiroshima, My Love [Hiroshima mon amour]*. France, Japan: Argos Films; Como Films; Daiei Studios; Pathé Entertainment; Pathé Overseas. [DVD: 2003. New York: The Criterion Collection].

Rouch, Jean. 1958. *Me, a Black [Moi, un noir]*. France: Films de la Pléiade. [DVD: 2012. Australia: Ronin Films].

Rouch, Jean. 1959. *The Human Pyramid [La pyramide humaine]*. France: Films de la Pléiade.

Rouch, Jean, and Edgar Morin. 1961. *Chronicle of a Summer [Chronique d'un été]*. France: Argos Films. [DVD: 2013. London: British Film Institute].

Schnabel, Julian. 2007. *The Diving Bell and the Butterfly [Le Scaphandre et le Papillon]*. France: Pathé; France 3 Cinéma. [DVD: 2008. US: Walt Disney Studios].

Waters, John. 2000. *Cecil B. Demented*. US, France: Polar Entertainment; Le Studio Canal+. [DVD: 2001. UK: Momentum Pictures].

Wegener, Paul, and Stellan Rye. 1913. *The Student of Prague [Der Student von Prag]*. German Empire: Deutsche Bioscop. Available at: https://www.youtube.com/watch?v=OuvIvwSi1gI. [Accessed 10 March 2017].

Wexler, Haskell. 1969. *Medium Cool*. US: H&J (distributed by Paramount Pictures).

Index

Note: Page numbers followed by 'n' refer to notes.

For Product Safety Concerns and Information please contact our EU
representative GPSR@taylorandfrancis.com
Taylor & Francis Verlag GmbH, Kaufingerstraße 24, 80331 München, Germany

www.ingramcontent.com/pod-product-compliance
Ingram Content Group UK Ltd.
Pitfield, Milton Keynes, MK11 3LW, UK
UKHW020008200926
475702UK00015B/2534

* 9 7 8 1 0 4 1 1 0 8 6 8 9 *